SERVING CHILDREN AND FAMILIES THROUGH COMMUNITY-UNIVERSITY PARTNERSHIPS: Success Stories

OUTREACH SCHOLARSHIP

Editor:

Richard M. Lerner
Boston College
Chestnut Hill, Massachusetts, U.S.A.

Forthcoming books in the series:

Lerner, R., Sparks, E., and McCubbin, L.
Family Diversity and Family Policy
Ralston, P., Lerner, R., Mullis, A., Simerly, C., and Murray, J.
Social Change, Public Policy, and Community Collaboration: Training Human Development Professionals for the 21st Century

SERVING CHILDREN AND FAMILIES THROUGH COMMUNITY-UNIVERSITY PARTNERSHIPS: Success Stories

Edited by

Thomas R. Chibucos
Bowling Green State University

and

Richard M. Lerner
Boston College

Forewords by
Lonnie R. Sherrod and James C. Votruba

Afterword by
Sidney A. Ribeau

KLUWER ACADEMIC PUBLISHERS
Boston / Dordrecht / London

Distributors for North, Central and South America:
Kluwer Academic Publishers
101 Philip Drive
Assinippi Park
Norwell, Massachusetts 02061 USA
Telephone (781) 871-6600
Fax (781) 871-6528
E-Mail <kluwer@wkap.com>

Distributors for all other countries:
Kluwer Academic Publishers Group
Distribution Centre
Post Office Box 322
3300 AH Dordrecht, THE NETHERLANDS
Telephone 31 78 6392 392
Fax 31 78 6546 474
E-Mail <services@wkap.nl>

Electronic Services <http://www.wkap.nl>

Library of Congress Cataloging-in-Publication Data
Serving children and families through community-university partnerships: success stories / edited by Thomas R. Chibucos and Richard M. Lerner; forewords by Lonnie R. Sherrod and James C. Votruba; afterword by Sidney A. Ribeau.
p. cm.-- (Outreach scholarship; 1)
Includes bibliographical references and index.
ISBN 0-7923-8540-3 (alk. paper)
1. Community and college--United States. 2. Family services--United States. 3. Children--Services for--United States. I. Chibucos, Thomas R. II. Lerner, Richard M. III. Series.
LC238.S47 1999
378.1'03'0973--dc21 99-24717
CIP

Printed on acid-free paper.
Printed in the United States of America

TABLE OF CONTENTS

LIST OF CONTRIBUTORS

L. Annette Abrams, University Outreach Office, Michigan State University, East Lansing, MI 48824

Charlie Adams, Department of Education, Nutrition, and Restaurant and Hotel Management, Texas Tech University, Lubbock, TX 79409-1162

Elaine A. Anderson, Department of Family Studies, University of Maryland, College Park, MD 20742

Dita G. Andersson, Department of Counseling, Developmental and Educational Psychology, Boston College, Chestnut Hill, MA 02167-3813

Mary Andrews, College of Human Ecology, Michigan State University, East Lansing, MI 48824

Joyce Armstrong, Department of Family Sciences, Texas Woman's University, Denton, TX 76204-5769

Laura Bates, Department of Family and Child Ecology, Michigan State University, East Lansing, MI 48824-1030

Nancy J. Bell, Department of Human Development and Family Studies, Texas Tech University, Box 41162, Lubbock, TX 79409-1162

Daniel Bibeau, Department of Public Health Education, The University of North Carolina at Greensboro, Greensboro, NC 27412-5001

Charles A. Blackman, Professor Emeritus, College of Education, Michigan State University, East Lansing, MI 48824

Ann P. Blackwell, School of Family and Consumer Sciences, The University of Southern Mississippi, Box 5035, Hattiesburg, MS 39406-5035

Craig Blakely, Public Policy Research Institute, Texas A&M University, College Station, TX 77843-4476

Marilyn R. Bradbard, Department of Human Development and Family Studies, Auburn University, Auburn, AL 36849-5604

April Brown, Psychological Services and Education, Florida State University, Tallahassee, FL 32306

Robert Brown, United Way of Michigan and University Outreach Partnerships, Michigan State University, East Lansing, MI 48824

Martha J. Buell, Northern Delaware Early Head Start, University of Delaware, 101 Alison Hall, Newark, DE 19716

Judith R. Butterfield, Florida Cooperative Extension Service, Duval County 4-H, Jacksonville, FL 32254-2083

Ron Cameron, Psychological Services and Education, Florida State University, Tallahassee, FL 32306

Elizabeth A. Carroll, Department of Child Development and Family Relations, East Carolina University, Greenville, NC 27858-4354

Carol A. Cartwright, President, Kent State University, P.O. Box 5190, Kent, OH 44242-0001

Karen McKnight Casey, Department of Family and Child Ecology, Michigan State University, East Lansing, MI 48824

Deborah J. Cassidy, Department of Human Development and Family Studies, P.O. Box 26170, University of North Carolina at Greensboro, Greensboro, NC 27402-6170

Jo Cato, Georgia Department of Human Resources, Atlanta, GA 30303

Thomas R. Chibucos, School of Family and Consumer Sciences, Bowling Green State University, Bowling Green, OH 43403-0254

Marilyn Coleman, Human Development and Family Studies, University of Missouri-Columbia, Columbia, MO 65211

Linda L. Dannison, Family and Consumer Sciences, Western Michigan University, Kalamazoo, MI 49008

Catherine R. DeMason, Rockingham County Student Health Centers, Eden, NC 27288

Tamara B. Dinkins, Florida Cooperative Extension Service, Duval County 4-H, Jacksonville, FL 32254-2083

Tracy K. Dranginis, Department of Rural Sociology, University of Missouri, Kansas City, MO 64113

Martha Farrell Erickson, Children. Youth and Family Consortium, University of Minnesota, 12 McNeal Hall, 1985 Buford Avenue, St. Paul, MN 55108

Joan E. Esser-Stuart, College of Human Environmental Sciences, University of Alabama, 100 Doster, Box 870158, Tuscaloosa, AL 35487-0158

La Nelle Ethridge, Parents as Teachers, 515 N. Zenith Avenue, Lubbock, TX 79403

Richard Fabes, Department of Family Resources and Human Development, Arizona State University, P.O. Box 872502, Tempe, AZ 85287-2502

Jay Faron, Executive Director, Boys and Girls Clubs of Pitt County, Inc., 621 Firetower Road, Winterville, NC 28590

Ginny Felstehausen, Department of Education, Nutrition, and Restaurant and Hotel Management, Texas Tech University, Lubbock, TX 79409-1162

Mark A. Fine, Department of Human Development and Family Studies, University of Missouri-Columbia, 31 Stanley Hall, Columbia, MO 65211-7700

Celia B. Fisher, Department of Psychology, Fordham University, Dealy Hall, 441 East Fordham Road, Bronx, NY 10458

Hiram E. Fitzgerald, Department of Psychology and Applied Developmental Science Programs, 6 Kellogg Center, Michigan State University, East Lansing, MI 48824-1022

Karen Freeman, Jordan Family Development Center, 812 N. College, Bowling Green, OH 43402

Sara Gable, Human Development and Family Studies, Extension, University of Missouri-Columbia, Columbia, MO 65211

Michael Gamel-McCormick, Individual and Family Studies, and Center for Disabilities Studies, University of Delaware, 101 Alison Hall, Academy Street, Newark, DE 19716

Lawrence H. Ganong, Human Development and Family Studies, University of Missouri-Columbia, Columbia, MO 65211

Deborah B. Gentry, Department of Family and Consumer Sciences, Illinois State University, Normal, IL 61790-5060

Alisa S. Ghazvini, Florida's Children's Forum, Florida State University, Tallahassee, FL 32306-1490

Sylvia Grogan, Director of Marketing, Morehead Memorial Hospital, Eden, NC 27288

Janice Grover, Department of Human Development and Family Studies and the Birmingham Early Learning Center, Auburn University, Auburn, AL 36849-3501

Robert P. Haigh, Department of Public Welfare, Room 308 Health and Welfare Building, Harrisburg, PA 17120

Elizabeth G. Haley, College of Human Sciences, Texas Tech University, Lubbock, TX 79409-1162

Alice Henderson Hall, Human Development and Family Studies, University of North Carolina at Greensboro, Greensboro, NC 27402-6170

Rena Hallam, Northern Delaware Early Head Start, University of Delaware, 101 Alison Hall, Academy Street, Newark, DE 19716

Marilyn J. Halusky, Florida Cooperative Extension Service, Duval County 4-H, Jacksonville, FL 32254-2083

June Henton, Department of Human Development and Family Studies, Auburn University, Auburn, AL 36849-3501

Susan A. Hicks, Extension, Cornell University, Ithaca, NY 14853-2801

Leigh Curtis Higgins, Choice Middle Schools Program, Baltimore, MD 21220

Ann Higgins-D'Alessandro, Department of Psychology, Fordham University, Dealy Hall, 441 East Fordham Road, Bronx, NY 10458

Gladys J. Hildreth, Department of Family Sciences, Texas Woman's University, P.O. Box 425769, Denton, TX 76204-5769

Tracey L. Hurd, Department of Education and Human Services, Simmons College, 300 The Fenway, Boston, MA 02115

Shirley Hymon-Parker, Department of Human Ecology, University of Maryland Eastern Shore, Princess Ann, MD 21853-1299

Jean Ispa, Human Development and Family Studies, University of Missouri-Columbia, Columbia, MO 65211

Golden Jackson, Department of Consumer and Textile Science, The Ohio State University, 1787 Neil Avenue, 231 Campbell Hall, Columbus, OH 43210-1295

Charles Johnson, Department of Psychology, and Public Policy Research Institute, Texas A&M University, College Station, TX 77843-4476

Cynthia E. Johnson, Department of Child Development and Family Relations, East Carolina University, Greenville, NC 27858-4354

Susan R. Jones, School of Educational Policy and Leadership, The Ohio State University, 1787 Neil Avenue, Columbus, OH 43210-1295

Alesa H. Judd, Bibb County Child Caring Foundation Policy Board, Centreville, AL 35042

Joanne G. Keith, Young Spartan Program and Department of Family and Child Ecology, Michigan State University, 203 Human Ecology, East Lansing, MI 48824-1030

Judith Peck Key, Mott Children's Health Center, Flint, MI 48503

Sally Kilmer, School of Family and Consumer Sciences, Bowling Green State University, Bowling Green, OH 43403-0254

Sally A. Koblinsky, Department of Family Studies, University of Maryland, College Park, MD 20740

J. Lee Kreader, Illinois Department of Human Services, Chicago, IL 60604

Anne Larkin, Education Department, Lesley College, Cambridge, MA 02138-2790

A. Fredericka Larsen, WSOS Child Development and Head Start, 109 Front Street, Fremont, OH 43420.

Richard M. Lerner, Center for Child, Family, and Community Partnership, Boston College, Chestnut Hill, MA 02467-3813

Ronald F. Levant, Center for Psychological Studies, Nova Southeastern University, 3301 College Avenue, Ft. Lauderdale, FL 33314

Kathleen A. Lodl, Cooperative Extension, and Department of Family and Consumer Sciences, P.O. Box 830801, University of Nebraska, Lincoln, NE 68583-0801

Dale Lucy-Allen, Student Volunteer Programs, Springfield College, 263 Alden Street, Springfield, MA 01109-3797

Tom Luster, Department of Family and Child Ecology, 101 Morill Hall, Michigan State University, East Lansing, MI 48824-1030

Carol Lynn Martin, Department of Family Resources and Human Development, Arizona State University, P.O. Box 872502, Tempe, AZ 85287-2502

Nancy Martland, Eliot-Pearson Department of Child Development, Tufts University, 105 College Avenue, Medford, MA 02155

Donna Massie, Mott Children's Health Center, Flint, MI 48503

Susan Maxwell, Georgia Child Care Council, Atlanta, GA 30318

Charles McClintock, College of Human Ecology, Cornell University, Martha Van Rensselar Hall, Ithaca, NY 14853-4401

Raun D. Melmed, Southwest Autism Research Center, Phoenix, AZ 85006

Jacquelyn Mize, Department of Human Development and Family Studies, Auburn University, Auburn, AL 36849-3501

Judy Jolley Mohraz, President, Goucher College, Baltimore, MD 21204-2794

Virginia Molgaard, Institute for Social and Behavioral Research, Iowa State University, Ames, IA 50011-0002

Johnetta Morrison, Human Development and Family Studies, University of Missouri-Columbia, Columbia, MO 65211

Greg Muller, School to Careers, Snow College, 150 E. College Avenue, Ephraim, UT 84627

Ann K. Mullis, Department of Family and Child Sciences, Florida State University, Tallahassee, FL 32306-1490

Ronald L. Mullis, Department of Family and Child Sciences, Florida State University, Tallahassee, FL 32306-1490

Richard N. Nader, Public Policy Research Institute, Texas A&M University, H. C. Dulie Bell Bldg., Room 316, College Station, TX 77843-4476

Cathy Nathan, Child Development Research Center, Texas Tech University, Box 41162, Lubbock, TX 79409-1162

J. Jay Ney, Cooperative Extension System, University of Idaho, 1239 Idaho Street, Lewiston, ID 83501

Barbara O'Donnel, School of Family and Consumer Sciences, Bowling Green State University, Bowling Green, OH 43403-0254

Carol Painter, Psychological Services and Education, Florida State University, Tallahassee, FL 32306

Tracy M. Palmer, College of Community Health Sciences, University of Alabama, Tuscaloosa, AL 35487

Daniel F. Perkins, Department of Family, Youth, and Community Sciences, 3041 McCarty Hall, P.O. Box 110310, University of Florida, Gainesville, FL 32611-0310

Margaret M. Petruska, Howard Heinz Endowment, 30 CNG Tower, 625 Liberty Avenue, Pittsburgh, PA 15222

Loretta P. Prater, School of Family and Consumer Sciences, Eastern Illinois University, Charleston, IL 61920-3099

William H. Quinn, Department of Child and Family Development, The University of Georgia, Dawson Hall, Athens, GA 30602-3622

Celeste Sturdevant Reed, Institute for Children, Youth, and Families, Michigan State University, East Lansing, MI 48824

Sidney A. Ribeau, President, Bowling Green State University, Bowling Green, OH 43403

Jose Ribeiro, Cambridge Public Schools, and Department of Education, Lesley College, Cambridge, MA 02138

Robbie Roberts, Department of Human Development and Family Studies and the Birmingham Early Learning Center, Auburn University, Auburn, AL 36849-3501

Kathleen Boyce Rodgers, Department of Human Development, Washington State University, P.O. Box 64636, Pullman, WA 99164-6236

Stephen A. Rollin, Department of Human Services and Studies, 215 Stone Building, Florida State University, Tallahassee, FL 32306-4468

Fred Rothbaum, Eliot-Pearson Department of Child Development, Tufts University, 105 College Avenue, Medford, MA 02155

Roberta Rubin, Psychological Services and Education, Florida State University, Tallahassee, FL 32306

Lorilee R. Sandmann, University Outreach, 6 Kellogg Center, Michigan State University, East Lansing, MI 48824-1022

Shelly E. Schadewald, Jackson Non-Profit Support Center, 325 West Michigan Avenue, Jackson, MI 49201

Stacey Scheckner, Psychological Services and Education, Florida State University, Tallahassee, FL 32306

Cindy K. Schneider, Southwest Autism Research Center, Phoenix, AZ 85006

Jennifer Seydel, Teacher Preparation and Certification Department, Springfield College, 263 Alden Street, Springfield, MA 01109-3797

Lonnie R. Sherrod, William T. Grant Foundation, 570 Lexington Avenue, 18th Floor, New York, NY 10022-6837

Lou Anna Kimsey Simon, Provost and Vice President for Academic Affairs, 438 Administration Building, Michigan State University, East Lansing, MI 48824-1046

Stephen A. Small, Department of Child and Family Studies, University of Wisconsin at Madison, Madison, WI 53706

Andrea B. Smith, College of Education, Western Michigan University, 2333 East Beltline S.E., Grand Rapids, MI 49546-5936

Edward A. Smith, Department of Human Development and Family Studies, 110 Henderson Building South, The Pennsylvania State University, University Park, PA 16802-6504

Michael Smyer, Graduate School of Arts and Sciences, Boston College, Chestnut Hill, MA 02467-3813

Richard L. Spoth, Center for Family Research in Rural Mental Health, Iowa State University, 2625 N. Loop Drive, Suite 500, Ames, IA 50010-8295

Anne M. Stanberry, Family and Consumer Sciences, The University of Southern Mississippi, Hattiesburg, MS 39406-5035

Georgia L. Stevens, Cooperative Extension, and Department of Family and Consumer Sciences, University of Nebraska, P.O. Box 830801, Lincoln, NE 68583-0801

Donald Stricker, WSOS Community Action Commission, 109 S. Front Street, Fremont, OH 43420

Kathy R. Thornburg, Department of Human Development and Family Studies, University of Missouri-Columbia, Columbia, MO 65211

Christine M. Todd, College of Family and Consumer Sciences, Outreach, University of Georgia, 224 Dawson Hall, Athens, GA 30602-3622

Lynne Vernon-Feagans, College of Health and Human Development, The Pennsylvania State University, 201 Henderson Building, University Park, PA 16802-6501

Francisco Villarruel, Department of Family and Child Ecology, Michigan State University, East Lansing, MI 48824

James C. Votruba, President, Northern Kentucky University, Highland Heights, KY 41099-0001

Lenore E. Walker, Domestic Violence Institute, 50 S. Steele St., #850, Denver, CO 80209

Mary E. Walsh, Department of Counseling, Developmental and Educational Psychology, Boston College, Chestnut Hill, MA 02467-3813

Daniel Ward, Psychological Services and Education, Florida State University, Tallahassee, FL 32306

Carol Weinberg, Education Department, Goucher College, 1021 Dulaney Valley Road, Baltimore, MD 21204-2794

Richard A. Weinberg, Advisory Council on Adolescent Health Programs, University of Minnesota, St. Paul, MN 55108

Anne Wharff, Illinois Department of Human Services, Springfield, IL 62701

John R. Wheat, College of Community Health Sciences, University of Alabama, Tuscaloosa, AL 35487

Quincy White, Housing Authority of Lubbock, 1708 Avenue G, Lubbock, TX 79401

Deborah Wilkes, Georgia Department of Human Resources, Atlanta, GA 30303

Steven K. Wisensale, School of Family Studies, U-58, University of Connecticut, Storrs, CT 06269-0001

John Wright, Psychological Services and Education, Florida State University, Tallahassee, FL 32306

Raymond K. Yang, Department of Human Development and Family Studies, Gifford Building, Colorado State University, Fort Collins, CO 80523-1570

FOREWORD

Lonnie R. Sherrod
William T. Grant Foundation

The social-behavioral sciences are not currently fulfilling their role as the "social intelligence of society" (Prewitt, 1995); as a result, a paradigm change may be needed in the social-behavioral sciences. There are, of course, several methods by which people try to understand and describe the human condition; art and religion are as valid as science. However, traditionally these different methods of gathering information on the human condition have been used for different purposes. Art and religion, for example, provided guidance for daily living, values formation, inspiration, and other kinds of personal soul-searching. Social science was viewed as providing the information needed for social decision-making, and for explaining social situations, and phenomena. That is, information generated by social scientific inquiry provided the fuel for the design of the social policies and social institutions that constitute our society. The social-behavioral sciences were viewed to be useful in part because they provided tools to accomplish behavior change—to increase the likelihood that people led productive, healthy lives. Science, furthermore, has been viewed as useful to society because ideally it provides objective information not contaminated by social values, ideology, or other subjective interests.

However, this situation is changing, or in some cases has already changed, and science is no longer viewed to provide a basis for informed decision-making about society. I have written elsewhere about one example of this: The disassociation between science and philanthropy. Around the turn of this century, philanthropy emerged to identify the core causes of social problems; it sought to use science's ability to separate cause and effect as a tool. As philanthropy increasingly concerned itself with social reform, beginning in the 1960s, it lost this connection to research (Sherrod, 1998). Another equally important example is the perceived demise of public education and the increasingly widespread belief that the current educational system does not educate youth even to read and write. Indeed, the educational system, at every level including higher education, which is based on social scientific ideas and findings, is not believed to prepare young people adequately for their role as active, productive citizens in the modern world (Bloom, 1987; Cremin, 1990; Hamburg, 1994; Howe, 1993). A third example is offered by the long history of evaluation of social programs designed to improve the life circumstances of disenfranchised individuals and families; most such research shows that such programs have little or no long-term impact (Walker & Vileela-Velez, 1992). All these examples point to the fact, I believe, that the social-behavioral sciences are failing to fulfill their role as the "systematic social intelligence of society" (Prewitt, 1995). As a result, important policy decisions are being made without adequate information or are being based on subjective forms of information such as ideology.

Certainly the social-behavioral sciences have made important contributions to society in terms of "inventions." Testing for an array of personal attributes is one good example. Although many people would argue that IQ testing is a failure not a success, it does offer an important and socially meaningful technology. Psychotherapy and other means of treating mental illness are further examples. Even research on self-concept and self-efficacy has proved useful in preventing HIV infection (Bandura,1992). Scientists, including social scientists[1], have, in fact, differentiated efficacy, referring to statistical significance or change in test scores, from effectiveness, which denotes meaningfulness in terms of the functioning of the individual, family or institution. A program may, for example, show a statistical effect, but this may translate into a small and meaningless contribution to individual well-being. That is, science has been generally successful in demonstrating efficacy, but this efficacy has rarely been translated into effectiveness.

University-community partnerships provide one means, not the only one, of accomplishing a paradigm shift in the social-behavioral sciences. First, the approach to research that is advocated is both new and of increasing social relevance. The work that characterizes these partnerships is based on contextualism, includes concerns for ethnicity and culture, attends to diverse populations (by race, class, region, age, and other individual attributes), relies on multiple methods, and cuts across traditional disciplines (Fisher & Lerner, 1994). All of these characteristics of research are new and ground-breaking and carry the potential to truly change the face of social-behavioral science research in ways that increase its usefulness and relevance to the non-scientific world.

Second, reaching out to communities and involving non-researchers in the research process has the potential to revitalize research as well as increase its social relevance. These approaches bring fresh perspectives not just to the topics of research but also to methods. They directly tackle challenging, real-world problems, traditionally avoided by scientists because they were too difficult to handle in scientifically valid ways. Through their pronounced concern for dissemination, they get the word out about the results from science. This can contribute to renewing the public's faith in the social sciences as a vehicle for addressing social problems.

Hence, these university-community partnerships have the potential to restore the social-behavioral sciences as the "social intelligence of society." They can develop a science that increases its effectiveness without compromising efficacy. They can forge new connections to philanthropy, revitalize education in terms of its relevance to society, develop new approaches to evaluating social programs, and provide a solid base of information relevant to making important policy decisions and designing effective programs (Sherrod, 1998).

The partnerships described in this volume in various stages of development represent an emerging field, too young for its worth to be fully evaluated. However, its potential is great–for its impact on education as well as on science. Only time can tell if this potential will be fully realized. Nonetheless, as volumes such as this one showcase such examples and, in so doing, promote the creation of new examples, the field will grow. And as it grows, we will learn. And as we learn, the prospects of realizing this potential will increase.

ENDNOTE

1. The biological, medical, and physical sciences, indeed, have a larger array of contributions that do inform and impact individual lives.

REFERENCES

Bandura, A. (1992). A social cognitive approach to the exercise of control over AIDS infection. In R. J. DiClemente (Ed.), *Adolescents and AIDS: A generation in jeopardy.* San Francisco, CA: Sage.

Bloom, A. (1987). *The closing of the American mind.* New York: Simon and Schuster.

Cremin, L. (1990). *Popular education and its discontents.* New York: Harper and Row.

Fisher, C., & Lerner, R. (Eds.). (1994). *Applied developmental psychology.* New York: McGraw-Hill.

Hamburg, B. (1994). Education for a Changed America: The Need for Stronger Basics and an Additional "3-R's." President's Report in *The Annual Report of the William T. Grant Foundation.* New York: Citation Graphics.

Howe, H. (1993). *Thinking about our kids.* New York: The Free Press.

Prewitt, K. (1995). Social sciences and private philanthropy: The quest for social relevance. *Essays on Philanthropy, 15.* Series on Foundations and their Role in American Life. Indiana University Center on Philanthropy.

Sherrod, L. (1998). The common pursuits of modern philanthropy and the proposed outreach university: Enhancing research and education. In R. M. Lerner & L. A. K. Simon (Eds.), *University-community collaborations for the twenty-first century: Scholarship for youth and families* (pp. 397-417). New York: Garland.

Walker, G., & Vileela-Velez, F. (1992). *Anatomy of a demonstration: The Summer Training and Education Program (STEP) from pilot through replication and post program impacts.* Philadelphia, PA: Public Private Ventures.

FOREWORD

James C. Votruba
Northern Kentucky University

In his last essay, published posthumously in 1996, Dr. Ernest L. Boyer challenged universities to become more vigorous partners in the search for answers to our most pressing social, civic, economic, and moral problems, and to reaffirm their commitment to what he called the scholarship of engagement (Boyer, 1996). This volume is a ringing response to that challenge. The successful partnerships described herein demonstrate that universities and communities, working together, can have a profound impact on improving the lives of children and families while, at the same time, moving the university to a larger sense of its own mission and purpose.

Over the past decade, I have had the privilege of knowing many of the authors represented in this volume. In some cases, I have had the opportunity to participate in their work and help celebrate their success. These are special people characterized by passion and persistence, courage and commitment. In the process of building community-university partnerships, they have often had to challenge traditional views of scholarship and the role of the university in society. At times, they have even placed their careers at risk because of a lack of both understanding and support for their work among department chairs, deans, and promotion and tenure committees. The result is that, far too often, the building of community-university partnerships takes place at the periphery rather than at the center of academic life.

There is a growing voice on behalf of strengthening the university's public engagement. Most recently, NASULGC's Kellogg Commission on the Future of State and Land-Grant Universities issued its third report entitled, *Returning to our Roots: The engaged institution* (1999). The report asserts that "In the end, the clear evidence is that, with the resources and superbly qualified professors and staff on our campuses, we can organize our institutions to serve both local and national needs in a more coherent and effective way. We can and must do better."

Doing better will require university leaders to build campus environments that support community-university partnerships and the effort that it takes to achieve them. In my experience, those universities that support the development of partnerships have several characteristics in common.

First, they have developed an intellectual foundation that supports the scholarship of engagement as an integral part of the institution's overall academic mission. From this perspective, community-university partnerships are viewed as opportunities to enhance the discovery, transmission, and application of knowledge through scholarship that occurs within the context of communities. Far from being peripheral to the life of the campus, these partnership are viewed as central to the university's mission and are reflected in the campus mission statement and other efforts to describe the institution's vision and purpose.

Second, they have developed the organizational infrastructure necessary to support the development of community partnerships. Over the past decade, we have seen a relatively large number of universities create centers and institutes designed to support interdisciplinary problem-focused scholarship in partnership with communities. These units generally include not only faculty members but also professional staff who are experienced in the complex process of designing and maintaining community partnerships. Agility and adaptability in their community relationships generally characterize those units that are successful in building community partnerships.

Third, these universities have made commitment to the scholarship of engagement an important standard for hiring and evaluating presidents, provosts, deans, and chairs. Do those who occupy these key leadership positions understand and support the scholarship of engagement? Are they demonstrating that support through the priorities that they set and the projects that they choose to support? For community-university partnerships to flourish there must be supportive leadership at every level of the institution.

Fourth, those universities that support community partnerships nurture the scholarship of engagement through faculty socialization and development. They offer young faculty members opportunities to experience the scholarship of engagement through mentoring relationships with faculty experienced in this work. At the same time, they offer opportunities for faculty members at all levels to renew and refocus their careers by engaging in community-based scholarship.

Fifth, they make the scholarship of engagement an integral part of the annual university planning and budgeting process. On far too many campuses, the rhetoric of public engagement is not accompanied by resource support. As with funding for research and teaching, funding for public engagement must be ample, stable, and performance driven. Units should receive resource support for community-university partnerships that are a priority for the campus and they should be held accountable for achieving agreed upon outcomes. At the public policy level, states should consider funding community-university partnerships that address issues of public priority. There is ample precedent for this in the funding of the Cooperative Extension Service.

Sixth, universities that support partnerships acknowledge excellence in the scholarship of engagement through the annual evaluation of unit-level and faculty performance and in the faculty promotion and tenure process. Universities that support the scholarship of public engagement have developed standards by which this scholarship is measured and evaluated. Nothing sends a stronger message that this work is important than when it is seen as important in salary, promotion and tenure decisions. Additionally, some universities have created resource incentives for units that make a collective commitment to the scholarship of engagement through the development of community-university partnerships. Unit-level incentives and rewards have enormous potential for enhancing this form of scholarly work.

Finally, universities that support the scholarship of engagement have worked to deepen their understanding of how to create and sustain community-university partnerships. They have developed "principles of good practice" that are used to develop, administer, and evaluate these partnerships on an on-going basis. For example, principles of good practice emphasize the need for both community and university to be very clear from the outset concerning what each brings to the relationship in terms of human and financial resources. They emphasize the need to clearly define the purpose of the partnership and the outcomes to be achieved. They make clear how the partnership will be evaluated and by whom. They emphasize the need for progress benchmarks against which the partnership will be evaluated. Finally, they anticipate the day when the partnership will end and they agree upon a process of disengagement.

The growth of applied developmental science as a field of graduate study in American universities offers great opportunity for the next generation of professors to practice the scholarship of engagement as an integral part of their graduate education. Many of the authors represented in this book are leaders in applied developmental science and regularly involve graduate students in their community-based scholarship as a way of training them to engage in this new and exciting form of scholarship.

American universities have historically received such enormous public support because the public has viewed universities as being aligned with the public interest. Whether it was bringing science to agriculture, providing the workforce for industrial expansion, supporting national defense, or providing intergenerational mobility through near universal access, American higher education has been viewed as integral to our nation's future. The partnerships described herein are further evidence that America's universities continue to address the broader needs of communities that we serve. These partnerships reflect the commitment of faculty and staff to addressing some of society's most complex and formidable challenges through community partnerships in which each partner is both teacher and learner. For American universities, a return to public engagement as an integral part of our academic mission is a return to our roots and to the source of our public support.

REFERENCES

Boyer, E. L. (1996). The scholarship of engagement. *Journal of Public Service and Outreach*, *1*, 11-20.

Kellogg Commission on the Future of State University and Land-Grant Colleges. (1999). *Returning to our roots: The engaged institution*. Washington, DC: National Association of State Universities and Land-Grant Colleges. February.

PREFACE

A major challenge facing contemporary higher education is to enhance its relevance and connectedness to the issues and problems faced by the broader society—as these problems are defined by community members, and not by academics acting independently of the views of non-academic community members. Indeed, perhaps the most consistently identified "problem" in higher education, as reflected in the comments and behavior of taxpayers, legislators, governing boards, funders, parents, students, and businesses, is that the academy is not playing a visible role in contributing to the improvement of the lives of people in the community.

Such contributions may not seem to be a part of the mission of colleges and universities, as such missions may be generally understood today. Nonetheless, as both Peter Magrath (1993, 1998) and Ernest Boyer (1994), among others (e.g., Graham Spanier, 1997, and James Votruba, 1996), remind us, there is a long and rich history of directing scholarship to address the "practical" problems of life, as those problems are defined by the communities within which these lives are lived. This is true in both public universities, especially land-grant ones, and several private institutions (for example, those, such as institutions in the Jesuit tradition, founded to have a direct role in the promotion of social justice in communities). Simply, there has been a long tradition of "outreach scholarship" (Lerner and Simon, 1998) in America. This tradition, while perhaps dimly remembered in some quarters in modern academe (e.g., see Bonnen, 1998) is gaining renewed attention.

Even given this long tradition, however, a key contemporary reason for attention to outreach scholarship and to collaborations between universities and communities concerns the pressures in and on higher education institutions that demand such work. For example, federal policy makers (e.g., Kennedy, in press) and national philanthropic organizations (Richardson, 1996; Sherrod, 1998, in press) are explicitly urging universities and colleges to use their learning resources, and to engage in scholarship, in ways that add value to the lives of youth, families, and communities.

Universities have listened to, and continue to heed, such appeals. Indeed, engagement in outreach scholarship by some universities has a long and uninterrupted history across the twentieth century. For other institutions, such work is emerging as a new focus. Nevertheless, whatever its history may be at a given college or university, numerous examples now exist of successful community-university collaboration and outreach scholarship. A key purpose of this book is to illustrate the diverse instances of such work.

We present several dozen exemplary "success stories" of community-university partnerships that serve to enhance the lives of children, youth, and families. These illustrations are drawn from collaborations across the breadth of the nation and reflect the work of large and small, public and private, research-intensive and liberal arts/undergraduate education-oriented colleges and universities. Moreover, these partnerships involve an array of target audiences, covering the individual life span from infancy through old age and involving a diverse set of groups and organizations (e.g., families, schools, formal and informal non-governmental organizations [NGOs], courts, professional organizations, and governmental organizations). In addition, this outreach scholarship takes many forms, for example, technical assistance, evaluation, training, program design and delivery, demonstration projects, action research, and dissemination.

The success stories are meant to be useful to two broad audiences: 1) Individuals in decision-making roles in academe that directly impact what gets done or does not get done in colleges and universities (presidents, vice presidents, provosts, deans, department chairs, governing board members, and faculty and student leaders); and 2) Persons outside of academe who are concerned with creating positive change across a wide-range of issues pertinent to the lives of youth, families, and communities (e.g., foundation leaders and philanthropists, business leaders, government and civic leaders, legislators, community program leaders, advocates, and lobbyists).

We believe that the illustrations of community-university partnerships presented in this volume will demonstrate to these audiences that successful scholarship (i.e., scholarship that is both fundable and publishable) and successful outreach (i.e., university facilitated knowledge that serves community-defined values and goals) can be woven throughout the fabric of the university. Our hope is that the breadth of examples of community-university partnerships provided in this volume will provide ideas to university and community leaders about how this work might be accomplished. For this reason we have asked the authors of each "success story" included in this book to discuss the bases of the success of their collaboration, the barriers to as well as the facilitators of such work that existed within their university and the community, and the lessons learned about building and sustaining such efforts. We hope that the information presented in this volume may help guide universities and communities to work together to promote positive development of the diverse children, families, and communities of our nation.

REFERENCES

Bonnen, J. T. (1998). The land-grant idea and the evolving outreach university. In R. M. Lerner & L. A. K. Simon (Eds.), *University-community collaborations for the twenty-first century: Outreach scholarship for youth and famlies* (pp. 25-71). New York: Garland.

Boyer, E. L. (1994, March 9). Creating the new American college. *Chronicle of Higher Education*, A48.

Kennedy, E. M. (In press). University-community partnerships: A mutually beneficial effort to aid community development and improve academic learning opportunities. *Applied Developmental Science*.

Lerner, R. M., & Simon, L. A. K. (Eds.). (1998). *University-community collaborations for the twenty-first century: Outreach scholarship for youth and families*. New York: Garland.

Magrath, C. P. (1993). *Comments to the Board on Home Economics on November 12, 1993*. Washington, DC: National Association of State Universities and Land-Grant Colleges.

Magrath, C. P. (1998). Foreword: Creating a new outreach university. In R. M. Lerner & L. A. K. Simon (Eds.), *University-community collaborations for the twenty-first century: Outreach scholarship for youth and famlies* (pp. xxi-xix). New York: Garland.

Richardson, W.C. (1996). A new calling for higher education. *The John W. Olswald Lecture*, The Pennsylvania State University, University Park.

Sherrod, L. (1998). The common pursuits of modern philanthropy and the proposed outreach university: Enhancing research and education. In R. M. Lerner & L. A. K. Simon (Eds.), *University-community collaborations for the twenty-first century: Outreach scholarship for youth and families* (pp. 397-418). New York: Garland.

Sherrod, L. (In press). Giving child development knowledge away: Using university-community partnerships to disseminate research on children, youth, and families. *Applied Developmental Science.*

Spanier, G. B. (1997). Enhancing the capacity for outreach. *Journal of Public Service and Outreach, 2*(2), 7-11.

Votruba, J. C. (1996). Strengthening the university's alignment with society: Challenges and strategies. *Journal of Public Service and Outreach, 1*(1), 29-36.

ACKNOWLEDGMENTS

To the extent that this book makes the kind of contribution we hope it will make a great debt is owed to several colleagues. The idea for the book arose as a consequence of the stimulating exchanges among the participants at the Third National Applied Development Science Conference at Florida State University (March 7-8, 1997). This meeting was sponsored by the American Association of Family and Consumer Sciences, by the Association of Administrators of Human Sciences, and by several colleges and universities across the nation. We are grateful to all of the colleagues at the meeting whose ideas and outreach efforts gave us the impetus to develop this book.

Many of these colleagues contributed chapters to this book. To them, and indeed to all the authors of this volume, we acknowledge our great debt. Their creativity and commitment to building new community-university partnerships serving youth and families are the vital ingredients supporting transformation of higher education in the direction of outreach.

We are deeply grateful as well to James C. Votruba, President of Northern Kentucky University, and to Lonnie R. Sherrod, Executive Vice President of the William T. Grant Foundation, for writing forewords to this book. Their vision and leadership in higher education and philanthropy, respectively, have framed the dimensions of systems change in higher education and outreach scholarship that are synergistically building new and sustainable bridges between universities and communities. We are grateful as well to Sidney A. Ribeau, President of Bowling Green State University, for generously contributing an afterword for this book. His administrative leadership exemplifies the efforts that must be made in higher education if community-university partnership building and outreach scholarship for youth and families are to be rewarded by and sustained in the academy.

We appreciate greatly the superb professional contributions of the editors at our respective institutions, Elaine Thomas and Sofia T. Romero. Their skills, organizational abilities, knowledge, and wisdom enabled this book to be developed and completed efficiently and productively. Final manuscript preparation was done by Judy Maxey and Sherry Haskins at BGSU, whose expertise, patience and guidance were (as always) outstanding. The editorial guidance for camera-ready preparation provided by Mary Panarelli and Melissa Fearon at Kluwer was outstanding. We also thank Dr. Robert Chametzky, editor at Kluwer Academic Publishers, for his support during the development and production of this book, and Scott Delman, Senior Publishing Editor at Kluwer, for his leadership in bringing this book to completion.

Finally, we are indebted to our families, and we dedicate this book to them. Their support was indispensable during our work. Their love reminded us why we care so deeply about making the institutions within which we work responsive to the hopes and aspirations of people living in real families, in real communities.

T.R.C./R.M.L.

1 SERVING CHILDREN AND FAMILIES THROUGH COMMUNITY-UNIVERSITY PARTNERSHIPS: A VIEW OF THE ISSUES

Thomas R. Chibucos
Bowling Green State University

Richard M. Lerner
Boston College

INTRODUCTION

A sea change is occurring in the way in which colleges and universities work with communities to promote the positive development of youth and families. Across both public and private institutions a model is emerging for the creation or enhancement of community-university collaborations and of university units devoted to "outreach scholarship" to better serve youth, families, and communities. New, university-wide centers or institutes devoted to integrating the university's ability to generate, transmit, preserve, or apply knowledge with the strengths, vision, values, and voice of the community are being established (Lerner & Miller, 1998). In turn, units whose traditional mission has been community collaboration (such as the Cooperative Extension Service) have a new vigor as they find impetus for weaving their work throughout the fabric of the institution (Votruba, 1992).

These units are providing points of access (and accountability) to communities and, through co-learning collaborations with them, are creating partnerships that are increasing the life chances of young people, their families, and their communities. The emergence of such a model for community-university collaborations—for "outreach universities" (Lerner & Simon, 1998b; Sherrod, 1998, in press a, in press b; Spanier, 1997a, 1997b; Votruba, 1992, 1996, in press)—could not come at a better time in the history of the United States.

Challenges to the overall positive development of American youth and their families exist today at historically unprecedented levels (e.g., Carnegie Corporation of New York, 1995; Dryfoos, 1990, 1994; Hamburg, 1992; Lerner, 1995). Yet, universities have not been a central part of the systems change needed to empower individuals, families, and communities to use their capacities to envision, enact, and sustain effective and appropriately scaled programs and policies addressing these challenges (Lerner & Simon, 1998c). Indeed, some leaders of higher education have warned that if universities do not undertake such actions as central parts of their missions they will be in danger of becoming "Jurassic Parks:" Enclaves housing people whose activities and skills may be of largely historical interest but seem of little value for addressing and resolving some of the key issues of contemporary concern to society (Richardson, 1996).

To become part of the solution to the problems confronting youth, universities must use their abilities to generate, transmit, preserve, and apply knowledge to address issues that communities define as meaningful and in ways that communities value. In other words, universities must undertake as core parts of their mission a commitment to outreach scholarship (Lerner & Simon, 1998b, c). They must also demonstrate a strong commitment to building sustainable community-university partnerships. The growing commitment to such systems change that is occurring across the United States is precisely the basis for our belief that we are on the threshold of a new era of collaboration between higher education institutions and the communities they serve.

For example, in a recent book (Lerner & Simon, 1998a), university administrators, faculty leaders, foundation heads, and leaders of community and state organizations expressed a shared view that systems change is needed in America to enhance the life chances of our nation's youth. There was agreement also that universities must be incorporated into this change for two particular reasons: 1) In order to increase the probability of its success; and 2) To rekindle the spirit within universities, and the belief in society, that higher education institutions must, and actually do, contribute to the lives of people in ways that citizens define as valuable. The contributors to the book emphasized also that there is a fortunate convergence of societal and intellectual events such that, if decisive action is taken, a means exists to bring universities into a new system of community-wide, multi-institutional, and integrated collaborations. Such partnerships are seen as providing perhaps the essential and the best chance of building and sustaining programs and policies effectively promoting positive youth development.

CHANGES IN HIGHER EDUCATION

One set of events promoting a window of opportunity for this systems change involves the increasing social, economic, and political pressure for universities to provide improved access to communities and, as well, to be more accountable to them. Leaders of higher education (e.g., Boyer, 1990, 1994; Magrath, 1993, 1998) have noted that universities can no longer remain enclaves of ethereal intellectual isolation, removed from the ebb and flow of the larger society surrounding them, *if* they are to expect public support and elicit public trust. Universities must find ways to use their talents and resources to contribute to the public good—as defined by the public and not just by universities themselves—if they are to survive and thrive as contributing institutions into the next century.

For example, the newly-created Kellogg Foundation Commission, involving university presidents across the nation, represents an invaluable source of energy for creating such a sea change in the way universities envision and enact their relationships with communities (Richardson, 1996; Spanier, 1997). The Commission may be a vital impetus for promoting the systems change that will result in the enhancement of outreach scholarship for youth, families, and communities.

Clearly, presidents and provosts can foster differences in university climate and culture pertinent to outreach scholarship and to community-university partnership-building, and can have major impacts on the faculty reward system. However, the strength of the disciplines and the traditions of academic freedom in America require that systems change involves innovations at the level of faculty activity (e.g., scholarship, graduate training, and supervision of undergraduate education, for instance, involving service learning) (Lerner & Simon, 1998 b, c; Votruba, in press). We must capture the minds as well as the hearts of faculty if we are to institutionalize among these agents of research, teaching, and service a commitment to engage in outreach scholarship and partnership-building for youth and families. We must create a point of influence effecting this systems change that acts synergistically with the one that may be promoted by actions such as the creation of the Kellogg Commission. This additional influence should promote among faculty members discussion and actions regarding criteria and issues pertinent to outreach scholarship and community-university collaboration that parallel the ideas being forwarded by university administrators. Administrative vision and faculty culture must be seamlessly linked in order that the scholarly merit of the outreach and partnership building roles of the university become central forces shaping the university for the next century.

NEW SYSTEMS MODELS OF HUMAN DEVELOPMENT

The need for this linkage between trends in higher education toward outreach collaboration, and faculty-based intellectual activity is where a second set of events converges with those fostering institutional change. These events are linked to the evolution of a person-context relational (systems) model of human development that integrates developmental and ecological data and theory. The model has become increasingly important in scholarship in human development (Lerner, 1995, 1998a, 1998b). The model also provides a frame for the integration of basic and applied research and, in effect, indicates that interventions (policies or programs) represent a means to test theory-guided ideas about how to configure the person-context system to promote healthy development within the actual ecology of human development (Lerner, 1998b). Thus, the evaluation of these interventions provides not only important information about "best practice" in community-based policies and programs but, at the same time, offers key empirical insight into theoretical ideas about the core relational process of human development.

This developmental systems, or developmental contextual, perspective has come to provide an organizing framework for basic theoretical issues in human development, as well as for: 1) a new text in human development (Fisher & Lerner, 1994); 2) a new outreach scholarship journal, *Applied Developmental Science*; and 3) the formation of a coalition of several scholarly societies and numerous public, land-grant, and private universities: The National Task Force on Applied Developmental Science (Fisher, et al., 1993). The net effect of this scholarship and collaboration is to both support and foster the *Zeitgeist* for viewing community-collaborative scholarship pertinent to youth and families as the cutting-edge of developmental science.

There is a convergence, then, in (a) the societal and academic pressures pushing universities to provide access for and accountability to the youth, families, and communities they serve; and (b) intellectual trends in the human developmental sciences that foster outreach scholarship promoting healthy youth and family development. In an important sense, the emergence of applied developmental science facilitates the systems change that, through initiatives such as the Kellogg Foundation Commission, is furthering a vision for outreach scholarship and community-university collaboration within American universities.

GOALS FOR THE BOOK

Numerous examples now exist of successful community-university partnerships and outreach scholarship. A key purpose of this book is to illustrate the diverse instances of such work. These illustrations demonstrate that successful scholarship and successful outreach can be woven throughout the fabric of the university. That is, faculty, students, and staff from any discipline, profession, or field can work productively within the frame of this model. These examples demonstrate as well the importance of capitalizing on the expertise of those facets of the university already embedded in communities (e.g., the Cooperative Extension Services of land-grant universities).

Further, invaluable lessons are available to members of the academy by listening to the voices of individuals and organizations external to it. Communities are expert systems that have unique knowledge about the nature of development in their ecology and about the needs and resources pertinent to the healthy functioning and future of its youth. Thus, the university, as an expert system as well, must respect the knowledge of the community and must not dictate either the substance or time frame of collaborative activities. Universities need to be certain not to over-promise, or to claim an ability to contribute to a focus where no faculty expertise is available. But, the university must be ready to do what it is uniquely capable of doing. That is, providing its knowledge resources through activities such as technical assistance, needs assessment, program design and evaluation, continuing education, or demonstration research to collaboratively pursue community-defined and community-valued goals for youth development.

In addition, the illustrations of community-university partnerships and outreach scholarship in this book provide other key learnings about such work. One is that productive outreach scholarship requires a compelling intellectual model for the integration of multiple disciplines and multiple professions with the community. Further, the commitment of university central administration (and other key university stakeholders, such as boards of trustees, alumni groups, legislators, and funders/donors) to the support of this model is critical to its usefulness and ultimate success. Despite the political pressures for resources from more traditional, disciplinary-based programs, specific support to sustain a commitment to community-university partnerships and outreach scholarship is essential (Lerner & Miller, 1998). This commitment will be enhanced by delivering to these administrators evidence that the criteria for quality outreach scholarship are being realized in an array of units from a diverse set of universities. Accordingly, a major audience for the examples of successful, youth- and family-serving partnerships and outreach scholarship presented in this book is university administrators—and the other key stakeholder groups we have mentioned.

The need to persuade such audiences of the importance *and feasibility* of promoting community-university collaboration and outreach scholarship at their colleges and universities is crucial at this time in the history of our nation and of the American University system. There is excellent outreach scholarship being conducted across the nation (Lerner & Simon, 1998b); and there is a growing commitment among administrative and faculty leaders to this work, and to the development of community-university collaborations. Nevertheless, the interrelated problems of broader, nation-wide dissemination of the outreach scholarship model, of the sustainability of outreach units, of long-term institutionalization of outreach scholarship, and of an enduring commitment to community-university partnerships remain to be solved. It is clear to us that these problems must be solved within the context of a substantive agenda open to the values and developing capacities of the communities with which universities collaborate. Less certain are the precise ways in which effectiveness and scale, as well as sustainability, will be attained. Each college or university will need to find its own way of adapting the outreach scholarship model to its specific institutional and community cultures.

Our hope is that the breadth of examples of community-university collaborations in this volume will provide ideas about how this work might be accomplished. Accordingly, the authors of each "success story" included in this book discuss the bases of the success of their collaboration, the barriers to as well as the facilitators of such work that existed within their university and the community, and the lessons learned about building and sustaining such efforts. Across these discussions of why collaborations may succeed and fail we believe that readers may discern general ideas pertinent to building productive partnerships. For example, ideas such as co-learning (Lerner & Simon, 1998c), bringing all stakeholder voices to the "collaborative table" (Weiss & Greene, 1992), and building on community strengths and assets (Benson, 1997; Kretzmann & McKnight, 1992) are emphasized repeatedly across the diverse instances of community-university collaboration presented in this volume. It is useful to discuss briefly the diverse examples of collaboration presented in the book.

THE ORGANIZATION OF THIS BOOK

As shown in Table 1, the illustrations of community-university collaboration contained in this book are drawn from work conducted across the breadth of the nation. In addition to this geographical diversity there is, as well, institutional diversity. Large and small, public and private, research-intensive and liberal arts/undergraduate education-oriented colleges and universities provide examples of community-university collaborations serving children, families, and communities.

Table 1. *Examples of Community-University Collaborations: Geographic and Community Settings, Target Groups, and Substantive Foci*

Chapter #	State	First Author	Setting	Target Group	Substantive Focus
2	Alabama	Bradbard	Urban community	Children and parents	Child care
3		Esser-Stuart	Health system	Children	Health
4	Arkansas	Fabes	Medical clinic	Child and parents	Austism
5	Colorado	Yang	University	Children and families	Child care
6	Connecticut	Wisensale	State government	Professionals	Family development
7	Delaware	Hallam	Social services agencies	Women and infants	Family support
8	Florida	Mullis, A.	Schools	Grades 2-8	Literacy
9		Mullis, R.	Counties throughout state	Preschool children and staff	Rural child care
10		Perkins	4-H	Youth	Youth assets
11		Rollin	Boys/Girls Clubs	Elementary and middle school children	Positive youth development
12		Walker	Courts	Defendants	Mental health services
13	Georgia	Quinn	Courts	First offenders and their families	Juvenile justice
14	Idaho	Ney	Communities throughout state	Youth	Community support for youth
15	Illinois	Gentry	Schools	Elementary school students	Mediation curricula
16		Prater	Community college	Adult students	Training early childhood education specialists
17		Cato	Community agencies	Professionals and agencies	Child care
18	Iowa	Spoth	Communities throughout state	Family outreach personnel	Youth and family development
19	Maryland	Hymon-Parker	University	College students	Early childhood education
20		Koblinsky	Community surrounding university	Homeless families	Head Start services
21		Mohraz	Community surrounding university	Youth at risk for dropping out	School behavior and success

Table 1, *continued*

22	Massachusetts	Hurd	Urban school	Disadvantaged students	Improved attainment in higher education
23		Lucy-Allen	Schools	University students	Community revitalization
24		Martland	World wide web/Internet	Youth, agencies, and the media	Public education
25		Walsh	Community surrounding university	Children and families	Child and family development
26	Michigan	Bates	Medical center	Teenage mothers	Family services
27		Fitzgerald	Communities throughout state	NGOs (United Way)	Training in program evaluation
28		Keith	State and city government	College and elementary school students	Achievement and career development
29		Sandman	Communities throughout state	Families	Community center development
30		Schadewald	State Department of Public Health	Adolescents	Adolescent risk-taking
31		Smith	Social service agency	Grandparents	Support for custodial grandparents
32	Minnesota	Erickson	Communities throughout state	Individuals and community groups	Enhance community impact of university
33	Mississippi	Blackwell	Public schools	Teachers and other school personnel	Enhance school-university partnerships
34	Missouri	Dranginis	Community agencies	University students	Prepare students to work collaboratively in communities
35		Fine	Courts	Divorcing families with children	Adjustment to divorce

Table 1, *continued*

36	Nebraska	Stevens	State and local agencies	State and local agencies	Coalition building
37	New York	Higgins-D'Alessandro	University and community surrounding the university	University students and community groups	Develop expertise for enhancing partnerships
38		McClintock	Local and state government	Professionals	Continuing education
39	North Carolina	Cassidy	Child care centers	Child care providers	Child care
40		Johnson	Community agencies	Non-profit agencies and youth	Building community linkages
41	Ohio	Cartwright	Preschools	Children with disabilities and their teachers	Improved use of technology
42		Chibucos	University	Children and parents	Child care/Head Start
43		Jackson	Neighborhood groups	Neighborhood residents and groups	Community capacity building
44	Pennsylvania	Smith	Hospitals and social service agencies	Adolescents	Rural health care
45		Vernon-Feagans	Communties throughout state	Pregnant women	Prenatal care
46	Texas	Bell	Communities throughout state	Community residents	Technical assistance
47		Hildreth	Schools	Multi-ethnic parent groups	Parent education and child achievement
48		Nader	Community agencies	Community agencies	Enhance community grant-writing capacity
49		Nathan	Housing authority	Residents in subsidized housing	Enhance self-sufficiency
50	Wisconsin	Boyce-Rodgers	Communities across the nation	Adolescents	Youth-empowerment

Moreover, these partnerships involve an array of target audiences. For example, they cover all periods of the individual life span—from the prenatal period and pregnancy through infancy, youth, and old age. In addition, the collaborations concern a diverse set of groups and organizations such as families, schools, formal and informal NGOs, courts, professional organizations, community agencies, and governmental organizations. There is an even greater degree of diversity in regard to the substantive focus of the collaborations. Indeed, Table 1 illustrates that outreach scholarship can take many forms, for example, technical assistance, evaluation, training, program design and delivery, demonstration projects, action research, and dissemination.

We believe that the illustrations of collaboration contained in this book and summarized in Table 1 provide support for the thesis that higher education institutions with diverse missions can work productively with community partners having a broad range of interests to promote positive outcomes for children and families. Indeed, as illustrated in this book, there is functionally no clear limit to the combination of settings, groups, and substantive issues that may be interrelated successfully.

CONCLUSIONS

Together, the several dozen examples of successful community-university collaborations serving youth and families presented in this book demonstrate that the contemporary culture of American universities can be changed. In fact, these examples—from 23 states and over 40 different colleges and universities—provide a window to a transformation process that is quantitatively increasing and qualitatively enhancing its benefit to society. However, both the administrative and other stakeholder groups enabling this systems change, and the faculty, staff, students, and community partners enacting it, require the sustenance provided by political, financial, and intellectual resources for their work to proceed effectively.

We hope that the information presented in this volume will motivate stakeholders to work for the allocation of such resources. In addition, by indicating how community-university partnerships can be developed at a pace and at a scale requisite to address the needs of our communities, we believe that the book illustrates ways in which university expertise can be brought to bear on significant issues of youth, family, and community life. Finally, we sincerely hope that the book may provide a path for learning how, together, universities and communities can promote the positive outcomes for children and families that are moral and practical imperatives for all citizens of our diverse democracy.

REFERENCES

Benson, P. (1997). *All kids are our kids: What communities must do to raise caring and responsible children and adolescents.* San Francisco: Jossey-Bass.

Boyer, E. L. (1990). *Scholarship reconsidered: Priorities of the professoriate*. Princeton, NJ: Carnegie Foundation for the Advancement of Teaching.

Boyer, E. L. (1994, March 9). Creating the new American college. *Chronicle of Higher Education*, A48.

Carnegie Corporation of New York. (1995). *Great transitions: Preparing adolescents for a new century*. New York: Carnegie Corporation of New York.
Dryfoos, J. G. (1990). *Adolescents at risk: Prevalence and prevention*. New York: Oxford University Press.
Dryfoos, J. G. (1994). *Full service schools: A revolution in health and social services for children, youth, and families*. San Francisco: Jossey-Bass.
Hamburg, D. A. (1992). *Today's children: Creating a future for a generation in crisis*. New York: Time Books.
Fisher, C. B., Murray, J. P., Dill, J. R., Hagen, J. W., Hogan, M. J., Lerner, R. M., Rebok, G. W., Sigel, I., Sostek, A. M., Smyer, M. A., Spencer, M. B., & Wilcox, B. (1993). The national conference on graduate education in the applications of developmental science across the life-span. *Journal of Applied Developmental Psychology, 14*, 1-10.
Fisher, C. B., & Lerner, R. M. (Eds.). (1994). *Applied developmental psychology*. New York: McGraw-Hill.
Kretzmann, J. P., & McKnight, J. L. (1993). *Building communities from the inside out: A path toward finding and mobilizing a community's assets*. Chicago: ACTA Publications.
Lerner, R. M. (1995). *America's youth in crisis: Challenges and options for programs and policies*. Thousand Oaks, CA: Sage.
Lerner, R. M. (1998). *Theoretical models of human development* (Vol.1). *Handbook of child psychology* (5th ed.), Editor in chief: W. Damon. New York: Wiley.
Lerner, R. M. (1998a). Theories of human development: Contemporary perspectives. In R. M. Lerner, (Ed.), *Theoretical models of human development* (Vol.1). *Handbook of child psychology* (5th ed., pp. 1-24), Editor in chief: W. Damon. New York: Wiley.
Lerner, R. M., & Miller, J. R. (1998). Developing multidisciplinary institutes to enhance the lives of individuals and families: Academic potentials and pitfalls. *Journal of Public Service and Outreach, 3*(1), 64-73.
Lerner, R. M., & Simon, L. A. K. (Eds.). (1998a). *University-community collaborations for the twenty-first century: Outreach scholarship for youth and families*. New York: Garland.
Lerner, R. M., & Simon, L. A. K. (1998b). The new American outreach university: Challenges and options. In R. M. Lerner & L. A. K. Simon (Eds.), *University-community collaborations for the twenty-first century: Outreach scholarship for youth and families* (pp. 3-23). New York: Garland.
Lerner, R. M., & Simon, L. A. K. (1998c). Directions for the American outreach university in the twenty-first century. In R. M. Lerner & L. A. K. Simon (Eds.), *University-community collaborations for the twenty-first century: Outreach scholarship for youth and families* (pp. 463-481). New York: Garland.
Magrath, C. P. (1993). *Comments to the Board on Home Economics on November 12, 1993*. Washington, D.C.: National Association of State Universities and Land-Grant Colleges.
Magrath, C. P. (1998). Foreword: Creating a new outreach university. In R. M. Lerner & L. A. K. Simon (Eds.), *University-community collaborations for the twenty-first century: Outreach scholarship for youth and families* (pp. xxi-xix). New York: Garland.
Richardson, W. C. (1996). A new calling for higher education. *The John W. Olswald Lecture*, The Pennsylvania State University, University Park.
Sherrod, L. (1998). The common pursuits of modern philanthropy and the proposed outreach university: Enhancing research and education. In R. M. Lerner & L. A. K. Simon (Eds.), *University-community collaborations for the twenty-first century: Outreach scholarship for youth and families* (pp. 397-418). New York: Garland.
Sherrod, L. (In press a). Funding opportunities for applied developmental science. In P. Ralston, R. M. Lerner, A. K. Mullis, C. Simerly, & J. Murray (Eds.), *Social change, public policy, and community collaboration: Training human development professionals for the twenty-first century*. Norwell, MA: Kluwer.
Sherrod, L. (In press b). Giving child development knowledge away: Using university-community partnerships to disseminate research on children, youth, and families. *Applied Developmental Science*.
Spanier, G. B. (1997a). Enhancing the capacity for outreach. *Journal of Public Service and Outreach, 2*(2), 7-11.
Spanier, G. B. (1997b). Enhancing the Quality of Life for Children, Youth, and Families. Unpublished manuscript, The Pennsylvania State University, University Park.
Votruba, J. C. (1992). Promoting the extension of knowledge in service to society. *Metropolitan Universities, 3*(3), 72-80.

Votruba, J. C. (1996). Strengthening the university's alignment with society: Challenges and strategies. *Journal of Public Service and Outreach, 1*(1), 29-36.
Votruba, J. C. (In press). Afterword. In P. Ralston, R. M. Lerner, A. K. Mullis, C. Simerly, & J. Murray (Eds.), *Social change, public policy, and community collaboration: Training human development professionals for the twenty-first century*. Norwell, MA: Kluwer.
Weiss, H. B., & Greene, J. C. (1992). An empowerment partnership for family support and education programs and evaluations. *Family Science Review, 5*, 131-148.

2 BUILD IT AND THEY WILL COME . . . THE BIRMINGHAM EARLY LEARNING CENTER: CREATING A VISION FOR THE FUTURE OF ALABAMA'S CHILDREN

Marilyn R. Bradbard
June Henton
Jacquelyn Mize
Janice Grover
Robbie Roberts
Auburn University

In the popular baseball movie, *Field of Dreams*, the character played by Kevin Costner hears a voice urging, "Build it and they will come . . . " Although the purpose behind the message was unclear, he knew he should begin by building a baseball field on his Iowa farm. A similar situation occurred in Birmingham, Alabama in 1994, except that the cast of characters was different, and instead of a baseball field, the vision was a community-university partnership to build a world-class child care center.

In February 1994 a representative from the Birmingham Urban Revitalization Partnership, a group of business and civic leaders from Birmingham, AL, organized by Mayor Richard Arrington, Reverend John Porter, and Elmer Harris, CEO of Alabama Power Company, presented a group of faculty from Auburn University's Department of Human Development and Family Studies with a challenging proposal to join a team of architects and interior designers to design a world-class child care facility. This was a once in a lifetime opportunity for the faculty to plan a building with the goal of creating a national model for quality day care. However, we were quite cynical about whether the community would actually invest in a center of this caliber when confronted with the reality of how much it would cost. We were astonished when, after 10 months of discussions, planning and visiting leading child care facilities in several states, a 6.5 million-dollar center opened its doors to the public in August 1995. Auburn University's Department of Human Development and Family Studies was asked to invest in this endeavor as a partner and to manage the program for the next decade. This fantasy to "build it and they will come . . . " became a reality.

THE NATURE OF THE PARTNERSHIP: OUR PURPOSES AND GOALS

In 1994 the Birmingham Urban Revitalization Partnership had a vision to rebuild an area of downtown Birmingham, Alabama that had been taken over by drugs, vandalism, and other crime. Although Birmingham is a dynamic and prosperous community, city leaders realized that areas of the community were economically depressed and critically underused. This group proposed that community revitalization was essential to ensure Birmingham's long-term economic prosperity. Further, the group members believed that a public-private effort was the best organizational framework for meeting their community development goals. With this information in mind, the Birmingham Early Learning Center (BELC) was conceptualized by the Birmingham Urban Revitalization Partnership and, with the monetary help and support of corporate and community partners, was built in the heart of the city's Greater Civil Rights District. To fund the capital construction of the building, each of the 18 "founding partners" purchased between one and 50 slots for their employees at a cost of $3,500 per slot per year for 10 years or an initial lump sum of $25,000. "Contributing partners" provided monetary support to fund outreach efforts, scholarships for low income children, and parent education programming.

Table 1

The Partners - Employer Sponsors Who Invested in the Building and Have Reserved Spaces for their Employee's Children:

Alabama Power Company
AmSouth Bank of Alabama
Arthur Andersen and Company
Banks, Finley White and Company
Berkowitz, Lefkovits, Isom & Kushner, P.C.
The Children's Hospital of Alabama
City of Birmingham
Compass Bank
First Alabama Bank
London & Yancey
Maynard, Cooper & Gale, P.C.
Merrill Lynch
Sirote & Permutt
Sonat, Inc.
Southern Company Services
Southern Nuclear Operating Company
SouthTrust Bank

Contributing Sponsors Who Made Contributions to Help Accomplish the Center's Scholarship, Community Training, Parent Education, and Other Goals:

Alabama Gas Corporation
Alabama Power Foundation
Auburn University
Balch & Bingham
BellSouth Foundation
BellSouth Telecommunications
Birmingham Area Chamber of Commerce
Borden, McKean and Payne, Architects
Brasfield & Gorie General Contractors
Drummond Company, Inc
EBSCO Industries, Inc.
Economic Development Partnership of Alabama
Energen Corporation
Ernst & Young
Bill Harbert Construction Company
Crawford T Johnson, III

Table 1, *continued*

Mercedes-Benz U.S. International	Southern Research Institute
Metropolitan Development Board	Trademark Interiors
Operation New Birmingham	

As the partner designated to operate the BELC, Auburn University's Department of Human Development and Family Studies provides a curriculum that not only educates children, but also fosters their developing social and practical skills. The Center's two directors—the Director of Children's Programs and the Director of Teacher Training and Outreach—are members of Auburn's faculty and, as such, their salaries are contributed by the University. The inclusion of Auburn in this partnership ensures that the Center's child care practices reflect current research, as well as accepted theory.

The BELC is designed to accommodate 200 children, ranging from six weeks to five years of age. Along with the two directors with advanced degrees, the Center employs approximately 40 teachers, with bachelor's or master's degrees in child development and/or early childhood education, and assistant teachers with specialized training in child development (e.g., CDA, associates degree). The Center is one of only a small number (5%) of centers across the nation that is accredited by the National Academy of Early Childhood Programs to ensure the application of developmentally appropriate practice (DAP) in children's programming (Bredekamp & Copple, 1997).

DAP classrooms are organized with learning centers, where activities, equipment, and materials are available for creating and exploring. Each classroom has a loft, a computer, and a tiled wet room for art, animal and plant care, as well as for sand and water play. The teacher's role is to provide a challenging and stimulating environment where children can freely explore their surroundings and engage in problem-solving as they learn mathematics, science, language and literacy, art, music, and self-help skills. The teachers offer children a variety of real experiences and extend those experiences in many ways through projects.

The Center's 16 spacious classrooms are located on the outer perimeters of a square "figure eight" design, with two large playgrounds located in courtyards in the center of each half of the "eight." As a safety precaution, these playgrounds cannot be viewed from the street. They are equipped with trike trails, state-of-the-art water play apparatuses, climbing equipment, and recycled/poured tire soft surfaces. The wide corridors surrounding the interior of the building also are designed as trike trails and named after popular preschool storybooks. A large indoor play area located in the center of the building, the Chicka-Chicka Boom Boom Room, also named after a storybook, contains a working child-sized kitchen and can serve as a meeting space for 200. An excellent security system, with video cameras throughout the building and grounds, enables parents and teachers to constantly monitor their children's classrooms and playgrounds. An apartment complex for visiting faculty members and up to six teacher trainees is available on-site along with state-of-the-art research facilities.

Nursing mothers have a room of their own and can stop by to nurse their infants whenever they wish. The Center also provides take-home dinners one night every week for busy working parents who need a break from cooking. As part of its ongoing mission, the Center provides outreach programs that offer assistance to other child care centers and workers who are striving to improve quality, as well as a quarterly satellite series for parents and child care workers entitled, "Principles of Parenting," and monthly community seminars on child and family development issues. Each of these features is impressive in its own right; however, the most unique aspect of the Center is the integrated teaching, research, and outreach functions resulting from the ingenuity of a university-corporate-government partnership committed to "raising the bar" of standards for quality child care.

ANALYSIS OF THE PROCESS

How Does the University Benefit from this Partnership?

Other than by helping preschool children develop a solid educational foundation, how does a university benefit from the type of partnership we describe above? Auburn, like all land-grant universities, has the tripartite mission of teaching, research, and service, and the Center allows us to be more effective in each of these areas. Specifically, this collaboration has provided:

- Opportunities for students to observe and practice state-of-the-art teaching methods in a model program.
- Internship placements for students that lead to full-time preschool teaching positions after graduation.
- Supervision of student teachers by on-site master teachers with degrees in child development/early education.
- Child care administrative training for students in a cutting-edge nationally accredited program.
- Research subject pool for faculty and graduate students; honors thesis opportunities for undergraduates.
- State-of-the-art urban research laboratory that provides opportunities for faculty to seek grant funds that require an urban population.
- Enhanced opportunities to form collaborative partnerships with other colleges and universities in the State, as well as throughout the United States.
- Opportunities to interface with area businesses and industries to promote work/family research, educational programming, and outreach activities.
- Opportunity to contribute to economic development efforts in the State by showcasing the Center to companies thinking of locating in Alabama.
- Visibility for Auburn University as a participant in one of the most innovative models in the nation.

How Do the Other Partners Benefit from this Collaboration?

The corporations and the City of Birmingham benefit from this Partnership in several important ways. First, because Auburn University manages the Center, the Partnership is eligible for tax exempt status and, consequently, benefits financially. Second, as the largest state university in Alabama and the only university in the state with a doctoral program in Human Development and Family Studies, the

Partnership's credibility is enhanced by our involvement. Perhaps most important, however, is the fact that Auburn University, as a state land-grant university, is committed to its outreach mission and views opportunities such as this collaboration as integral to that mission. As such, Auburn University administrators from the President to the Provost to the Vice President for Development have committed their time, resources, and fund raising personnel to advance the goals of this Partnership.

LESSONS WE HAVE LEARNED

Economic Challenges

In planning for a project of this scope, it is easy to "think big." A "model" approach suggests that no cost would be spared in creating this optimal quality child care center. In reality, however, child care as an industry will always have to face hard economic facts about limited resources. In particular, there are real limits to what parents can and will pay for even the best program, and in the final analysis, somebody has to fund the difference in costs between what parents can pay and the high utility, maintenance, and personnel costs required to manage such a facility. The challenge of raising private funds to supplement parent fees while, at the same time, maintaining our standards of quality, is one that few academics are prepared to face. We are slowly coming to terms with the need for continuous fund-raising efforts to supplement parent fees and corporate contributions.

High Expectations

Many parents of young children are, of course, new to the challenges of parenting and are feeling their way through the very personal process of balancing work and family demands. Some of them still view child rearing in a very idealized way. When offered "state of the art" child care, they may have unrealistic expectations about the ways a child care center can or should attempt to reduce their stresses. Even in the best centers, there will be sniffles, bumps, bites and, on occasion, hurt feelings, and misunderstandings. The true test of quality is not to ensure that these events never occur but rather to (a) reduce and manage these unavoidable problems, and (b) interpret and explain the developmental appropriateness of these problems for parents, using current child development theory and practice. During the first two years of the Center's operation, parents, staff, and the corporate community came to grips with the fact that although a very high standard of practice was being implemented, it would not be without a few problems. Only in the past year have we seen the development of a mutual trust among parents, the corporate community, and the staff who have all come to realize they are working together in the best interest of the children.

World-view Differences

A university-community partnership is not an easy collaboration. The corporate community often has an agenda that differs from that of university faculty, and our "world views" are not always compatible. One simple example that describes this difference was brought to our attention when we staffed the Center. From the university perspective, hiring outstanding teachers at a "worthy wage" was the central focus of how we defined quality child care. We were more than willing to compromise on extra computers in the classrooms, special carpeting, or tiled walls if these compromises would allow us to invest more money in teachers' salaries. The corporate partners, on the other hand, were very interested in how the Center looked to corporate visitors. Thus, the computers, the custom-made carpeting, and the overall aesthetic appeal of the building were central concerns. From the corporate perspective, the "eye appeal" of the Center was what would convince other companies to move to Alabama or invest in this or similar revitalization efforts. We now know that both of these world views have merit and, in the process of coming to terms with these different perspectives, have learned some valuable lessons.

Communication is the Key

Another lesson we have learned is that communication is difficult at a distance. Our campus is located 150 miles from Birmingham. Although our two faculty members are located in Birmingham, they do not have the daily support or collegiality of the department; rather, they are more likely to be involved with Partnership activities. As such, we have had to devise ways to ensure that our three-way communication (Auburn campus ↔ Center faculty; Center faculty ↔ Partnership; Partnership ↔ Auburn campus) is functioning in top form. Specifically, when travel is inconvenient or impossible, we make an effort to phone, e-mail, or FAX.

Besides the day-to-day communication, Auburn faculty frequently participate in lunchtime brown-bag seminars on child and/or family development issues in Birmingham, consult on developmental issues at the Center, or use the Center for other meetings. In turn, the Birmingham faculty and the Partners visit Auburn frequently to participate in outreach programming via satellite, meetings, or athletic events. Teachers at the Center are encouraged to seek advice from Auburn faculty, logon to the library via the Internet, and use any resources on the campus that are available to them. In the future, we hope to have teacher exchanges between the BELC and our on-campus child care facility and, perhaps, to have Internet exchanges between the children and families from both locations. In short, we have learned a great deal from this collaboration, and the learning is ongoing. If communication remains open, we are convinced our collaboration will continue to be a success.

PROSPECTS FOR LONG-TERM SUSTAINABILITY AND SUCCESS

We are nearing the end of our third year of a (minimum) 10-year agreement to manage the educational programs of the Birmingham Early Learning Center. As a partner in this endeavor we have achieved several important goals. The Center was accredited in 1997. Professionals from around the world have visited the Center, and at least three other cities/universities are interested in replicating our model. Our satellite programs have been viewed in most states in this country, as well as in several countries around the world. We have trained several hundred child care providers in Alabama. And, we have made great strides in providing a "worthy wage" for our teachers. Most important, our children and parents are pleased with the developmentally appropriate experiences we provide.

Our most immediate goal is to include a larger segment of the university in the operations of the Center—in other words, to make the Center a teaching/research/outreach laboratory for each college unit on our campus. In the past year we have involved our Nutrition and Food Sciences Department in our activities by engaging one of the faculty members as a dietary consultant. One of our engineering departments has offered to work with us to solve an acoustical problem. In a similar fashion it is possible to involve departments and programs such as early childhood education, rehabilitation and special education, health education, building science, landscape architecture, interior design, veterinary medicine, nursing, pharmacy, communications, communication disorders, and journalism. In fact, the latter two departments have the expertise to solve one of our more immediate and pressing needs: developing and implementing a mass media plan to bring the Center to the attention of those individuals and organizations who have both the ability and the monetary resources to implement similar programs in their own communities, as well as a belief system that places the development of preschool children as a top priority.

Finally, in the future we plan to conduct systematic evaluations of our programming efforts to ascertain (a) the cognitive and social gains made by the children who attend the Center, (b) teaching competency improvements that result from our ongoing caregiver training programs, and (c) parenting knowledge and behavior improvements that have resulted from our satellite broadcasts. We also intend to develop measures of community satisfaction that will allow us to assess how the Center, as a part of a larger urban revitalization effort, has affected the greater Birmingham area.

As in the *Field of Dreams*, it is as yet unclear what direction the Birmingham Partnership will take. What is clear, however, is that all the pieces are in place to establish a national model program to make a tremendous difference in the lives of children and families.

REFERENCES

Bredekamp, S., & Copple, C. (Eds.). (1997). *Developmentally appropriate practice in early childhood programs* (Rev. Ed.). Washington, DC: NAEYC.

3 THE BIBB COUNTY CHILD CARING FOUNDATION (BCCCF): A STORY THAT NEEDS TO BE SHARED

Joan E. Esser-Stuart
University of Alabama

Alesa H. Judd, Chair
Bibb County Child Caring Foundation Policy Board

Tracy M. Palmer
John R. Wheat
University of Alabama

Health care policy makers and health reformers have become increasingly concerned with improving access to health care for children. Health insurance, often referred to as an "enabling factor," is a crucial component of health care access. Health insurance facilitates the use of health services by providing financial access to the health care system (Simpson, Bloom, Cohen, & Parsons, 1997). Nearly 11 million children went without health insurance in 1996—the highest number and proportion of uninsured children since 1987 (Bennefield, 1997; General Accounting Office, 1996).

In the past decade, the proportion of persons in the United States insured privately has decreased from 74% to 66%; the proportion of persons enrolled in Medicaid increased from 16% to 26% during the same period (Federal Interagency Forum on Child and Family Statistics, 1997). Despite Medicaid expansions, the rate of uninsured children has remained unchanged over the last decade. More than three million uninsured children (30% of all uninsured children) are eligible for Medicaid or other public insurance. These children, however, remain unenrolled due to a variety of factors including lack of outreach efforts, complicated eligibility requirements, and cultural differences (Bennefield, 1997; General Accounting Office, 1996; Families USA, 1997).

It is interesting to note that uninsured children frequently come from families with working parents earning moderate incomes of $17,280 to $28,000 annually (Families USA, 1997). Many of these children go uninsured because parents work for employers who either do not provide coverage, or require parents to pay most, if not all, of premium costs. These premium costs can easily exceed $1500 dollars annually (Swartz, 1997). Families with lower incomes often forego health insurance coverage to meet family needs such as food, shelter, utilities and clothing.

Many child advocates have become increasingly concerned that the lack of employer-based health insurance coverage for the children of working parents places these children and their families in an extremely vulnerable position and at-risk for poorer health. A recent report by Families USA (1997) revealed that there are an estimated 23 million uninsured children if children who have gaps in their coverage are included. Children who experience gaps in their health coverage are similar to uninsured children with regard to overall health status and utilization of health care services. These children are less likely than insured children to have a personal primary care provider, less likely to seek care from a physician, and less likely to receive basic, preventive care and on-time immunizations (Newacheck, Stoddard, Hughes, & Pearl, 1998; Mustin, Holt, & Connell, 1994). Additionally, uninsured children are four times more likely than insured children to go without needed medical services, such as dental or vision care, and prescription medications (Simpson et al, 1997).

Uninsured children and their families have been a concern for quite some time. Innovative programs have been implemented to meet the health care needs of uninsured children. Blue Cross and Blue Shield insurance companies throughout the United States have developed several programs and these programs often share "Child Caring" as a part of their designation. We discuss here a successful public-private partnership between Blue Cross and Blue Shield of Alabama (BCBS of Alabama), the University of Alabama College of Community Health Sciences (CCHS), and the civic-minded Bibb County community. The partnership was designed to expand the scope of the Alabama Child Caring Foundation and was initiated to address a pivotal question, "What would happen if every child within a community was assured access to medical care?"

NATURE OF PARTNERSHIP

BCBS of Alabama established the Alabama Child Caring Foundation in the fall of 1987 to provide insurance coverage of primary and preventive health care services to uninsured school age children in Alabama. The Alabama Child Caring Foundation is a non-profit foundation that accepts contributions from businesses, congregations, civic organizations, charitable foundations, individuals and families. BCBS of Alabama matches on a one-to-one basis each dollar contributed to the foundation and provides the administrative support for the foundation to ensure that all of the contributions are used to provide health coverage for uninsured children.

PURPOSES AND GOALS

The first participants in the partnership were invited into a small, rural community approximately 40 miles from the university for the pilot project. Participants wanted to address the following questions:

- What would happen if every child in the community had access to medical care?

- What would be the impact of universal access to health care on attendance and performance in school?
- How would the community as a whole benefit from a child's knowledge of personal health and hygiene?
- Does access to medical care really make that much difference in a child's life?

ANALYSIS OF THE PROCESS

The pilot project was initiated and later successfully implemented based upon relationships. Relationships between the project stakeholders, including a major donor with family ties in the community, led to the implementation of the project in Bibb County, Alabama. The University of Alabama CCHS and members of the Rural Alabama Health Alliance (RAHA), an organization of rural health care providers and community leaders, established an ongoing working relationship. Later, community leaders from Bibb County secured needed people and other resources to implement the project successfully based upon relationships between and among Bibb County community members, health care providers, social service agencies and the Bibb County School System.

During early phases of implementation, each of the partners became aware of the needs and concerns of other participants in the change effort. They were united by common goals and made a commitment to maintaining open lines of communication. The openness was facilitated through the development of a local policy board to guide and coordinate activities while promoting respect for one another and opportunities to learn from each other. Meetings were arranged on various stakeholders' home turfs to increase participation. Participants used regular and frequent communication to build trust and understanding between and among partners.

RAHA, established to enhance rural health care and to promote medical and health education in rural communities, joined the original partners in the implementation of the pilot project. The University of Alabama CCHS faculty worked with the members of RAHA to establish the Bibb County Child Caring Foundation (BCCCF) Policy Board. The BCCCF Policy Board, which became the driving force central to the project, is responsible for defining community needs, acquiring needed resources, formulating policies and overseeing program development.

The heart of the partnership is a community-centered approach to health and well being. At the policy level, the partnership supports the Bibb County Child Caring Foundation, a policy board involving local community members, to evaluate child health needs, provide needed services, and to provide insurance monies for medically uninsured children. At the organizational level, the program works with providers and agencies to develop needed primary care and community services. At the individual level, the program provides children with preventive health assessments and appropriate referrals to health care providers through school-wide health assessments.

RAHA members from Bibb, Fayette, and Pickens counties meet every six weeks to network with one another and to engage in creative problem solving to ensure that the residents of these three rural counties receive health care services. RAHA members contributed advice, knowledge and expertise to the project and provided useful insights. In addition, RAHA provided the 501-C-3 status that facilitated the receipt of funds from the Alabama Child Caring Foundation for the BCCCF project. RAHA also provides other forms of financial administration and financial assistance to the project.

The Policy Board has worked with its partners to launch successful fundraising necessary to provide dental services to the community's children and has negotiated lower and discounted rates for dental services with local dental care providers. Vision services have been provided to the children through an alliance with the Alabama Child Caring Foundation and its relationship with the Vision Service Plan.

The project provided opportunities for co-learning. Rural Health Scholars, Rural Medical Scholars, third-year medical students, students from the University of Alabama Capstone College of Nursing, and local high school students enrolled in the Health Science Technology Program administered the health screenings. These students were afforded additional learning opportunities and received invaluable "real world" community health learning experiences.

ACHIEVEMENTS RELATED TO GOALS

Both qualitative and quantitative assessments were used in the evaluation of the Bibb County Child Caring Program. Initially, a rapid ethnographic assessment was conducted using personal interviews with key community informants. This assessment afforded opportunities for both the university research team and the local policy board to gain information about the community's perceptions and knowledge of the local health care system. An evaluation of the project based upon qualitative interviews with the community leaders and project stakeholders was conducted at the close of the second year.

The Policy Board determined that annual school-based health fairs and parent surveys would be used to identify uninsured children, assess their health status, and make referrals for additional services. These uninsured children have been enrolled in either Medicaid or the Alabama Caring Program for Children. The Policy Board has ensured that the community's children are enrolled in an insurance program. In addition, the Policy Board has formed relationships with local health care providers and established a child health status baseline. The Policy Board determined that these baseline data would be used to assess the impact of the project on the community and will be used to evaluate child health longitudinally. The annual school health fairs provide important longitudinal data about the overall health of the community's children. Demographic variables, health status indicators, self-reported personal health information, health care utilization characteristics and social behavioral data, and information on the number and type of referrals from the health screenings are compiled on an annual basis into a child data book.

The evaluation process is an integral component of the project. The local policy board reviews progress on a monthly basis. Collaborative reports and child data books are prepared annually. In addition, student surveys, client satisfaction questionnaires and qualitative interviews with stakeholders and community members have been used as formative evaluations of the project.

PROSPECTS FOR LONG-TERM SUSTAINABILITY

Taken collectively, the evaluation components provide evidence of the community's ownership of the program, while also providing information that will be beneficial to other communities as they develop and implement programs to meet their individual community needs. Fayette and Pickens counties are currently designing community interventions to meet the needs of their community residents and may choose to replicate aspects of the BCCCF project during the next year.

WHY WAS THIS A SUCCESSFUL PARTNERSHIP

This collaborative project is an excellent example of synergy since the whole is much greater than the sum of the individual parts. All of the partners in the collaborative relationship have unique roles, responsibilities and stakeholders that are important and contribute to the overall success of the community project. They are united in a common goal of ensuring access to medical care to all the community's children. The unity is assured and purpose maintained by the coordinating activities of the local Policy Board, composed of people who live and work in the community and among the children for whom insurance is so needed.

REFERENCES

Bennefield, R. (1997). Health insurance coverage: 1996. Current Population Reports, U.S. Bureau of the Census, Series P60, No. 199. Washington, DC: Government Printing Office.

Families USA. (1997). *One out of three: Kids without health insurance, 1995-1996*. Washington, DC.

Federal Interagency Forum on Child and Family Statistics. (1997). *America's children: Key national indicators of well-being*. Washington, DC: Government Printing Office.

General Accounting Office. (1996). *Health insurance for children: Private insurance coverage continues to deteriorate*. Washington, DC: Government Accounting Office/HEHS-96-129.

Mustin, H., Holt, V., & Connell, F. (1994). Adequacy of well-child care immunizations in U.S. infants born in 1988. *Journal of the American Medical Association, 272*, 1111-1115.

Newacheck, P., Stoddard, J., Hughes, D., & Pearl, M. (1998). Health insurance and access to primary care for children. *New England Journal of Medicine, 338*(8), 513-519.

Simpson, G., Bloom, B., Cohen, R. A., & Parson, P. E. (1997). Access to health care part 1: Children. National Center for Health Statistics: *Vital Health Statistics, 10*(196). Washington, DC: Government Printing Office.

Swartz, K. (1997). Volunteerism and children's health insurance: Expand coverage. *Inquiry, 34*, 103-105.

4 ARIZONA STATE UNIVERSITY AND THE SOUTHWEST AUTISM RESEARCH CENTER: PARTNERS IN HELPING CHILDREN WITH AUTISM AND THEIR FAMILIES

Richard A. Fabes
Carol Lynn Martin
Arizona State University

Raun D. Melmed
Cindy K. Schneider
Southwest Autism Research Center

When Maria and Nick of Phoenix discovered that their first child, Matthew, had developed autism they were devastated. Until the age of two, they were unaware that anything was wrong with his development. At that time, Matthew stopped talking, lost motor skills, and began to avoid physical contact with others. Now 4 years old, Matthew has difficulty relating to people, adapting to new environments and sleeping, has severely impaired communication skills, has limited intellectual ability, engages in repetitive movements, and often is irritable and aggressive. Maria and Nick are determined to improve their son's prospects. Fortunately, in the Phoenix metropolitan area there is a group of physicians and university child development researchers who are collaborating to bring together services and interventions for children like Matthew and their families. Because of the collaborative efforts of these community and university professionals, Nick and Maria are participating in research investigating new treatments for the problematic symptoms of autism, are attending parent support groups, and have a resource where they can obtain information on autism, its causes, and its treatment.

BACKGROUND AND PURPOSE

Autism is a developmental disability characterized by difficulties and abnormalities in communication, social relationships, cognitive functioning, sensory processing, and behavior. Approximately 10-15% of individuals with autism have average or above average intelligence, including some in the superior range. Another 25 to

35% have IQs in the borderline to mild mental retardation range, and the remainder are moderately to profoundly mentally retarded (Cohen & Volkmar, 1997). As such, autism appears to be a complex neurobiological disorder that often is complicated by hyperactivity, sleep disturbances, aggression, mental retardation, eating disorders, and self-injury. Some children appear to be autistic from birth, whereas others like Matthew seem to develop normally until some point between the first and third years of life.

Autism occurs in approximately one per 2,000 children and is four times more prevalent in boys than girls. It is the third most common childhood disability, and its incidence appears to be increasing (Campbell, Cueva, & Hallin, 1996). When statistics include other closely related disorders (such as pervasive developmental disorder and Asperger syndrome), a much higher incidence is found—affecting nearly 400,000 people in the US today.

Autism is not a mental illness, nor is it caused by bad parenting. Although the precise pathogenic mechanisms are unclear, they appear to involve both chemical and structural abnormalities in the brain. There is a genetic predisposition to the disorder and this may possibly make some individuals more susceptible to aggravating environmental factors than others. This is where the relationship between child development researchers at Arizona State University and concerned physicians in the Phoenix metropolitan area came together to form the Southwest Autism Research Center (SARC), a nonprofit community-based organization devoted to the scientific study of autism and to helping children and families who are afflicted with the disorder.

The increase in the number of cases of autism led two local physicians to search for some of the factors that might be involved in the symptomatic variations associated with autism and its increasing incidence. They noticed that many of the children with autism had a history of frequent upper respiratory, ear, and gastrointestinal infections which were frequently treated with antibiotics.

Recurrent and/or prolonged use of antibiotics is known to increase the incidence of yeast overgrowth, particularly *candida albicans*. This form of yeast exists in various parts of the body in low levels, but the doctors noticed that autistic children seemed to suffer from increased levels of intestinal yeast. This overgrowth of yeast may release toxins in the body that can impair the functioning of the nervous system and the immune system (Edelson, 1998). In case studies, overgrowth of yeast also has been linked to hyperactivity, short attention span, irritability, fatigue, sleep problems, allergies, and stomachaches (Crook, 1996)—all common symptoms reported by parents and physicians of children with autism. The question was whether treatment of the yeast overgrowth might in any way improve the symptoms of children with autism.

ANALYSIS OF THE PROCESS

The physicians were well aware that there are several safe, effective, and relatively inexpensive ways to treat yeast overgrowth. For example, the anti-fungal medication Nystatin has been proven to be effective in treating yeast infections (Blaschke-Hellmessen, Buchmann, & Schwarze, 1996). The physicians began recommending that parents of children with an appropriate history try this medication and the anecdotal feedback they received confirmed their observations—that yeast overgrowth may be frequent in autism and may aggravate its symptoms. After treatment, parents were reporting that their autistic children were more attentive, responsive, less irritable, and more capable of engaging in self-care behaviors.

Of course, anecdotal reports and observations are not rigorous enough to pass scientific scrutiny. What was needed was a controlled study in which children were given Nystatin or a placebo. Then any resulting behavioral changes could be measured and monitored. Although the physicians knew they needed a more rigorous test of their treatment plans, they had limited experience regarding how best to carry the research out, what issues they were likely to face, how to manage and analyze the data, and how to interpret the results. This is where the connection between the physicians and the ASU researchers began and the structure of the SARC was enhanced. Together, the team set out to find better ways to understand autism and help children and their families cope with the various symptoms of the disability.

With physicians' knowledge of autism, the metabolic aspects of yeast and its treatment, together with the developmental and research expertise of the ASU team, SARC initiated a rigorous study of the effects of Nystatin on the symptoms of autism. Together, SARC and ASU developed and designed the study, recruited children, and began data collection. Over 50 autistic children, their parents and siblings, and some nonrelated, non-autistic children have participated. The research is funded in part out of the collaboration—fund raising efforts of SARC and seed money from ASU have covered the considerable expenses from the study. The ability to raise funds from multiple sources clearly is a strength of the collaborative arrangements between SARC and ASU.

ASU faculty provided their expertise in working with children and families in research, in conducting and evaluating interventions, and in reviewing and interpreting the existing literature and resulting data. They also recruited several graduate students to join the project, some of whom conducted their thesis projects using data from the study. Thus, one outcome of this relationship is that a number of young professionals in child development became aware of the issues related to autism and how families adapt to the demanding stressors associated with it. Their interest and involvement increases the likelihood that these students become professionals who are committed to addressing the needs of their communities during their graduate training, as well as after they graduate.

LEARNINGS FROM THIS PARTNERSHIP

No university-community collaboration is without its share of differences of opinion, differences in approaches to research and dissemination of information, and differences in regard to priorities and needs. Research does not take place in a vacuum and research agendas are driven by individuals' motivations, backgrounds, and perceptions of the problems and the questions to be asked (McCall, 1996). Practitioners, researchers, and community members often have different world views and the boundaries between them may be rigid. In the case of SARC, it was important to break down these barriers and communicate the views and needs of each orientation to better serve the population in need. For example, parents of children with autism eagerly, almost obsessively, want to find ways to help their children and families. This eagerness often leads these parents to become frustrated by the slow pace with which new research findings and treatments become available. Practitioners face these parents and children everyday and must deal with their desires and demands for treatment and information. Families also face frustration when what appears to be a new and promising treatment does not turn out to be effective.

Early on, we saw both types of frustration in the parents who belong to the local autism support groups. Parents of young autistic children were enthusiastic about our study and their participation. They saw this project as a new and exciting approach to treating some of the problem symptoms of autism and were eager to be part of the study. All of them, of course, wanted to be certain that they would be in the experimental group (the one that received the Nystatin). Several of them withdrew from the study or went out and got a prescription and immediately put their child on it, thereby complicating the study and its design.

In contrast, parents of older autistic children were more reticent and pessimistic about the study and its potential. They said that they have had their hopes raised many times, only to be dashed and disappointed. They were reluctant to participate and did not particularly want to go through the disappointment of having their hopes raised again. From a research perspective, we were faced early on with the issue of sampling and volunteer bias.

Additionally, it was critical that we recruit non-autistic, non-related children and families as the control comparison for our studies. This has been a point of divergence for the practitioners and researchers at SARC. Practitioners often are more focused on the target group in question. In this case, it was imperative that control participants be recruited. Because this research involved drawing blood, it became clear that there would need to be serious and continuing recruitment efforts devoted to convincing parents of the normal children to participate. With limited funding and personnel, the recruitment of control participants was delayed because of the emphasis on serving the target population. As the research progressed, and data began coming in, the discussions between the members of SARC brought out the critical importance of the control group. As a result, heightened attention and efforts were devoted to this.

The gaps between the priorities of the researchers and practitioners at SARC have been narrowed with continued dialog and discussion. In this case, we are evolving into a group in which service, evaluation, and science go hand in hand. The willingness to evolve has enhanced the level of cooperation and trust among those involved. Increased emphasis on obtaining control participants is just one of the outcomes, the others include increased mutual respect and involvement, cross-fertilization of ideas and issues, and increased commitment to serving both the scientific community and the public at large. This level of collaborative interaction is probably more influenced by the positive and honest interpersonal relationships developed among the core members of SARC than by scientific principles alone (Siegel, 1998).

The practitioners, however, are not the only ones who had to make adaptations to conducting research and service in real life environments. The ASU researchers also had to come to grips with the fact that conducting this kind of research meant giving up some of the ideas and notions about control they are accustomed to having. Because this research was conducted in the context of the physicians' practices, the researchers' notions of control were challenged in at least two important ways. First, the fact that this study included parents and children who are trying to cope with the severe and chronic problems related to autism meant that many of these families were already seeking a number and variety of interventions for their children. Thus, the impact of Nystatin itself may be difficult to ascertain given that the children were receiving so many different interventions. In addition, the recruitment of participants and the implementation of the procedures were conducted by the practitioners and their staff. Many researchers may be uncomfortable turning over critical aspects of the study to others, particularly practitioners who have less experience in these areas. Once again, the trust developed among the core members of SARC enhanced the confidence of all involved.

The second sense of control that was lost for the researchers was more psychological than scientific. This research was practitioner-initiated—the practitioners had the desire to study autism, its possible causes and resulting behaviors. To do this, they needed a working relationship with researchers. The ASU researchers brought with them expertise in developmental research (i.e., design, methods, analysis, etc.). However, because the practitioners were the "experts" in the topic under study, the usual sense of being the one looked to for most answers to the questions that arise was somewhat lost for the researchers. Thus, a true partnership was necessary and the success of this partnership depended on the development of shared goals. In this case, the desire to help children with autism and their families served as a catalyst for the development of a successful partnership.

Because the practitioners turned to ASU researchers for their expertise in design, data management, data analyses, interpretation, and write up, they too must deal with a loss of control once the data leave their hands. This loss of control over the research process has the potential to be a problem because of the length of time it takes to carry out a research project. Practitioners are eager to find out the results of the study and often are under pressure from parents to find out if the treatment is successful. In addition, access to the data can sometimes be a problem when the data are collected and analyzed in two different locations (the physician's office and ASU). The luxury that researchers usually have in carefully managing and analyzing the data and reflecting over the findings may be compromised due to the urgency of the problems under study and the different demands placed upon SARC members.

SUCCESSFUL OUTCOMES AND PARTNERSHIPS

The establishment of SARC and the partnership developed with ASU has broadened the scope of involvement for all participants. For the physicians, the knowledge gained from the research has led to other research questions and plans for future collaborations and studies. The partnership has brought them in contact with graduate students and other university personnel and organizations that may contribute to the cause. For example, the mental health clinical training sites at ASU offer SARC families low-cost therapy to help them deal with stress and the demands of family life and to cope with the chronic and pervasive disorder of autism. For the ASU researchers, it has meant a broadening of their professional goals with greater emphasis on meeting the immediate and long-term needs of families and children with autism. For the families and children who participate in the SARC projects, it has led to an increased understanding of the importance of research and science in answering questions about autism and a feeling that they are contributing to the advancement of the understanding and treatment of autism. It also has meant having a resource to turn to for information and support. For SARC itself, it has meant a broadening of its goals—providing support groups, fund raising, working with the media, and making contacts with other organizations (both locally and nationally).

WHY THIS PARTNERSHIP WAS SUCCESSFUL

SARC was established by the dedication and hard work of two local community physicians. Their efforts and commitment served as the basis from which all of the work developed and they continue to be the cornerstone for the center. Without their guidance, perseverance, and dedication, this project would not have been started. The establishment of the partnership was initiated at their request and the success of the relationship between SARC and ASU also rests on their willingness to involve others in their campaign to assist children and families with autism.

The success of this partnership derives from the mutual respect developed among its core participants. From this respect, common goals and visions are being constructed. In addition, the communication and discussions fostered by this mutual trust facilitate interdisciplinary learning for all participants. In our case, trust and respect resulted from the core participants' willingness to listen to the concerns of each other, the acknowledgment of different skills and points of view, and a recognition of the competencies that each member had to offer to the ultimate goal of helping families and children with autism. Additionally, the success of the partnership is due to the partners' willingness to expand their own sphere of comfortableness and become involved in issues and problems that typically are beyond their areas of expertise. For the members of SARC, this entails becoming "science practitioners"—dealing with real-life problems and the scientific endeavors devoted to understanding and intervening in these (Weissberg & Greenberg, 1998). Thus, successful university-community partnerships such as ours involve the willingness to take a risk and evolve professionally and personally.

REFERENCES

Blaschke-Hellmessen, R., Buchmann, H., & Schwarze, R. (1996). Effect of orally administered animycotics on the intestinal colonization with yeasts. *Mycoses*, *39*, 33-39.

Campbell, M., Cueva, J., & Hallin, A. (1996). Autism and pervasive developmental disorders. In J. M. Weiner (Ed.), *Diagnosis and psychopharmacology of childhood and adolescent disorders* (pp. 151-192). New York: Wiley.

Cohen, D., & Volkmar, F. R. (1997). *Handbook of autism and pervasive developmental disorders*. New York: Wiley.

Crook, W. G. (1996). *The yeast connection handbook.* New York: Free Books.

Edelson, S. M. (1998). *The candida yeast-autism connection.* Philadelphia: Center for the Study of Autism.

McCall, R. B. (1996). The concept and practice of education, research, and public service in university psychology departments. *American Psychologist*, *51*, 379-388.

Siegel, I. E. (1998). Practice and research: A problem in developing communication and cooperation. In W. Damon, I. E. Sigel, & K. A. Renninger (Eds.), *Handbook of child psychology* (Vol. 4, pp. 1113-1132). New York: Wiley.

Weissberg, R. P., & Greenberg, M. T. (1998). School and community competence-enhancement and prevention programs. In W. Damon, I. E. Sigel, & K. A. Renninger (Eds.), *Handbook of child psychology* (Vol. 4, pp. 877-954). New York: Wiley.

5 CHILD CARE ON CAMPUS: A TRUE PARTNERSHIP BETWEEN AN ACADEMIC PROGRAM AND VENDOR

Raymond K. Yang
Colorado State University

Child-care services were provided for working mothers long before World War II. Some "company towns" provided these services to workers during the 19th century (Kamerman & Kahn, 1987). Although the specific content of these services may not have resembled what we now call child-care (e.g., group care in a single location), they assisted parents whose other obligations made it difficult for them to be with their children. Hernandez (1993, p. 152) has estimated that during the 1930s, over 300,000 infants and children (0-5 years) had both parents working full-time; these children required some form of child care. Over the years, the Women's Bureau of the U.S. Department of Labor (1953, 1971, 1979, 1989) conducted detailed surveys of employed women's need for child care and how it was being met. Out-of-home child care for working parents has been a small and sporadic component of employee benefits, except for occupations employing large percentages of women, such as apparel manufacturing (Collins, 1989; LeBlanc & Hennon, 1979; Perry, 1978). During the last 30 years, as women entered the workforce at-large in unprecedented numbers, child care has become a broad political issue affecting business, legislation, and child development researchers (e.g., Advisory Committee on Child Development, National Research Council, 1976; Hernandez, 1995; Krcmarik, Yang, & Fritz, 1994; Zigler, Kagan, & Klugman, 1983).

As businesses employing and serving large numbers of people, universities reflect and interact with their communities: Many faculty and staff live in the community proximal to campus; many students are from nearby communities; many community members support the university's athletic teams and attend cultural events (e.g., theater, lectures); and the university plays a direct role in the economic development of an area. In addition to its role as a business and corporate entity, many in the university feel that it bears an additional unique responsibility: Exemplifying, translating, and bringing to the commonweal the benefits of intellectual endeavor (teaching and research).

Colorado State University is a Land Grant, Carnegie Research I university. The University is located in a growing metropolitan area of about 100,000, enrolls 22,000 students (20% of whom are between 26 and 49-years-of-age, and who could have child care needs) , and employs 6,500 faculty, professionals, and staff. Like other comparable universities, a percentage of the Colorado State community needs and uses child care services. The city in which the university is located (Fort Collins), has sufficient private vendors to meet the community's needs for preschool-aged care for children, but not for infants and toddlers. A university-operated facility, which serves as the practicum/internship site for students majoring in human development and family studies, enrolls preschool children[1] of university members. About four applications are received for every opening in the university's program.

THE EFFORT TO BRING CHILD-CARE TO CAMPUS

The university's first program for pre-school aged children was started in 1929 as a part of its home economics program. The children's program served as a practicum and internship site and a setting in which children's curricula could be developed. The program retained its academic mission, eventually becoming a part of the Department of Human Development and Family Studies. In the early-1980s the department expanded the program in response to growing campus-wide need for child care services. This gave the program a dual mission—one academic, the other service-related. This expansion inevitably led to departmental resources being increasingly allocated to this service. For example, the center director, a member of the tenured faculty, spent progressively more time in the center with children and student-teachers. Because this occurred informally, no costs were reassigned, that is, a larger percentage of the director's salary was not transferred to the center's budget.[2] In three years, the department ended this campus-wide service, and returned to a smaller program serving the original practicum/internship functions.

On many campuses, an on-site facility has been the preferred child-care option.[3] There are several reasons for this: (a) Convenience of location is one of two primary criteria used by parents in selecting child-care.[4] Access to a facility at the work-site decreases transportation time; (b) Parents have convenient access to their children during the day, and can visit or easily reach them in case of an emergency; and (c) Considerable evidence indicates that work-site child-care boosts employee morale and performance, and decreases absenteeism in the manufacturing industries (Burud, Aschbacher, & McCroskey, 1984; Chapman, 1987; Galinsky & Hughes, 1987; Magid, 1983; Milkovich & Gomez, 1976; Ransom, Aschbacher, & Burud, 1989; Thomas & Thomas, 1990; Youngblood & Chambers-Cook, 1984), and, possibly, in higher education institutions (Anderson, Getz, & Siegfried, 1995).

In 1990, the university president's staff decided to explore the matter of child-care services for the university community (faculty, staff, students). Following an initial discussion of legal liability issues, a campus-wide survey was conducted, verifying the need for and probable use of a facility located on campus.[5] Thereafter, a task force was formed to develop recommendations regarding the provision of child-care services to the university. The task force membership comprised students, staff, faculty, and administrators (whose responsibilities encompassed child-care-related matters, e.g., legal counsel).

The task force recommended that the university partner with an outside vendor to provide child care, and that the vendor work closely with the academic department specializing in early childhood education (human development and family studies). A request for proposals was announced, public hearings held, and proposals accepted. Several proposals were submitted from local vendors and national corporations. Faculty from human development and family studies were very involved in evaluating the proposals.

The involvement of the academic department in the entire process was important. The intent was to select a vendor who would work closely with the department's academic program and serve as a practicum/internship setting for students. It was believed that a partnership would ensure the quality of the child-care offered by the vendor, and remove from the academic department the burden of providing a university-wide service. The partnership was not viewed as making superfluous the activities of the department's extant early childhood center. Rather, it was seen as an opportunity for the department's program to move into more experimental areas, for example, developing techniques for offering therapeutic services to families via activities in classrooms with children of heterogeneous developmental levels (i.e., including children with moderate developmental delays).

This partnership between the vendor and academic department raised a concern in the community: The university was ostensibly providing an unfair competitive advantage to the selected vendor by sending skilled practicum/internship students into its classrooms.[6] This concern was ultimately precluded by the university's contention that the service was only for persons associated with the university, that is, faculty, students, and staff. It was not available to the community. This matter took 18-months to resolve and required involvement of the president's office and legal counsel.

A second concern raised on campus involved insurance liability. A partnership is a joint venture where all partners hold some amount of liability. The university, in protecting its own interests, was uncomfortable with this potentially ambiguous situation, and some advisors recommended that the partnership not be pursued (Trissel, 1989).

After evaluating proposals, the task force selected a vendor. One requirement in the request for proposals was that the vendor construct a facility on university property adjacent to the Department of Human Development and Family Studies. The university intended to lease the property to the vendor for a nominal sum. Unfortunately, the vendor was unable to secure a construction loan from local banks because none were willing to have only the building as collateral. They wanted the land, but couldn't have it, because it was owned by the university. This unanticipated problem brought the process to a halt.

Five years later, the university re-instituted its effort to bring child-care to campus. Another survey was conducted, re-establishing the need for and probable use of a child-care center.[7] Another task force was appointed, and another request for proposals released. The critical difference between this second effort and its unsuccessful predecessor was the provision of a facility: The university committed to reassign the use and renovate one of its existing buildings to make it suitable for the successful bidder's needs. The cost of renovation was estimated at $217,000. The request-for-proposals process was repeated. With the exception of the commitment to renovate an existing building, no change was made from the original request. In spite of this attraction, this time, fewer bidders submitted proposals. The bidders who five years prior had been selected during the first bidding submitted another proposal. However, their proposal was not selected as the most competitive in this second round.

At this writing, a contractual agreement has been signed by the university and vendor. The lease will reflect the unique relationship with the vendor and will contains aspects of a landlord/tenant document. Parents who are employees at the university have first access to the child-care center. The center is guided by a board including parents, university faculty, and center staff. This board will be the setting for creating the collaboration between the academic program and the vendor in curricula and other activities.[8]

A NEW AND UNIQUE PARTNERSHIP

Most often, universities provide on-site child-care services to employees and students in one of two ways. First, existing programs (e.g., child and family development, early childhood education, administrative services, student services) may be colligated and funded to expand their capabilities.[9] For example, during the 1980s, the California State University did this on their campuses. Legislative encouragement[10] was an important aspect of this, as was support by students on specific campuses.[11] Second, service may be offered by a private vendor or an independent, non-profit agency.[12] For example, KinderCare® currently provides child-care services on seven higher-education campuses (M. Anderson,[13] personal communication, February 4, 1998).

Colorado State University used neither of these options, but started with the premise that a truly collaborative relation between a vendor and an academic program would produce the highest quality service at the most competitive overall cost. Recalling its earlier failure, the university elected to create from the outset a partnership: The academic department would bring its expertise and skilled students, while the vendor would bring its business sensibilities to the service. This collaboration was explicitly stated in the request for proposals, and codified in the composition of the board of directors. To make this explicit at the outset was important. In her extensive report on child-care services on university campuses in 1995, Thomas (1995) noted that on campuses having more than one center (one-third of campuses), relationships between the centers ranged from "...openly competitive, hostile or disrespectful to friendly but no relationship" (p. 4) to collaborative.[14] Collaborative relations were most frequent when the centers were administered within the same unit or had the same advisory board.

Thomas's (1995) finding that competitiveness, hostility, or no interaction can comprise the range of relationships between on-campus child care centers denotes the importance of attending early to this problem. These type of relations seem predisposed to duplicating services, making parents unhappy, and keeping staff from sharing valuable information. Anecdotal reports suggest that even on campuses with centers that collaborate, interaction is minimal (S. Burk, personal communication, March 31, 1998; J. Li, personal communication, March 30, 1998). Our own experience taught us that an academic department does not have the administrative infrastructure to sustain a campus-wide service. Our department's missions in instruction and research were eroded by the task (costed and in-kind) of offering child care to the entire campus. To us, a partnership seemed ideal, but Thomas's description of relations between programs was a clear warning of what could happen if attention were not given early to structuring a truly collaborative relationship.

BROADER LESSONS LEARNED

About half of higher education institutions offer child care services to their faculty, staff, and students (Anderson, Getz, & Siegfried, 1995). One of two methods is typically used when providing child-care services to a university community: (a) administratively locating it in an office with "auxiliary service" responsibilities (e.g., student services, business/finance) or the academic vice president/provost's office, and contracting to a vendor; or, (b) locating the service entirely within an academic department (Anderson, Getz, & Siegfried, 1995). Only 12% of institution-run programs are associated with an academic program (Anderson, Getz, & Siegfried, 1995, but compare Thomas, 1995, whose estimate is 39%). When an academic program is not associated with the service, an outside contractor is usually used, since the auxiliary service does not have the content expertise to provide it. This is what makes Colorado State's method atypical. Neither method was selected. Rather a method that brought expertise together from on- and off-campus was chosen.

With the addition of one novel aspect, this equal partnership is an example of Lerner, Ostrom, and Freel's (1995) concept of outreach scholarship. They argue that a generous appreciation of a community's ability to articulate its bonafide strengths, needs, and goals establishes "...a sound basis for a co-learning approach to university-community collaboration" (p. 490). Lerner, et al. note that community-specified needs often require multi-disciplinary solutions—something that university faculty are uneasy offering from their discipline-specific programs. Lerner, et al. believe that discipline-specific offerings are often ineffective solutions, and their concept of outreach scholarship is an attempt to change the paradigm to improve the long-range effectiveness of these types of collaborations.

The novel aspect of Colorado State's collaboration is that expertise was brought from off campus onto campus, the net effect being an improvement of services to the university community. The direction of movement was opposite to that presumed by Lerner, et al. The collaboration recognized at the outset that the university could not efficiently provide child care services to its entire faculty, staff, and students. Contracting with a private vendor could efficiently bring those services to campus. An important part of the efficiency included the real costing of expenses; hidden and in-kind costs (such as those mentioned earlier) would be minimized or accurately costed and budgeted.

University early childhood centers typically have the highest quality programs and best trained staff; this is where those who become contractors are trained. To us, bringing together the business pragmatism (e.g., accuracy in costing) of a contractor and the content expertise of faculty specializing in child development created a complementary relationship. To the extent that complementary abilities were emphasized, the negative relationships described by Thomas (1995) can be precluded. From a broader perspective, this collaboration could be viewed as a recognition that for "outreach scholarship" there is a counterpart that reaches from the community into the university. This counterpart can be as enriching as what the university brings to the community, and could strengthen the context for real rather than ostensible co-learning.

ENDNOTES

1. The program serves between 85 and 105 children in half- and full-day programs.
2. Thomas (1995) estimated that parent fees cover 50% of a campus child-care center's costs. The rest she estimates are covered by subsidies and in-kind donations (31%), and other sources (19%, e.g., grants).
3. Other campus child-care options can be available for university employees: For example, vouchers for parents to use at off-campus centers of their choice; pre-tax deductions to fund in-home care (as a part of a "cafeteria benefits" selection for salaried employees); or university subsidization of an off-campus center giving discounted prices to university employees.
4. The other primary criterion is cost.
5. 3,051 surveys were distributed to a stratified random sample of faculty, staff, and students. Thirty-seven percent of faculty and staff and 12% of students returned surveys.
6. State law prohibits state agencies (e.g., the university) from competing unfairly with private vendors in public services.
7. This survey was sent to a random sample of 5,000. Forty-two percent of employees (faculty and staff) and nine percent of students returned surveys. The improvement in return-rate is probably attributable to "reminder" notes being sent to survey recipients. The survey was administered by Michael E. Kennedy, Division of Administrative Services, Colorado State University.
8. In August, 1998, the University Children's Center opened, serving a full clientele of infants, toddlers, and pre-school children.
9. The majority of on-campus child-care is administratively located in these types of units. Thomas's (1995) estimate is 68%. Anderson, Getz, and Siegfrieds' (1995) estimate is 88%.
10. California Senate Bill 764, passed in 1980, requires state universities to include provisions for employee child-care services in their master plans. In 1987, the California State University Board of Trustees reaffirmed its earlier commitment that student-parents should have child care services available to them. In 1989, the Academic Senate supported child care services for faculty (Academic Senate Resolution 1831-88/FA). The New York State Legislature also funded the State University of New York campuses to provide child care services to student-parents on their campuses.
11. For example, on the San Luis Obispo campus, the Associated Students, Inc., helped fund a construction loan for child care services (Resolution #88-21 and Bill #88-03).
12. Twelve percent of on-campus child care services are administratively located in these types of units (Thomas, 1995).
13. Anderson works for KinderCare® At Work, a division of KinderCare® Learning Centers, Inc.
14. Thomas (1995) notes that one-third of campuses offering child care have more than one center. If these centers are located in different administrative units, the stage is set for poor relationships among them.

REFERENCES

Advisory Committee on Child Development, National Research Council. (1976). *Toward a national policy for children and families*. Washington, DC: National Academy of Sciences.

Anderson, C., Getz, M., & Siegfried, J. (1995, May) Who's minding the kids: A survey of college child care services. *NACUBO Business Officer*, *28*, 46-52.

Burud, S. L., Aschbacher, P. R., & McCroskey, J. (1984). *Employer supported child-care*. Boston: Auburn House.

Chapman, F. S. (1987, February 16). Executive guilt: Who's taking care of the children? *Fortune*, *126*, 30-37.

Collins, L. (1989, May 1). Employers offering child care benefits that few use. *Business Insurance*, *23*, 23-24.

Galinsky, E., & Hughes, D. (1987). *The Fortune magazine child care study*. New York: Bank Street College.

Hernandez, D. J. (1993). *America's children*. New York: Russell Sage.

Hernandez, D. J. (1995). Changing demographics: Past and future demand for early childhood programs. *The Future of Children*, *5*(3), 1-12.

Krcmarik, S. F., Yang, R. K., & Fritz, J. J. (1994). Employer obstacles to child care. *Child and Youth Care Forum*, *23*, 413-428.

LeBlanc, D., & Hennon, C. B. (1979). On-site child care and other child care policies of business firms and their impact on everyday life. Paper presented at the annual meeting of the National Council on Family Relations, Boston, MA.

Lerner, R. M., Ostrom, C. W., & Freel, M. A. (1995). Promoting positive youth and community development through outreach scholarship . *Journal of Adolescent Research, 10*, 486-502.

Magid, R. Y. (1983). *Child care initiatives for working parents: Why employers get involved* (pp. 37-40). New York: American Management Association.

Milkovich, G. Y., & Gomez, L. R. (1976). Day care and selected employee work behaviors. *Academy of Management Journal, 19*, 111-115.

Perry, K. S. (1978). Survey and analysis of employer-sponsored day care in the United States. Unpublished Ph.D. dissertation. University of Wisconsin, Milwaukee. *Dissertation Abstracts International, 39*(1979), 5305A.

Thomas, L. T., & Thomas, J. E. (1990). The ABCs of child care: Building blocks of competitive advantage. *Sloan Management Review*, (Winter), 31-41.

Thomas, J. A. (1995). *Child care and laboratory schools on campus: The national picture*. Paper presented at the annual meeting of the National Association for the Education of Young Children, Washington, DC.

Trissel, S. L. (1989, July/August). Employer-provided child care: A risk worth taking? *Public Risk, 3*, 21-22, 26.

Women's Bureau, U.S. Department of Labor. (1953). *Employed mothers and child care*. (Women's Bureau Bulletin 246, U.S. Department of Labor). Washington, DC: U.S. Government Printing Office.

Women's Bureau, U.S. Department of Labor. (1971). *Day care services: Industry's involvement*. (Women's Bureau Bulletin 296, U.S. Department of Labor, No. 19710-419-843). Washington, DC: U.S. Government Printing Office.

Women's Bureau, U.S. Department of Labor. (1979). *Community solutions for child care*. (Office of the Secretary, U.S. Department of Labor, No. 1979 0-620-014/4498). Washington, DC: U.S. Government Printing Office.

Women's Bureau, U.S. Department of Labor. (1989). *Employers and child care: benefiting work and family*. (Office of the Secretary, U.S. Department of Labor, No. 1989-192-311/00189). Washington, DC: U.S. Government Printing Office.

Youngblood, S. A., & Chambers-Cook, K. (1984). Child care assistance can improve employee attitudes and behavior. *Personnel Administrator, 29*, 44-45.

Zigler, E. F., Kagan, S. L., & Klugman, E. (1983). *Children, families, and government*. New York: Cambridge University Press.

6 PARTNERING WITH THE STATE LEGISLATURE: CONNECTICUT'S FAMILY IMPACT SEMINAR

Steven K. Wisensale
University of Connecticut

PURPOSES AND GOALS

In December, 1996 the School of Family Studies at the University of Connecticut, in cooperation with the Connecticut General Assembly, organized and presented a Family Impact Seminar, "Youth Violence: The Role of Families, Schools, and Communities." The purpose of the seminar was to bring together key Connecticut legislators, representatives of the Executive and Judicial branches, human service providers, community activists, young people, policy experts, and academic researchers for a one-day discussion designed to inform policy makers about youth violence prior to the start of the legislative session in January.

The purpose of this chapter is to present an overview of Family Impact Analysis in general and the Family Impact Seminar in particular, to describe how the Connecticut seminar was funded and organized, to identify some of the obstacles that had to be overcome as well as recognize the stepping stones that proved helpful, to explain how the one-day seminar was evaluated, and to discuss the impact of the seminar one year later. Each topic is presented below.

THE PROCESS: WHAT IS FAMILY IMPACT ANALYSIS?

Family Impact Analysis is a process by which proposed laws or existing policies are assessed to determine their particular impact on families. Patterned somewhat after the Environmental Impact Statement, which was initiated in the 1970s to determine to what extent the environment could be harmed or helped by specific public policies, Family Impact Analysis operates under a similar assumption. That is, the family is viewed as a sensitive and, perhaps, fragile ecological unit that may be especially vulnerable to particular public policies.

Having originated in Western Europe and several Scandinavian countries in the 1960s, Family Impact Analysis was first introduced in the United States in the 1970s. Since then it has received bipartisan support from Democrats and Republicans alike. It was endorsed by Presidents Carter and Reagan, by Senators Mondale (D-MN) and Hatch (R-UT), and by child development experts Urie Bronfenbrenner of Cornell and Edward Zigler of Yale (Steiner, 1981). It was also adopted overwhelmingly by the 1980 White House Conference on Families (Dempsey, 1981).

Family Impact Analysis consists of at least two different models. The Family Impact Seminar is primarily an educational model. Prior to the start of a legislative session a specific policy is chosen and key legislators, policy experts, and human service providers meet in a seminar format to discuss how the particular issue relates to families. Based on the input and outcome of the seminar, legislation may be designed and introduced accordingly (Ooms & Preister, 1988).

The other approach takes the shape of the Family Impact Statement. That is, prior to enacting legislation or implementing a given policy by an appropriate agency, an effort will be put forth to gauge both the positive and negative effects such a policy may have on families. A formal written document, consisting of responses to prearranged questions, will be filed in the form of a Family Impact Statement (similar to an Environmental Impact Statement) prior to the adoption or implementation of legislation. Such a statement may be filed by a legislative committee, a public agency, an interest group, an independent research organization, or other interested parties (Wisensale & Waldron, 1991). Of the two models, the University of Connecticut selected the Family Impact Seminar.

ACHIEVING THE GOAL: FUNDING AND ORGANIZING THE CONNECTICUT SEMINAR

At least three important questions had to be addressed prior to moving forward on the Family Impact Seminar. First, what should be the topic? Second, how should it be organized? And third, how could it be funded? With respect to the first question, Connecticut had one of the highest youth homicide rates in New England, if not the country. Gang warfare in Hartford, New Haven, and Bridgeport had become particularly violent by the mid-1990s. The fact that families and schools were not only impacted by such violent behavior, but were also in a position to prevent it, made the selection of the topic fairly easy.

In organizing the Family Impact Seminar, several things were clear. First, it was agreed that it had to come before the legislative session began in January. Otherwise, it would be too late to convert any proposals produced by the Seminar into legislation. Second, it was also decided that a half-day seminar would not be sufficient. In order to include all of the key actors, a one-day session was necessary. Third, it was determined that an expert on youth violence would be the keynote speaker in the morning session, followed by a panel discussion among four major state commissioners representing the departments of Health, Social Welfare, Education, and Children and Families. The afternoon session would be devoted to a roundtable discussion among 20 key people, including legislators, human service providers, policy experts, academic researchers, young people, and community activists. One week in advance, all 150 participants in the Seminar were mailed a copy of the 20-page policy paper that served as the reference point for the day's discussions.

The Seminar was funded by a $30,000 grant from the William Caspar Graustein Memorial Fund of New Haven. The Graustein Foundation has a long history of funding projects related to children and youth, and therefore, was very enthusiastic about supporting the Family Impact Seminar. The funds were used to cover the fee of the keynote speaker (including transportation), the University of Connecticut faculty member who supervised a graduate student in researching and writing the policy paper, and the Director of the Institute of Public Service who did much of the planning for the Seminar. Also covered were the costs of publishing and mailing the policy paper and the free continental breakfast that was provided for the participants. There was no conference fee; lunch was available in the Legislative Office Building at cost.

LESSONS LEARNED: OVERCOMING OBSTACLES AND FINDING STEPPING STONES

In order to create and implement the Family Impact Seminar on youth violence, several significant obstacles had to be overcome. First, to prevent any turf battles among schools and departments within the University, the School of Family Studies and the Institute of Public Service (the University's outreach arm and conference organizer) reached out and included the Schools of Social Work, and Education. Both had experts on youth violence who were willing to participate in the Seminar.

Second, the selection of seminar participants became quite political in the sense that every effort was made to make it as bipartisan and representative as possible. Thus, legislators from both parties were included and so too were policy experts who had different views as to how to address the problem of youth violence. Because of scheduling conflicts the Republican Governor could not make opening remarks. However, the Speaker of the House, a Democrat, did so willingly. This proved to be particularly fortunate for both the Speaker and the organizers of the Seminar because just two weeks earlier the Speaker announced that the upcoming session of the legislature would devote itself to a "Prevention Budget." That is, more funds would be set aside for children and youth now in an effort to prevent problems in the future. Because the entire focus on the Family Impact Seminar would be on prevention, the Speaker became our stepping stone. In return, he used the occasion to gain much positive publicity for himself before announcing that he would run for Governor.

The third obstacle to overcome concerned the number of participants that could be accommodated by the Seminar. Seating capacity and costs limited it to 150 participants. At least another 50 applicants were turned away. However, even these 50 were at least given access to the policy paper that was written especially for the Seminar. Also related to numbers was the problem of balancing the 20-member roundtable for the afternoon discussion. Many more legislators, interest groups, and community activists wanted to participate than was manageable under such a format. Consequently, this created some animosity among a few people who could not be involved.

WAS IT SUCCESSFUL? EVALUATING THE SEMINAR, MEASURING THE IMPACT

As organizers, we felt compelled to evaluate the Seminar as soon as possible to gather immediate feedback. We also were committed to measuring its impact over the next year. Regarding our first objective, we asked each Seminar participant to complete a one-page questionnaire prior to departing at the end of the day. Questions were asked about the quality and relevance of the keynote address, the morning panel discussion among commissioners, and the afternoon roundtable. As a result, we learned what worked, what did not, and who was effective and why.

With respect to the second concern, we monitored two legislative committees (Public Health, and Education) in particular throughout the legislative session to determine to what extent specific bills related to youth violence were either heard or adopted by the General Assembly. No major pieces of legislation related to our topic were passed but existing funding earmarked for addressing violent behavior in public schools was increased.

But beyond any legislative activity, the Family Impact Seminar produced at least three positive outcomes. First, it brought together three different schools (Family Studies, Education, and Social Work) of the University of Connecticut in a cooperative and collaborative effort to address a major social problem. Second, it clearly put the University of Connecticut front and center before the State Legislature. Such recognition is extremely important in this era of budget cuts in higher education. And third, the Seminar gave the University much positive media coverage. Plans are in the works to secure funding for another impact seminar during the next legislative session.

But equally important, the positive impact of the Seminar extended well beyond the University campus and into the broader community. Specifically, it helped draw attention to the issue of youth violence that otherwise may have been placed much lower on the legislative agenda. That is, confronted with a suburban-dominated General Assembly, representatives from the state's three major cities, where an overwhelming majority of youth violence occurs, often find it difficult to induce their legislative colleagues to address urban problems. Youth violence is such a problem.

The Seminar was also beneficial to the community of social service providers, including school teachers, social workers, police officers, youth counselors, and family specialists. The Seminar not only provided a platform for these participants to present their views, but it also served as a catalyst for future networking activities among such individuals and the organizations they represent.

In short, the Family Impact Seminar fostered collaboration among the schools and departments at the University of Connecticut, opened the eyes and ears of key legislators, and brought together a diverse group of human service providers from the broader community who focused on an important issue that continues to grow more problematic for the nation as a whole.

REFERENCES

Dempsey, J. (1981). *The family and public policy*. Baltimore: Brookes Publishing Co.

Ooms, T., & Preister, S. (1988). *A strategy for strengthening families: Using family criteria in policymaking and program evaluation*. Washington, DC: The Family Impact Seminar.

Steiner, G. (1981). *The futility of family policy*. Washington, DC: The Brookings Institution.

Wisensale, S., & Waldron, R. (1991). Applying the family impact statement to DRGs: Implications for future policymaking. *Lifestyles: Family and Economic Issues, 12*(1), 1991.

7 NORTHERN DELAWARE EARLY HEAD START: AN INTERAGENCY APPROACH TO SUPPORTING CHILDREN AND FAMILIES

Rena A. Hallam
Martha J. Buell
Michael Gamel-McCormick
University of Delaware

NATURE OF PARTNERSHIP

Northern Delaware Early Head Start (NDEHS) is a collaborative interagency program designed, implemented, and evaluated by a consortium of Delaware agencies committed to empowering and supporting pregnant women, infants, and toddlers, and their families. The consortium is comprised of six agencies including New Castle County Head Start, Wilmington Head Start, Easter Seal Society of Del-Mar, Children and Families First, Delaware Association of Child Care Professionals, and the Center for Disabilities Studies and the Department of Individual and Family Studies at the University of Delaware. The University serves as the grantee and coordinator of the consortium. The program was funded in October 1997 during the third national wave of federal support to develop Early Head Start programs. The NDEHS consortium of agencies represents an innovative collaborative model bringing together the university with a diverse group of non-profit community agencies to provide direct services to 95 children and families in the local area. The consortium also works to have an impact on many more families and service providers as a result of its capacity-building approach in the areas of child care, family support, and service coordination.

PURPOSE AND GOALS

The goals and activities of NDEHS are driven both by the needs of the children and their families in the target service area as well as by the Head Start program philosophy of family empowerment. The primary goals of the program emphasize the four cornerstones of Early Head Start: Child development, family development, community building, and staff development (Health & Human Services, 1994). NDEHS provides quality, comprehensive services to low-income pregnant women, infants, toddlers, and their families. The types of services provided are needs-driven and unique to each family being served. Although the program focuses on creating individualized services for children and families, the critical aspects of the program include the provision of high quality child care for infants and toddlers, health and development intervention services, service coordination among all service providers working with a family, prenatal support to pregnant women, and supports for parents in obtaining adult education and job training.

In addition to these primary services, the program also seeks to build local community capacity via innovative service partnerships and enhancement of existing services within local agencies. For instance, some families in the program prefer in-home family child care for their infants and toddlers. In an effort to address this need, NDEHS child development services may be offered through partnerships with individual licensed family child care providers. In this model, family child care providers care for children enrolled in Early Head Start and the consortium provides enhancements and supports to family child care providers including on-site technical assistance, access to materials and equipment, a family child care resource network, and opportunities to advance their professional credentials at no cost. A similar model is in place for center-based child care programs.

ANALYSIS OF THE PROCESS

Northern Delaware Early Head Start is founded on the principle of collaboration. For NDEHS, the collaborative process began in response to the federal call for the development of Early Head Start programs. The Department of Health and Human Services' request for proposals highlighted the need for flexible program models. During the proposal development period the interagency consortium was formed. Initial meetings focused on creating a shared philosophy of services to families and developing ideas for the actual implementation of the project. Through both formal and informal conversations and planned meetings, a shared mission was identified. One of the primary philosophical statements developed during these initial meetings addressed the importance and need for egalitarian parent partnerships throughout all aspects of program design. The need to focus on the family as the context within which children would be served became the central theme of the program model.

During the intensive planning process, the need to develop working and supportive relationships was critical. This need for relationship-building has been noted in previous studies on interagency collaboration (Stegelin & Jones, 1991). Partnerships between universities and community agencies can be particularly difficult in that institutions of higher education may have negative histories with community agencies or no history at all. In the case of NDEHS, the university personnel worked to develop a sense of equality by listening and responding to the concerns of the community agencies. A concrete example of this was the development of both center-based and family child care service delivery models. Initially, the university personnel had envisioned only a center-based model.

ACHIEVEMENTS RELATED TO GOALS

Since the time NDEHS received funding, the collaboration among the university and community partners has intensified to the point of sharing common intake forms, budgeting procedures, and training strategies for child care and other personnel. However, the implementation of the program would not have been possible without the collaborative foundation built during the proposal development phase of the project. We hope to continue to build on these achievements and develop a seamless system of services and supports that will be a real benefit to the families of New Castle County, Delaware.

PROSPECTS FOR LONG-TERM SUSTAINABILITY

The complex nature of operating this program calls for the consortium to continually revisit its mission, create and recreate shared understanding around terminology and philosophy, modify plans to meet changing needs of both families and agencies, and confront organizational and systems barriers to program implementation (Stagner & Duran, 1997). The consortium and the program it supports will only remain viable to the extent that people from each agency remain committed both to the mission of the program and to the relationships that have been built. The actual NDEHS program has been awarded funding for five years. It is hoped that the program will continue beyond this initial funding period.

LEARNINGS FROM THIS PARTNERSHIP

The NDEHS collaborative process has been exciting, rewarding, and challenging. In reflecting on this process, a number of lessons have already been learned.

Egalitarian Relationships are the Foundation of Meaningful Partnerships

The most critical elements to the success of NDEHS have been the egalitarian relationships built among the partners involved in the consortium. These relationships have served as the foundation for the program and allowed the consortium to overcome various obstacles in program planning and service delivery. The establishment of such relationships requires time, mutual respect, and a shared commitment to the project (Haertel & Wang, 1997). Without shared respect for the individual culture of all the partner agencies the project would not be possible. Such a relationship is the foundation for co-learning.

Creativity Is Essential to Success

Early Head Start is a relatively new federal program. The flexibility that comes with newness has allowed the NDEHS partners to be more creative in thinking about types of services to children and families and the actual systems to be used to provide those services. The opportunity to be involved in developing new service options also has supported relationship-building among partnering agencies. The sense of "we're in this together" has promoted interdependence, commitment, and flexibility to discover new solutions to any barriers that develop. Possibly most importantly, the newness has also created a sense of mutual ownership.

The program model developed by NDEHS requires creative thinking to successfully confront complex systems issues. For example, few models exist that address the nature of partnerships between universities and family child care providers, particularly direct service models. By developing and adhering to a philosophy that is driven by the needs of families, the community and partnering agencies have been able to create a truly collaborative system. This collaborative system and culture has allowed the consortium to address unanticipated issues that have continued to emerge.

Collaborative Work Must Be Driven by the Needs of the Local Community and Not By the Needs of One Partner

The history of university and community partnerships is not always positive. Many community agencies feel that universities do not understand the needs of their agencies and the families they serve. In addition, many community agencies report feeling manipulated when participating in one-sided exchanges with universities, such as the placement of student teachers in classrooms without compensation or sharing of resources. Community agencies also often feel they do not receive benefits or knowledge from projects when they and their consumers are used for research purposes. Because of these past experiences, universities and community agencies often have barriers to working collaboratively.

NDEHS has addressed these barriers by focusing primarily on direct services to children and families. Research and particularly program evaluation are important components of the program; however, the collaboratively established mission of the consortium to support children and families in poverty is the driving principle adhered to by all partners. This shared philosophy has strengthened the collaborative process among community agencies and the university and has assisted in tearing down some of the barriers that sometimes exist between community agencies and universities.

Financial Resources Facilitate the Collaborative Process

Interagency work requires an abundance of time and skill (Sanders, 1996). Access to financial resources can relieve some of the burden on agencies in terms of allocation of personnel time, training of staff and development of collaborative products and plans (Stagner & Duran, 1997). Moreover, the stability of funds over time promotes continuity and allows the consortium agencies to develop an identity that will be sustained.

This longer term stability of NDEHS has provided another piece of the foundation for partners so that other issues can be addressed. For NDEHS, one case in point is the university becoming more attuned to the professional development concerns and needs of Head Start programs in the region. This awareness then serves as an impetus for increased university advocacy surrounding the need to provide more community based, responsive professional development opportunities and credentialing for Head Start staff and other early childhood educators.

The collaborative relationship that has been formed in order to begin the Northern Delaware Early Head Start program will continue to grow and change over time. All true partnerships are organic and dynamic. It is the hope of all the consortium members that the results of this program will far exceed its initial purposes, reaching far into the child care and family support structures throughout northern Delaware. The fruits of this program have strengthened, and will hopefully continue to strengthen, the community agencies, the university, and the service delivery system, and will likely lead to new initiatives among many of the partners.

REFERENCES

Department of Health and Human Services. (1994). *The statement of the advisory committee on services for families with infants and toddlers.* Washington DC: Author.

Haertel, G., & Wang, M. (Eds.). (1997). *Coordination, cooperation and collaboration: What we know about school-linked services.* Philadelphia: Temple University Center for Research in Human Development and Education.

Sander, M. (1996). Building family partnerships that last. *Educational Leadership, 54*, 61-66.

Stagner, M., & Duran, M. (1997). Comprehensive community initiatives: Principles, practice and lessons learned. *The Future of Children,* 7, 132-140.

Steglin, D., & Jones, S. (1991). Components of early childhood interagency collaboration: Results of a statewide study. *Early Education and Development, 2*, 54-67.

8 DEVELOPING A PARTNERSHIP MODEL TO ENHANCE LITERACY: FOCUSING ON A COMMUNITY'S FUTURE

Ann K. Mullis
Florida State University

NATURE OF THE PARTNERSHIP

Completion of one's education is dependent upon a number of factors including parents' education, employment opportunities, future career aspirations, and current level of academic success (Mullis, Mullis, & Gerwels, 1998). It is clear that academic success is not possible without a child achieving some level of literacy; and, without literacy, children are not able to make the most of their academic experiences. One Florida rural county became concerned about issues of literacy because of low test scores on the California Achievement Tests. In this county, 67% of second graders, 61% of third graders, and 66% of fourth graders fell below the norms on the reading test.

These scores, as reported by the school district, coupled with high rates of poverty (more than 60% of children in public schools are considered to be economically disadvantaged and 75% of public elementary school children are eligible for the subsidized school lunch program), raised community concern about the future of their children. The results of the standardized tests were discussed in a number of county meetings—fraternal organizations, school board, County Extension advisory board, Parent-Teacher Organization/PTO. One result of these separate meetings was a county consensus that something needed to be done to improve literacy of children and thus enhance educational and career opportunities, and that one youth-serving organization, the Cooperative Extension Service 4-H and Youth Development Program, would be the logical developer of that "something." The county Extension Office had served as an informal Youth Center for children between the ages of eight and eighteen and was seen by youth and parents as a site for programs, recreation, and personal support.

PURPOSES AND GOALS

Community Coordination

The county director and the 4-H program leader convened an advisory committee of community leaders and stake holders. This advisory group consisted of parents, teachers, representatives of the school district office, representatives from the County Commission, representatives from community clergy, and representatives of other youth serving organizations.

The formation of this group was coincidental with the availability of United States Department of Agriculture funds targeting programs for youth-at-risk. The advisory group believed that their chances for receiving these funds would be improved if representatives from higher education were invited to participate. Three state funded universities were contacted and all agreed to participate in writing a proposal for funding and conducting the project and its evaluation upon funding.

The advisory group agreed that a proposal writing team of the whole would be unwieldy and recommended that a subcommittee of three university representatives, two County Extension faculty, and one school board member be charged with preparing the proposal. The advisory group members had a long history of working together on community based projects. The subcommittee had less history and had to work out turf issues, in particular those related to funding. By the nature of the request for proposals, the issues related to funding, overhead, and other financial concerns were resolved with one university assuming leadership and oversight of funds.

The proposal writing subcommittee was concerned that the interests of the community be served and that the project be designed to touch as many members of the community as possible. The subcommittee presented ideas for advisory group review and comment. This served at least two functions. First, all segments of the community were represented (inclusion and diversity were encouraged) and second, major community partners made commitments and "bought in" to various parts of the proposal.

Program Activities

The purpose of the project was to improve literacy among youth in three target groups: second-, third-, and fourth-graders in a school enrichment program; fifth-, sixth-, seventh-, and eighth-graders in a summer camping program; and high school students who served as mentors for the youngest group. The program was designed to build literacy skills (reading and writing) through programs introducing youth to the world of technology and to careers utilizing technological innovations. Technology was the "hook" designed to capture the interest of children, their parents, and members of the advisory board. The project was funded by USDA for a period of five years. This permitted the purchase of hardware and software that became the nucleus for a traveling community computer laboratory, stocked with programs targeting children six to eighteen years of age, and focusing of reading and writing skills.

The next stage was enrollment of children. The school counselors provided consultation as to which children might benefit most from the after school program and the opportunity to serve as a mentor to a younger child. The school district provided transportation from schools to the computer laboratory which was housed in the County Extension Office. The County Extension staff provided curriculum, planning, day-to-day organization, and also conducted the program. University faculty trained mentors, developed assessment tools, and conducted pre- and post-evaluations of children and mentors. Focus groups, with parents and members of the advisory committee, were conducted by university personnel. Advisory Committee members served as storytellers, visiting the program on particular afternoons to read to and with individual children. Parents were encouraged to participate as storytellers and were offered programs in parenting by the County Extension faculty.

Evaluation

A lesson from this program was the value of planning ahead, and defining roles and activities. By the time the project was funded there had been several discussions about job descriptions and what to do if a partner failed in a commitment. This did not eliminate problems by any means. For example, advisory board members maintained their commitments to serve as storytellers for the first two months of the project and then other activities began to intrude on this time. A previous agreement that broken commitments would be discussed at future advisory board meetings meant that, when this was included on the agenda, it was not to punish but to problem solve. The solution to this problem was to increase the number of potential storytellers and to provide a substitute list. Everyone agreed that the important thing was to provide one-to-one adult contact with each child and this was accomplished through increasing the number of community volunteers. In the second year, members of the adult literacy program became storytellers.

The computer laboratory was a major community attraction. Children participating in the program were viewed by non-participating peers as lucky. Far from seeming to be labeled as a program for poor readers it was viewed as important enrichment. Parents of non-participating children called wanting to enroll their child. This led to the computer laboratory "visiting" schools in the county so that more children could have the opportunity to use software that was designed to enhance reading (even though it was viewed by some children as a video arcade).

Involving parents during the hours from 2:30 p.m. until 6:00 p.m. is never easy. This project did not differ from many others that try to engage parents in specific activities with their children during typical work hours. While some employers were willing to allow breaks or lunch so parents could participate in the literacy activities others were not as supportive. Transportation was another problem. Some parents lacked reliable transportation and the county did not offer public transportation. This was a particular problem in the more rural areas.

In an effort to compensate for these difficulties additional activities were added to the program during evening hours and on Saturdays. The computer lab was moved to other community centers and churches to increase opportunities for children to demonstrate to parents and other family members exactly what they were learning.

ACHIEVEMENTS RELATED TO GOALS

After each year of the project, participating children were administered the Peabody Picture Vocabulary Test, the Coopersmith Self-Esteem Inventory and the Bailer Locus of Control Scale. Children's scores improved in all areas. Perhaps most important, in the view of the Advisory Board and the School District, was that children's scores on the California Achievement Tests improved. The average CAT reading scores of the youngsters in spring 1990 was 23 percentile, 15 percentile, and 28 percentile, respectively for second, third and fourth graders. These scores increased at least ten percent for each grade level during the first year of the project (Halsey, Mullis, and Beaulieu, 1992). Additionally, the project linked with the Reading is Fundamental (RIF) program, and books were distributed to each child three times a year. Children who had never owned a book of their own were signing up for library cards and volunteering to read to kindergarten and prekindergarten children in their own schools. The high school mentors reported that the project emphasized the importance of school and education. A change in this group was the 56% increase in those reporting that they expected to go on to college.

The children were not the only beneficiaries of the project. Members of the advisory board were not sure about working with universities, or about what faculty and graduate students could contribute. Although this project drew to a close, faculty have been invited back to work on projects related to child care, engaging youth in agriculture careers, and serving as research mentors with high school students.

PROSPECTS FOR LONG-TERM SUSTAINABILITY

The funding for this project ended in 1995 but the activities have continued. This is due in part to a strong and invested local advisory board. Members of this group have remained involved with the County Extension faculty and encouraged continued outreach related to literacy and technology. All the training conducted focused on capacity building within the county. The equipment and software remained in the county office and have been up-dated as budgets have allowed. The curriculum related to this project became in integral part of the on-going 4-H and Youth Development program.

WHY WAS THIS A SUCCESSFUL PARTNERSHIP?

The project was successful because it was client centered. From its inception the focus was on the needs of children and enhancing the skill they would need to be successful academically and in other arenas. The collaborating adults were able to overcome issues and develop meaningful solutions by remembering the real reason for the program.

A second reason for the success was shared expertise. There was no single keeper of all the information. This was truly a team effort. All members of the team, from members of the advisory board to participating children, knew, understood, and were committed to their roles in the project. The university participants were invited members of the team and recognized and respected residents of the community as most knowledgeable about issues and solutions.

REFERENCES

Halsey, L., Mullis, A. K., & Beaulieu, L. J. (1992). Enhancing literacy through technology education and career exploration. In Watson, D. G., Zazueta, F. S., & Bottcher, A. B. (Eds.), *Computers in agricultural extension programs* (pp. 784-790). St. Joseph, MI: American Society of Agricultural Engineers.

Mullis, R. L., Mullis, A. K. & Gerwels, D. (1998). Stability of vocational interests among adolescents and young adults. *Adolescence, 33*, 699-707.

9 IMPROVING RURAL CHILD CARE: A COMMUNITY-UNIVERSITY PARTNERSHIP

Ronald L. Mullis
Alisa S. Ghazvini
Florida State University

NATURE OF PARTNERSHIP

The primary aim of this community-university partnership was to improve the quality of child care offered children and families in four sparsely populated rural counties in north Florida. Through the provision of training and technical assistance, the partnership sought to expand the comprehensiveness of early childhood programs to better meet the needs of clientele in their communities. A second aim of this partnership was to establish a mentoring system in these counties so that assistance to child care professionals would remain an on-going process. The partnership involved Florida State University faculty, county Cooperative Extension Service personnel, Florida Pre-Kindergarten staff, and local Head Start staff.

In rural north Florida counties there are few for-profit and not-for-profit child care programs, other than those funded by federal or state agencies, that have been accredited by the National Academy of Early Childhood Programs (a division of the National Association for the Education of Young Children). It is generally agreed, among early childhood professionals, that one way to ensure high quality of care and education in group programs is through the Academy's accreditation process. The National Academy notes that child care professionals who choose to work toward accreditation demonstrate a commitment to self evaluation and self improvement. The process involves lengthy self study by center staff and parents, planning and implementing improvements where needed, and finally, seeking accreditation. In the rural counties targeted by this project there were no accredited programs.

Given the child risk factors in the north Florida counties, the provision of high quality, developmentally appropriate child care is particularly important. For example, racial composition of most rural north Florida counties range from 80% white and 20% non-white to 40% white and 60% non-white.The current per capita personal income ranges from $11,356 to $14,473, significantly below the state average of $19,711. The percentage of county citizens in poverty range from 15% to 23%. Indeed, the poorest counties in the state are in rural North Florida (Florida Department of Commerce, 1994). Unfortunately, these percentages increase more dramatically among families with preschool children. Twenty-one percent to 40% of North Florida rural families with children younger than age 6 live in poverty (Florida Kids Count, 1996).

PURPOSES AND GOALS

This project involved three major components:

1) Community Coordination
   - To develop local expertise and interest in activities and responsibilities related to accreditation of child care programs in the National Academy of Early Childhood Programs.
   - To provide on-going support, training and technical assistance to community based Cooperative Extension Sevice and child care personnel.
   - To obtain regular feedback and evaluation from county based personnel.
2) Center Accreditation
   - To recruit child care centers to participate in the accreditation program.
   - To assist at least 66% of participating centers in completing applications for accreditation to the National Academy of Early Childhood Programs.
   - To provide on-going support, training and technical assistance to participating centers.
   - To develop a group of community mentors who would assist centers in becoming accredited in the future, beyond the service span of this project.
3) Evaluation
   - To evaluate the effectiveness of the program on a regular basis.

ANALYSIS OF THE PROCESS

To accomplish the above goals and meet the needs of communities to enhance child care quality, accreditation consultants housed in the Family and Child Sciences Department at Florida State University worked with county Cooperative Extension Service personnel in each of four target counties. These individuals provided training and technical assistance to two child care centers in each county. This included introductory training, assistance in completion of a self study and the needed changes identified, preparing for the on-sight visits of Academy validators, and developing a system of local mentors to support other child care centers who might wish to seek accreditation. An advisory committee of 6-8 people representing project participants and child care professionals from all four counties was established. The advisory committee met quarterly, monitored project activities, and participated in the evaluation of the community-university partnership project.

To utilize Cooperative Extension Systems and Head Start's nationally developed programs and materials to match programs to local needs, two local Master Parent Involvement Educators were selected and trained by university personnel to carry out parent education programs to assist centers in their parent involvement efforts. Local county Head Start and Florida Pre-Kindergarten staffs were contacted for their assistance and involvement in these efforts.

Child care forums were established in each county for the discussion of and the development of solutions to child care and parenting issues, and to foster local capacity to continue project activities. County Extension staff were asked to nominate representatives to the forums from business, industry, agriculture, churches, agencies, organizations, and child care. These forums were held quarterly and included activities such as grant writing workshops, team building exercises, and coordination strategies.

ACHIEVEMENTS RELATED TO GOALS

The partnership project met its goals and objectives and, for the most part, exceeded expectations. Child care center staff who participated in the project carried out preparations for the accreditation process through self assessments and training. Project staff provided centers with technical assistance, practice validation visits, recommendations for center changes and evaluation activities in helping centers achieve accreditation. All centers submitted time lines for submitting their materials to the National Academy of Early Childhood Programs to begin the accreditation process and, ultimately, the validation visits. Once accredited, program staff served as mentors for centers in process. For some centers this provided motivation to continue the self study and helped them feel that their accreditation goals were attainable. Participants began to regard themselves as professionals, seeking out additional training opportunities and even forming a local affiliate of the National Association for the Education of Young Children in one county.

In addition to the above accomplishments, community participants identified county-specific parenting needs, purchased parenting materials, and developed plans for parenting programs. With the assistance of a Master Parent Involvement Educator, one county group developed a parenting survey designed for elementary school parents to determine the parent education needs at their school. Still another group planned a parenting newsletter for the county, produced a parenting resource directory, and incorporated parenting activities into local community events.

Child care forums in all counties were successful in organizing citizens from varied backgrounds and professions to address county-specific concerns, prioritize future activities, and set in motion implementation plans. Participants of one county requested help to prepare a grant proposal to an external source for financial support of an intervention program aimed at pregnant teens. One county worked on strategies to coordinate county activities by developing a coordinating council of different agencies and groups. This council continues its efforts after three years.

PROSPECTS FOR LONG-TERM SUSTAINABILITY

Accreditation activities continue after three years since this project began. Ten child care centers were either accredited or continued their efforts for accreditation beyond the project years. County Extension staff have been extremely diligent in efforts to support their child care center staff as they prepare for accreditation and post-accreditation activities. The university based program for child care accreditation, training, and technical assistance continues to work with these counties to sustain their efforts to complete and maintain accreditation activities.

LEARNINGS FROM THIS PARTNERSHIP

- Extension staff make good partners in up-grading child care center quality in rural areas.
- It is important to identify highly motivated, knowledgeable, and respected partners in each county so that the university/county bridge is a successful one. If these individuals see opportunities for their own professional development, then the likelihood for success is greatly magnified.
- It is important that both the center administrators and their staffs are fully involved at the same time. Any concerns need to be addressed quickly and fairly involving all partners.
- Don't be afraid to modify plans based on local initiatives. This will ensure that activities will be pursued and not abandoned after the outside consultants have left the county.

WHY WAS THIS A SUCCESSFUL PARTNERSHIP?

This was a successful partnership for several reasons. University consultants had relationships with county Extension Service faculty prior to the inception of this project. There was a level of trust that helped bridge the needs of the counties with the expertise of universities. The county agents were highly respected professionals in their respective communities, and understood the kinds of support and efforts it would take long before the proposal was written and implemented. They also knew the local politics of making changes in well established county systems. Above all, the partnership worked because the "experts" from the university listened and followed the guidance of local leaders before they instituted plans for helping child care center staff decide whether or not they wished to pursue accreditation and how the process would take place in their counties. Each county was different and we never forgot this when it came to working with center staff, parents, and other local professionals.

Furthermore, the collaborations established during the project successfully overcame turf issues and realized accomplishments that benefited the community. Staff from Prekindergarten, Head Start, and private child care programs discovered that working together enabled them to serve more of the county's children in appropriate environments. Business, civic, and government leaders realized the importance of their role in caring for the community's children and began to look for ways they could be supportive to families.

REFERENCES

Florida Department of Commerce. (1994). *Florida county comparisons*. Tallahassee, FL: Author.
Florida Kids Count. (1996). *Key facts about children, 6*. Tallahassee, FL: Florida Center for Children and Youth.

10 A PARTNERSHIP FOR YOUTH IN FLORIDA COOPERATIVE EXTENSION[1]

Daniel F. Perkins
University of Florida

Marilyn J. Halusky
Judith R. Butterfield
Tamara B. Dinkins
Florida Cooperative Extension Service, Duval County 4-H

> The problems confronting communities require that the academy be open to input from, and available to be influenced by, communities and by the diverse youth and families within them. (Lerner & Simon, 1998, p. 13)

America's communities are facing complex social issues, such as poorly educated children, teenage pregnancy, and family violence (Lerner, 1995). Many individuals and groups recommend working together to form strong problem-solving collaborative relationships to improve the present status and future well-being of children, families, and the communities in which they live (Carnegie Council on Adolescent Development, 1992, 1995; Dryfoos, 1990, 1994; Keith & Perkins, 1995; Lerner, 1993, 1995; W. T. Grant Foundation, 1988). Land-grant universities as pioneers in outreach scholarship have an important role to play in collaborative relationships on behalf of children, youth, and families. According to Bonnen (1998), the land-grant university, by its very definition, is committed to the application of first-class science and excellent scholarship to the practical problems of society. This chapter presents an example of an extension partnership in action for youth.

AN EXTENSION PARTNERSHIP IN FLORIDA

Cooperative Extension is the formal system and major vehicle through which each land-grant university extends its knowledge into and gains insights from the community. How extension operates varies within each state. In Florida, the

Cooperative Extension is a partnership between the University of Florida and each of Florida's 67 counties. Generally, educational programs are implemented in each county by extension agents. These agents are generally focused in one of the following areas: Agriculture, marine, community development, family and consumer science, and 4-H youth development. At the university there are state specialists who provide support to county agents within the particular area. Specialists are applied scholars whose responsibility it is to conduct sound research that has direct implications for extension programming in their specific field.

A RESPONSE TO THE COMMUNITY

The historical commitment of the Cooperative Extension Service is the backdrop to the example presented in this chapter. The partnership presented here is between a county extension office and a state specialist. The project was begun in response to a need expressed by the community through extension county 4-H agents. County 4-H agents were being called upon by parents, county commissioners, and other youth serving agencies to demonstrate how to evaluate youth development programs. This is where the story begins.

A state specialist met with a group of 4-H agents who wanted to evaluate their 4-H Youth development programs in terms of Search Institute's asset model (Benson, 1990, 1997; Blyth, 1993). The group decided to begin an asset-based project in two counties. The project includes several major tasks: (1) conducting a baseline assessment of assets by surveying 4-H youth; (2) analyzing and reporting the major findings; and (3) developing, piloting, and evaluating an asset-based curriculum to be implemented into 4-H club programming for the targeted counties. Due to space limitations, this chapter will present the process and outcomes of this project for only one of the two counties.

POSITIVE YOUTH DEVELOPMENT AND 4-H

4-H initiatives can be categorized as prevention programs, that is, they are designed to help young people keep from engaging in risky, health-compromising behavior. However, this description does not capture the overall purpose of 4-H programs. These programs are more than prevention programs; they are positive youth development programs. That is, because problem free youth are not necessarily fully prepared youth (Pittman, 1992), 4-H is designed to help young people develop the kinds of skills needed to make positive, healthy decisions, now and in the future. Indeed, addressing problems facing youth (alcohol and substance abuse, antisocial behavior, early sexual activity, and teenage pregnancy) depends on emphasizing positive youth development strategies as much as problem prevention and intervention strategies (Lerner, 1995; Perkins, Haas, & Keith, 1997).

Positive youth development means providing youth with the necessary opportunities to acquire a broad range of competencies and demonstration of a full complement of connections to self, others, and the larger community (Benson, 1997; Lerner, 1995; Perkins et al., 1997; Pittman & Cahill, 1992; Pittman & Zeldin, 1994; Takanishi, 1993). According to the positive youth development philosophy, investments in both human resources and social capital must be made to create opportunities for youth to expand their own capacities as they journey to adulthood, and to prepare them to be productive citizens in the next millennium.

Moreover, research suggests that there are specific competencies and characteristics found within adolescents and their contexts that safeguard and promote success in both developmentally-enhancing- and developmentally-adverse-contexts, and are responsible for adolescent resiliency (Benson, 1990, 1997; Bernard, 1991; Blyth, 1993; Furstenberg & Hughes, 1995; Jessor, 1993; Keith & Perkins, 1995; Luthar, 1991; Rutter 1987; Werner & Smith, 1992). These competencies and characteristics are labeled "assets" (Benson, 1990, 1997; Blyth, 1993), and are viewed as the building blocks of positive youth development (Perkins et al., 1997). These assets may result from "external" factors such as positive relationships in families, friendship groups, schools and the community, or they may result from "internal" factors reflecting the teenager's personal competencies, values, and attitudes (Benson, 1990, 1997; Blyth, 1993). Forty assets identified by Search Institute are presented in Tables 1 and 2.

Table 1
Percentage of Internal Assets for Youth from Duval County and Search Institute

Asset Type	Asset Name and Definition	Duval County	Search Institute
Commitment to Learning	**Achievement motivation** - Young person is motivated to do well in school.	66%	63%
	School engagement - Young person is actively engaged in learning.	61%	64%
	Homework - Young person reports doing at least one hour of homework every school day.	33%	45%
	Bonding to school - Young person cares about her or his school.	58%	51%
	Reading for pleasure - Young person reads for pleasure three or more hours per week.	38%	24%
Positive Values	**Caring** - Young persons places high value on helping other people.	58%	43%
	Equality and social justice - Young person places high value on promoting equality and reducing hunger and poverty.	59%	45%

Table 1, *continued*

	Integrity - Young person acts on convictions and stands up for her or his beliefs.	79%	63%
	Honesty - Young person "tells the truth even when it is not easy."	65%	63%
	Responsibility - Young person accepts and takes personal responsibility.	69%	60%
	Restraint - Young person believes it is important not to be sexually active or to use alcohol or other drugs.	67%	42%
Social Competencies	**Planning and decision making** - Young person knows how to plan ahead and make choices.	25%	29%
	Interpersonal competence - Young person has empathy, sensitivity, and friendship skills.	51%	43%
	Cultural competence - Young person has knowledge of and comfort with people of different cultural/racial/ethnic backgrounds.	37%	35%
	Resistance skills - Young person can resist negative peer pressure and dangerous situations.	41%	37%
	Peaceful conflict resolution - Young person seeks to resolve conflict nonviolently.	40%	44%
Positive Identity	**Personal power** - Young person feels he or she has control over "things that happen to me."	42%	45%
	Self-esteem - Young person reports having a high self-esteem.	62%	47%
	Sense of purpose - Young person reports that "my life has a purpose."	68%	55%
	Positive view of personal future - Young person is optimistic about her or his personal future.	79%	70%

Table 2
Percentage of External Assets for Youth from Duval County and Search Institute

Asset Type	Asset Name and Definition	Duval County	Search Institute
Support	**Family support** - Family life provides high levels of love and support.	77%	64%
	Positive family communication - Young person and her or his parent(s) communicate positively, and young person is willing to seek advice and counsel from parent(s).	36%	26%
	Other adult relationships - Young person receives support from three or more nonparent adults.	53%	41%
	Caring neighborhood - Young person experiences caring neighborhoods.	50%	40%
	Caring school climate - School provides a caring, encouraging environment.	44%	24%
	Parent involvement in schooling - Parent(s) are actively involved in helping young person succeed in school.	41%	29%
Empowerment	**Community values youth** - Young person perceives that adults in the community value youth.	37%	20%
	Youth as resources - Young people are given useful roles in the community.	32%	24%
	Services to other - Young person serves in the community one hour or more per week.	62%	50%
	Safety - Young person feels safe at home, school, and in the neighborhood.	42%	55%
Boundaries and Expectations	**Family boundaries** - Family has clear rules and consequences and monitors the young person's whereabouts.	45%	43%
	School boundaries - School provides clear rules and consequences.	69%	46%

Table 2, *continued*

	Neighborhood boundaries - Neighbors take responsibility for monitoring young people's behavior.	60%	46%
	Adult role models - Parent(s) and other adults model positive, responsible behavior.	29%	27%
	Positive peer influence - Young person's best friend models responsible behavior.	74%	60%
	High expectations - Both parent(s) and teachers encourage the young person to do well.	72%	41%
Constructive Use of Time	**Creative activities** - Young person spends three or more hours per week in lessons or practice in music, theater, or other arts.	28%	19%
	Youth programs - Young person spends three or more hours per week in sports, clubs, or organizations at school and/or in the community.	74%	59%
	Religious community - Young person spends one or more hours per week in activities in a religious institution.	80%	64%
	Time at home - Young person is out with friends "with nothing special to do" two or fewer nights per week.	63%	50%

The purpose of this collaborative effort between Duval County 4-H staff and the state extension office was to examine the assets of youth in Duval County 4-H (i.e., the city of Jacksonville), and to utilize the information to develop and pilot a curriculum. This curriculum will be used in Duval County 4-H programming to address particular assets reported as low by these youth.

PHASE ONE: BASELINE ASSESSMENT OF ASSETS

The data for this study were gathered from a survey administered to 4-H'ers in Duval County. The survey included Search Institute's Attitudes and Behaviors Survey (Benson, 1990) and a specialized 4-H survey. In order to maximize our sample size, clubs with ten or more members were targeted for this study. A total of 167 youth from eleven 4-H clubs participated in this study. However, 151 of the surveys were used in the analysis of data. The other 16 surveys were considered invalid because they were missing too much information or had a high score on the lie assessment scale within the survey.

Overall, the sample consisted of slightly more females (52%) than males (48%). The majority of the youth sampled were seventh graders (35%), followed by tenth (27%), sixth (20%), and eighth graders (18%). It is important to note that ninth, tenth, and eleventh graders were combined into the tenth grader category to create an adequate size category for statistical analyses. Moreover, young people of color comprised 34% of the sample (22% African American, 9% Multi-racial, 3% Hispanic, and 1% Native American). The sample was mostly European American youth (66%).

The majority of youth (75%) reported being from the suburbs of Jacksonville compared with 25% of the youth that reported being from the inner city. The majority of youth (50%) involved in 4-H clubs were not associated with the home school or Expanded Food and Nutrition Education Program (EFNEP). Twenty-five percent of youth were home schoolers and 25% were part of EFNEP. The average 4-H youth who completed this study had been involved with 4-H for over two years.

Results

As previously mentioned assets can equip adolescents to make wise choices. Some assets are encouragingly common (75% or more youth possess it) among 4-H youth in Duval County, such as family support, a religious community (an asset within the constructive use of time category), integrity, and a positive view of one's personal future (see Tables 1 and 2). In general, a higher percentage of 4-H'ers report possessing each asset than youth from the Search Institute sample. (The Search Institute sample comprises more than 100,000 youth from 213 communities across the United States) (Search Institute, 1997).

However, fewer 4-H youth in Duval County report feeling safe than youth from the Search Institute sample (42% and 55%, respectively). In addition, compared to youth from the Search Institute study fewer 4-H youth in Duval County report planning and decision-making skills, peaceful conflict resolution skills, and personal power. Moreover, other assets are alarmingly rare (30% or less report possessing it) among 4-H'ers, such as adult role models, creative activities, and planning and decision-making.

The average 4-H'er in Duval County reports fifty-three percent of the external assets and fifty-five percent of the internal assets. On average, 4-H'ers in Duval County have 22 of the 40 assets. This average is higher than the average for the Search Institute sample of youth (18 of the 40 assets).

As youth get older and face tougher choices, the number of assets tends to decrease in all the categories except the external asset category of constructive time use. Generally, there is a decrease in the majority assets within seven categories—support, empowerment, boundaries and expectations, commitment to learning, positive values, social competencies, and positive identity. Finally, the social competency category had the fewest number of 4-H'ers reporting possession of those skills.

PHASE TWO: PROGRAMMING RESPONSE

This investigation furnished important information about assets that provided direction for future programming. Generally, 4-H youth are doing well in most asset categories. However as noted earlier, one category, social competencies, contains the lowest reported assets among the Duval County 4-H youth surveyed. As such, the collaborative project team (i.e., the state specialist and Duval County 4-H staff) decided that specific programming was needed to provide 4-H'ers opportunities to build and enhance their social competencies.

In order to address this issue, the team examined the data and selected three of the social competency assets (i.e., decision-making, cultural competency, and peaceful conflict resolution skills) that were reported by less than 40% of the 4-H'ers in Duval County. These assets were the targets of this effort because the project team believed that they could provide direct programming around these issues. The team developed a curriculum targeting these assets from the social competency category. Within the curriculum are brief learning sessions and experiential activities designed to afford youth opportunities to learn about and build their decision-making skills, peaceful resolution skills, and cultural competencies.

The asset-based curriculum was piloted within four already-existing 4-H clubs. There were ten learning sessions that were conducted in each club over a five-month period (February-May 1998). The county 4-H faculty provided training and technical assistance to the adult leaders within the participating clubs.

In addition, an evaluation of the program is being completed by the state specialist to assess the effectiveness of the curriculum in terms of increasing these specific assets within 4-H youth. The evaluation design consists of a brief paper-and-pencil instrument to be conducted as a pretest, post-test, and as a six-month follow-up. A comparison group has been established for the evaluation. The comparison group comprises 4-H'ers in a Duval County 4-H club that is not implementing the curriculum.

The data from the clubs participating in the curriculum and the nonparticipating clubs will provide a good foundation for assessing the impact of the curriculum. This work will provide an example of an asset-based program and evaluation that communities are requesting. In addition, formative information from the evaluation will be used to revise the curriculum and prepare it for voluntary use in all of Florida's 4-H clubs.

In addition to the development of a scientifically tested curriculum, several other unanticipated outcomes have arisen. First, the county 4-H faculty are now being recognized and considered the local youth development experts by the Jacksonville Children Commission (the city's funding agency for children, youth, and family programs, and initiatives). Second, at the request of the Jacksonville Children's Commission, the project team has developed and will pilot a youth development certification program for front-line youth workers. These additional outcomes demonstrate the success of this collaboration.

CONCLUSIONS

The work of university partnerships, and extension in particular, is expanding rapidly as an approach to reduce fragmentation of community relationships and to build social and intellectual capital on behalf of children and youth (Albert & Wilbur, 1995). This project is one such effort, and this chapter has described part of this effort, focusing upon the process. Through this partnership of extension at the local and the state level the university is able to apply its knowledge in an effective way. Although success and challenges are met daily, the compelling reasons for our continued involvement in this project are summarized by these words:

> ...the multiplicity of problems confronting and confounding America's youth... provides the venue for this enhanced outreach initiative, building on higher education's oldest tradition of public service. America simply must do a better job of preparing its coming generations for the responsibilities they will assume and the lives they will lead. The richness of the intellectual resources of higher education must be mobilized to this end. (Mawby, 1998, p. 387)

ENDNOTE

1. This study was supported by grants from the Lutheran Brotherhood Association and the Duval County 4-H Foundation. The authors wish to thank Jose Rivera for his review of this chapter.

REFERENCES

Albert, L., & Wilbur, F. (Eds.). (1995). *Linking America's schools and colleges*. Jaffrey, NH: Anker Publishing.

Benson, P. L. (1990). *The troubled journey: A portrait of 6th-12th grade youth*. Minneapolis, MN: Search Institute.

Benson, P. L. (1997). *All kids are our kids*. San Francisco, CA: Jossey-Bass, Inc.

Bernard, B. (1991). *Fostering resiliency in kids: Protective factors in the family, school, and community*. Portland, OR: Northwest Regional Educational Laboratory, Western Regional Center for Drug-Free Schools and Communities, Far West Laboratory.

Blyth, D. A. (1993). *Healthy communities, healthy youth: How communities contribute to positive youth development*. Minneapolis, MN: Search Institute.

Bonnen, J. T. (1998). The land-grant idea and the evolving outreach university. In R. M. Lerner & L. A. K. Simon (Eds.), *University community collaborations for the twenty-first century: Outreach scholarship for youth and families* (pp. 25-70). New York: Garland.

Carnegie Council on Adolescent Development. (1992). *A matter of time: Risk and opportunity in the nonschool hours*. New York: Carnegie Corporation.

Carnegie Council on Adolescent Development. (1995). *Great transitions: Preparing adolescents for a new century*. New York: Carnegie Corporation.

Dryfoos, J. G. (1990). *Adolescents at risk: Prevalence and prevention*. New York: Oxford University Press.

Dryfoos, J. G. (1994). *Full-service schools: A revolution in health and social services for children youth and families*. San Francisco, CA: Jossey-Bass.

Furstenberg, F., Jr., & Hughes, M., E. (1995). Social capital and successful development among at-risk youth. *Journal of Marriage and the Family, 57*, 580-592.

Jessor, R. (1993). Successful adolescent development among youth in high-risk settings. *American Psychologist, 48*, 117-126.

Keith, J. G., & Perkins, D. F. (1995). *13,000 adolescents speak: A profile of Michigan youth.* East Lansing, MI: Institute for Children, Youth, and Families.
Lerner, R. M. (1993). Investment in youth: The role of home economics in enhancing the life chances of America's children. *AHEA Monograph Series, 1*, 9-34.
Lerner, R. M. (1995). *America's youth in crisis: Challenges and options for programs and policies.* Thousand Oak, CA: Sage.
Lerner, R. M., & Simon, L. A. K. (1998). The new American university: Challenges and options. In R. M. Lerner & L. A. K. Simon (Eds.), *University-community collaborations for the twenty-first century: Outreach scholarship for youth and families*. New York: Garland.
Luthar, S. S. (1991). Vulnerability and resiliency: A study of high risk adolescents. *Child Development, 62*, 600-616.
Mawby, R. G. (1998). Boldness for our times: Mobilizing university expertise to meet youth needs. In R. M. Lerner & L. A. K. Simon (Eds.), *University community collaborations for the twenty-first century: Outreach scholarship for youth and families* (pp. 3-23). New York: Garland.
Perkins, D. F., Haas, B., & Keith, J. G. (1997). An integration of positive youth development within the runaway youth and homeless shelter system. *New Designs for Youth Development, 13*, 36-41.
Pittman, K. J. (1992). *Defining the fourth R: Promoting youth development. Center for Youth Development.* Washington, DC: Academy for Educational Development.
Pittman, K. J., & Cahill, M. (1992). *Youth and caring. Center for Youth Development*. Washington, DC: Academy for Educational Development.
Pittman, K. J., & Zeldin, S. (1994). From deterrence to development: Shifting the focus of youth programs for African-American males. In R. B. Mincy (Ed.), *Nurturing young black males: Challenges to agencies, programs, and social policy* (pp. 45-58). Washington, DC: The Urban Institute.
Rutter, M. (1987). Psychosocial resilience and protective factors. *American Journal of Orthopsychiatry, 57*, 316-331.
Search Institute. (1997). *The asset approach: Giving kids what they need to succeed.* Minneapolis, MN: Search Institute.
Takanishi, R. (1993). The opportunities of adolescence - research, interventions, and policy: Introduction to special issue. *American Psychologist, 48*, 85-87.
Werner, E., & Smith, R. (1992). *Overcoming the odds: High risk children from birth to adulthood.* Ithaca, NY: Cornell University.
William T. Grant Foundation Commission on Work, Family, and Citizenship. (1988). *The forgotten half: Pathways to success for America's youth and young families*. Washington, DC: William T. Grant Foundation.

11 A SUCCESS STORY OF A WORKING CONSORTIUM: PROJECT KICK

Stephen Rollin
Roberta Rubin
Daniel Ward
April Brown
John Wright
Carol Painter
Ron Cameron
Stacey Scheckner
Florida State University

INTRODUCTION

Eight years ago, Project KICK (Kids in Cooperation with Kids) at Florida State University (FSU) was developed in response to the need for a school-based drug education program. The specific purpose was to test a number of assumptions and models concerning alcohol and drug abuse prevention and its relationship to early intervention and health promotion. The program employed a community-partnership in drug education, parent involvement, and peer counseling. The objectives for achieving these goals were: teaching drug knowledge, drug refusal, and appropriate problem-solving skills; enhancing self-esteem and social skills; developing conflict resolution skills; and promoting increased family participation.

The current state of Project KICK has come into fruition through the collaboration of several key individuals: the project principal investigator at FSU; the FSU Project KICK director, and the consortium coordinator representing various organizations within the community. Through consistent funding from the city, Project KICK has been able to maintain a long-term delivery of services.

NATURE OF PARTNERSHIP

Project KICK evolved through a succession of several phases that has seen the program grow from a school-based to a community-based program. In 1990 (Rollin, 1992), FSU received a grant to work with elementary and middle school students.

The impetus for this grant was to provide a drug-prevention peer mentoring research program.

Originally, the program was set up at two adjacent schools, one school being an elementary and the other being a middle school. The target population comprised students from both schools. This effort was a collaboration of school administrators, teachers, counselors, parents, representatives of the community, and the members of Project KICK. Using a peer-mentoring paradigm, seventh graders were designated as mentors providing modeling for the younger third-grade children. The goal of the peer mentoring structure was to provide the seventh graders with increased self-confidence and self-esteem, while at the same time providing positive role modeling for the younger children.

Due to the success and positive results of the initial program, the United States Department of Education refunded an expansion into another local school environment (Rollin, 1994). Thus, we were able to replicate the program in a different environment and reproduce similar positive results. We were also able to conduct a longitudinal study to measure the staying power of the initial intervention.

Subsequent to this, a request for proposal (RFP) was let out by the City of Tallahassee, Florida. During this time, Project KICK had already begun to meet with the local Boys and Girls Club, Inc. organization to discuss possible collaborative efforts for creating a model to serve the local children and youth, families, and communities (Rollin, Rubin, Marcil, Ferullo, & Buncher, 1995). This RFP represented the perfect opportunity to get several agencies throughout the district together in order to implement such a model of service. The proposed model was unique in that it represented an organizational collaboration as well as a vision for going into the community to provide peer mentoring.

PURPOSE AND GOALS OF THE CONSORTIUM

As a result of this collaboration, a consortium composed of several local organizations was formed. Because of the special combination of an intact model along with a vision, Project KICK and the consortium were funded by the City of Tallahassee. This relationship continues to thrive today. The Project KICK program has evolved and flourished for so long specifically because of the successful transition it has made from receiving federal grant money to being funded through local, state, and city dollars. The program also receives donations from local organizations outside of the consortium.

The consortium itself consists of seven organizations: The Boys and Girls Club of the Big Bend, Inc.; Mothers In Crisis; The Girl Scouts; Department of Adult Education at Florida State University; Big Brothers/Big Sisters; Family Involvement & Community Development (FICD); and Project KICK. This unique partnership provides the communities of Tallahassee with a comprehensive package of services aimed at drug prevention, decreased crime, and the promotion of family involvement.

Even though each agency within the consortium has a special focus, all the agencies involved combined their efforts in order to successfully reach our main objective which is to serve the community. Furthermore, each organization works collaboratively to meet the social, emotional, educational, and physical needs of the participants of Project KICK and youth throughout the community.

The Boys and Girls Club acts as the focal point for the consortium since it is where most direct services to the youth are provided. The regional director of the Boys and Girls Club acts as the lead agency coordinator of the consortium and mediator among all affiliated organizations. Each month, individuals representing every organization meet to discuss pertinent issues regarding the implementation of services. It is through the coordinated effort of Project KICK and other organizations within the consortium that we are able to combat the obstacles facing the youth on a community level.

The stakeholders of Project KICK include: members of the organizations in the consortium; the City of Tallahassee; other human services organizations in the community and their volunteers; the Leon County school district; the staff members of Project KICK; and of course the children, youth, parents, and families involved in the program. All stakeholders are actively involved in decision-making regarding the implementation of Project KICK.

ANALYSIS OF THE PROCESS

The staff members of Project KICK deliver the services directly to the students incorporating the input of all the consortium members involved. Primarily, the students of Project KICK are of low socioeconomic status and are African American male and females between the ages of 6 and 16. These students reside in a northern region of the state of Florida. They all live within the same neighborhood and they participate in many of the Boys and Girls Club's activities. Many of the activities at the club are sponsored by community organizations outside of the club (e.g., Alpha Kappa Alpha [AKA] sorority, Junior League). However, Project KICK has been the most consistent organization that has sponsored activities at the club.

The staff of Project KICK is made up of counseling psychology graduate students. They are diverse in many areas such as education, professional experience, ethnicity, gender, and age. All of these characteristics allow the staff to portray different perspectives and experiences that enhance the interactions and interventions with students. Project KICK's stability over the past five years at the Boys and Girls Club has caused it to become an active and organized part of the club. Project KICK is looked upon as a permanent fixture within the community itself. In a sense, Project KICK has become institutionalized in the community.

The intervention of Project KICK centers on its curriculum (Rollin et al., 1995). The Project KICK curriculum is based upon the concept that drug prevention incorporates more than "just say no to drugs." The curriculum has nine units that represent the areas that are essential to incorporating the Project KICK model. These nine units are: Orientation and Rapport Building; Learning to Like Myself; Feelings; Drug Education/Awareness; Friendships, Trust, and Peer Pressure; Basic Communication Skills; Anger Management; Conflict Resolution; and Problem-Solving/Decision-Making. These units were determined to be highly associated with the promotion of drug refusal skills and health promoting behaviors. In these nine units, there is a brief description of the unit, objectives that children and youth should master upon completion, and worksheets and activities that can be used to teach the unit. In addition, field trips are integrated into the unit to bring reality into the curriculum.

Implementing the curriculum through Project KICK is based on a peer-mentoring model. Typically in a peer-mentoring program, an older person becomes a mentor for a younger person. However, since Project KICK is hosted in a community center (The Boys and Girls Club), that one-on-one set up is not feasible. Therefore, in Project KICK there is a group assignment of younger children to older children; it is not a one-to-one ratio. In our peer mentoring model, the Project KICK staff works mainly with the older youth (who are usually 12 years old and up) in the beginning of the week as the first part of a two-component interaction. The second component emphasizes preparing the older children to teach the curriculum to the younger children. In this training, the older children should understand how to talk appropriately to the younger children, show interest in them, and be able to listen to their concerns. In addition, the older children must realize that the amount of curriculum material that is learned depends upon their efforts in teaching the material. If the older children have any problems, they are taught to report it to the Project KICK staff. Thus, the older children are really serving as aides to the staff.

Since our peer-mentoring model is located in a community center, the children are not required to participate in Project KICK. Thus, to achieve a significant level of participation in our interventions (usually about 30 children on any given day), a motivational component has been added to the Project KICK intervention. This component is called the Project KICK Achievement Motivation Store. Each time a child participates in one of the interventions sponsored by Project KICK, the child gets a specified number of points. The child can store up the points to use for purchasing items in the Project KICK Store. The store contains a number of various educational, athletic, and creative items such as books, school supplies, athletic equipment, puzzles, and art materials. This Achievement Motivation Store has definitely been a thriving success for participation in Project KICK's interventions. However, Project KICK does not only rely on the Store for motivating the children to participate. Another motivating component in Project KICK is parental involvement.

In regard to parental involvement, a home visitation component of Project KICK was added to the program when additional funds were made available from the City of Tallahassee. It was our belief that as parental involvement increased so would the participation of children and youth. Furthermore, it was believed that in order to impact the children and youth, a systems approach (which targets the child, family, school, and community) is needed. University graduate students were hired to conduct the home visits. Areas of concentration include: acting as a liaison between parents and the consortium agencies; soliciting parental input; assessing family needs relative to the consortium services; determining parental knowledge and involvement with Project KICK; and soliciting parental interest in participating in enrichment and volunteer activities offered by Project KICK.

EVALUATION AND ACHIEVEMENTS RELATED TO GOALS

The evaluation component of Project KICK has been a major part of the program from its onset in the schools to its movement into the community. A pre-test/post-test design is utilized each year to determine the overall effectiveness and the impact of the program upon its participants. A battery of tests is used to examine the five major outcomes of self-concept, decision-making skills, conflict resolution skills, drug knowledge and refusal skills, and basic social skills. The battery consists of both standardized and experimenter-developed tests. The variables are measured by the following instruments: Piers-Harris Self-Concept Scale (Piers & Harris, 1984); Smart Moves Drug Knowledge Questionnaire (Boys and Girls Clubs, Inc., 1990); Social Skills Rating System-Student Form (Gresham & Elliot, 1990); Student Attitudes About Conflict-Revised (Jenkins & Smith, 1988); and the KICK Questionnaire (Rollin & Rubin, 1990). In an attempt to elicit direct feedback from the participants, a satisfaction questionnaire is given to each participant at the end of the program. Positive results have been reported in the outcome areas described above. In addition, there has been consistently positive results reported on the satisfaction questionnaires. For most cohorts served by Project KICK, 100% of the participants expressed satisfaction with the program.

LEARNINGS FROM THIS PARTNERSHIP AND PROSPECTS FOR LONG-TERM SUSTAINABILITY

The success of the Florida State University's Project KICK with the various community agencies can be attributed to the continuous involvement of all affiliated community groups and stakeholders. Key organizations were contacted and brought into the planning sessions at the inception of the program. The program appears to have great sustainability in that it is in its fifth year at the community center in Tallahassee, Florida. The uniqueness of the "consortium concept" which includes several agencies working as the group serving the community has helped to reduce duplication of services and enhance collaboration among all community agencies. Funding was forthcoming because of the consortium concept. Combining several community agencies along with Florida State University has proved to be a very successful partnership.

REFERENCES

Boys and Girls Clubs, Inc. (1990). *Smart Moves Drug Questionnaire*. (Available from the Boys and Girls Clubs, Inc., 327 Office Plaza Drive, Suite 203, Tallahassee, FL 32315).

Gresham, F. M., & Elliot, S. N. (1990). *Social skills rating system*. Circle Pines, MN: American Guidance Services.

Jenkins, G., & Smith, M. (1988). *School mediate program evaluation report*. Albuquerque, NM: Center for Dispute Resolution.

Piers, E. V., & Harris, D. B. (1984). *The Piers-Harris Children's Self-Concept Scale: Revised manual 1984*. Los Angeles, CA: Western Psychological Services.

Rollin, S. A. (1992). *Project KICK* (U.S. Department of Education, Division of Drug Free Schools and Communities—$244,000 grant). Washington, DC.

Rollin, S. A. (1994). *Project Sidekick* (U.S. Department of Education, Division of Drug Free Schools and Communities—$199,999 grant). Washington, DC.

Rollin, S. A., & Rubin, R., (1990). *Project KICK Questionnaire*. Unpublished questionnaire.

Rollin, S. A., Rubin, R., Marcil, R., Ferullo, U., & Buncher, R. (1995). Project KICK: A school-based drug education health promotion research project. *Counseling Psychology Quarterly*, *8*(4), 345-359.

12 MENTAL HEALTH ISSUES IN CRIMINAL COURT: COLLABORATION AMONG BROWARD COUNTY, FLORIDA COURTS, AND NOVA SOUTHEASTERN UNIVERSITY

Lenore E. A. Walker
Ronald F. Levant
Broward County and Nova Southeastern University

NATURE AND PURPOSE OF THE PARTNERSHIP

In June 1997 the Broward County Courts in Fort Lauderdale, Florida began an experimental new specialty court to handle mentally ill defendants who are arrested on suspicion of committing non-violent misdemeanor (lower level) crimes. Prompted by several high publicity cases where defendants spent long periods of time incarcerated in jail awaiting hearings on their charges, the Chief Judge accepted the findings of the Broward County Public Defender's Office, the Broward County Sheriff's Office, the State Attorney's office, the mental health community, and other concerned community leaders and formed the first Mental Health Court in the nation to deal with criminal matters. Determining that it would better serve the community interests to rehabilitate by mental health treatment rather than punish through incarceration these chronically mentally ill persons, a judge with considerable mental health training was assigned to the court along with representatives from the local mental health community.

It became clear immediately that these defendants would need trained mental health professionals to assist in providing psychological evaluations. At the same time there was no money in the budget to hire those with the highest level of training necessary. Nor were there any psychologists being systematically trained to work as clinical forensic psychologists even if money could be found. Thus, collaboration between current forensic psychologists who were working in the courts after obtaining their own clinical psychology training and new graduate students would serve the individuals and the community well for the future.

The first few months indicated that there were a sufficient number of chronically mentally ill defendants who could benefit from having their crimes, such as shoplifting, loitering, intoxication in a public place, juvenile drug cases and simple, non-domestic assaults handled in this court. Like most who are arrested for crimes, these people were often poor, homeless, and sometimes from the minority community who were without many resources. Most of those who were quickly identified and diverted to the Mental Health Court had long histories known to mental health agencies in the county. They did not have family or friendship networks that could be helpful to advocate for them. They often were floridly psychotic at the time of their arrest and admitted to not having taken their anti-psychotic medication. Many had dual diagnoses including substance abuse and organic brain involvement. Some were mothers of young children who were in and out of social services care while others had teens who were basically on their own. The most notable fact began to emerge quite quickly: Broward County had no place to put these people while their treatment needs were being evaluated or interventions begun.

Although defendants alleged to have committed felony or major crimes are entitled to be represented by an attorney even if they cannot afford to pay, those accused of misdemeanor crimes usually do not get an attorney appointed to represent them unless specified by the county. Part of the agreements worked out for this new court was for the public defenders to represent the clients and be an integral part of the Mental Health Court. Dr. Lenore Walker is a psychologist who has worked for the past five years as a contract employee for the Broward County Public Defender's Office, and developed and coordinated the new practicum. Dr. Ronald Levant is a psychologist who recently became the Dean of the Center for Psychological Studies at Nova Southeastern University, which administers a contract with the Broward County Department of Social Services for services to children and elders in need of protection from abuse, and also operates a state-certified Community Mental Health Center that provides a continuum of care to 4000 residents of Western Broward County annually. Both of these institutions—Broward County Public Defender's Office and Nova Southeastern University—have been an integral part of the planning for the Mental Health Court along with other community agencies, but together they formed a special collaboration to provide needed psychological services to defendants both in the Mental Health Court and to the general defendant population served by the Public Defender's office attorneys.

PURPOSE AND GOALS

1. Community Coordination

As might be expected with large agencies serving many functions, neither the Public Defender's Office nor the Center for Psychological Studies had the additional staff or the discretionary budget to be able to participate in a meaningful way to provide services for defendants identified and sent to the Mental Health Court. Broward County has a population of over one million people, many of whom have fled across the southern borders where Miami is located, hoping to escape from what they perceive is a greater risk of crime. According to crime statistics, that is not a realistic appraisal since there are comparable numbers of murders committed in Broward and Dade Counties, although Dade has a greater proportion of non-white immigrants. Broward also has a very large retirement population that came from the Northeast cities where they also wanted to escape from crime as well as cold weather. This population is rapidly growing, and includes those considered to be the very old—defined as those in their 80's and older who need many more health and mental health services that are affordable on their often meager fixed incomes. Few services are available and those that are there do not have the time or resources to follow-up on those who do not keep their scheduled appointments. For the chronically mentally ill this is virtually a guarantee they will not get the care that they need. To address this unmet need, the same community group that led Broward County to set up the special criminal Mental Health Court is now working on obtaining funds to develop a residential and out-client treatment center for the seriously mentally ill, including those who have been charged with misdemeanor crimes.

2. Center Accreditation/Goals

The program that was developed by Nova Southeastern University and the Broward County Public Defender's Office is an advanced practicum setting for graduate students who have experience in conducting mental health assessments for diagnosis and treatment. The students apply for the practicum in the same way that they make application for other practicum settings. Students are required to have a minimum of ten to fifteen hours per week at a practicum site in their second and third years of graduate study, respectively. They may also take other elective practicums in their third and fourth years. They are assigned to a core faculty supervisor as well as expected to get supervision from licensed psychologists at the practicum site.

The first set of four practicum students who registered for the new practicum were all in their third or fourth year of coursework, had taken the required courses in psychological assessment including interviewing, case formulation, and administration and interpretation of standardized psychological tests and were interested in forensic psychology as an elective. They all were seeing other clients through other practicum sites including Nova's Community Mental Health Center and the special program to help abuse victims heal—the Trauma Resolution Integration Program. Several had prior forensic experience such as working with police and sheriffs. Some had specific training in neuropsychological evaluations.

The Broward Public Defender's Office, which has a staff of over 100 attorneys and legal interns, typically uses the services of forensic psychology consultants to evaluate defendants and assist attorneys in developing viable defenses including those that require mental health testimony such as determining: (1) if someone was competent at the time of the commission of a crime or if that person is currently competent to assist his/her attorney to properly prepare for trial; (2) if a person was psychotic or had other mental disease or disorder to be considered insane or mentally ill at the time of the commission of a crime; or (3) if the person was justified in using force or was subjected to duress because of abuse issues. In major crimes where the death penalty is charged, the forensic psychologist also investigates mitigation issues. For court-ordered competency evaluations, the county clerk keeps a list of forensic psychology experts who can be used for quick, confidential evaluations.

It was unusual for these psychologists to be called to evaluate someone in the Mental Health Court because of the quick turn around time the judge required. A defendant seen on Monday through Wednesday was usually adjudicated on Thursdays, so 24 hours was typically the time the psychologist had to get to the jail, do a quick competency evaluation and write a short report for the court. Most of the time, the judge was basing her conclusions on prior treatment records or the assessment of social workers or other mental health workers with less training than would be desirable given the serious mental illnesses presented here.

Our Nova practicum students were placed in the court each day and at the request of the judge could do a quick assessment right there while the court was busy with another case. While it was not the ideal evaluation, it was better than what had been done and it permitted the judge to resolve some cases right then and there without having to send the defendant back to jail if there was a better alternative. In other cases, the judge could request a written report to be submitted at a later date.

To set up the practicum, the coordinator contacted nine (9) of the forensic psychologists who were typically used by attorneys from the Public Defender's Office and known to the Mental Health Court Judge. She inquired if they were willing to work with practicum students and supervise their work on the cases they were assigned. Psychologists would still be paid for their time on the case and students would receive graduate credits for the practicum experience. All nine psychologists agreed to participate in the program. In fact, the ninth psychologist had heard of the program from others in the community and worked hard to be included. All involved approved these particular psychologists.

There were a few perks that both students and psychologist supervisors received. The psychologist supervisors all were granted adjunct faculty supervisor appointments on Nova's Center for Psychological Studies faculty by NSU, which carried with it an email account that permitted them to use library facilities as well as access to the Internet. The students received parking permits that were considered very valuable for anyone visiting the courthouse and a Public Defender's "get-out-of-jail-free" card that facilitated entrance and exit from the three jails, and shortened the wait time for clients to be brought down to be evaluated. Actually, the contract psychologists benefited from this preferential treatment too.

Students were assigned cases in two ways. The judge in the Mental Health Court could ask a student to perform an evaluation and give her the results directly. Sometimes they did not have the benefit of speaking with a psychologist supervisor prior to having to report the results and so they were more hesitant and tentative in their conclusions initially. As they gained more experience, their confidence grew and they were more willing to make recommendations even in that situation. The second way was for an attorney in the Public Defender's office to hire one of the psychologists in the program to perform an evaluation. Then, either the attorney or the psychologist could initiate the negotiation for a student to work on the case too. If the attorney did not want a student involved, then it was not done, but only one attorney refused the student assignment, allegedly because he wanted to have direct contact with the student and the practicum was set up for all contact to go through the supervising psychologist. We felt this system would better protect the students from undue influence before they gained sufficient confidence and experience. In addition, this arrangement would better preserve confidentiality. The psychologist then contacted a student to work with him or her and the student also had turn-down rights if he or she were overloaded with other cases or, as happened in one case, the students did not wish to work with a particular supervisor for personal reasons.

Students were asked to attend a weekly 1 1/2 hour seminar that met in the Public Defender's Office. Some of the supervising psychologists also attended weekly although several only came when they did a presentation. The first 10 weeks had different supervising psychologists give presentations on specific topics. The next six weeks were case conferences where supervising psychologists and students presented one or more cases to the others for discussion purposes. Attorneys were invited to these case presentations to help students get used to oral reporting, which is required in criminal cases prior to submitting written reports, especially when working with the defense.

The students also submitted weekly updates of all their cases to the practicum coordinator via email as well as full discussion of specific cases that she was supervising. A social worker who worked at the Public Defender's office supervised when students attended the Mental Health Court. Students were also permitted access to Dr. Walker's office computer on which the test scoring programs were stored. Each student thus had a supervising adjunct faculty psychologist, social worker, a faculty supervisor, practicum coordinator, and attended the group seminar.

3. Evaluation

The usual practicum evaluation process was put in place for both Nova and the Public Defender's office. Nova requires written progress reports at the end of the semester and the Public Defender's office requires an exit interview with attorneys and psychologists. In addition, there was constant informal monitoring of the practicum by the coordinator and the internship director at the Public Defender's office.

Case Example #1

Juveniles who commit a crime are often subjected to psychological evaluation by the court or by the attorneys at the Public Defender's office in order to find ways to help remediate rather than punish the youth's behavior. This is becoming a less attractive alternative to the courts given the rising number of youth who are committing serious violent crimes for which youth are being charged as adults. Here, too, a psychologist's evaluation of the youth's cognitive and affective functioning levels may be useful in arguing for remediation rather than incarceration when charging a juvenile as an adult may be a question.

In one particular case, a 17-year-old girl was arrested for shoplifting. It was during the psychological evaluation that she disclosed that she was pregnant, had been an incest victim and had just learned that she was HIV positive prior to committing the crime for which she was charged. Rather than sentence her to spend time in jail, the court placed her on probation with the provisions that she obtain proper prenatal care, mental health treatment and get services for HIV that the county does provide. Had she not been involved with the practicum student, she may well have fallen through the cracks and not received any services at all. Now she is on proper medication to best protect her and her baby.

Case Example #2

A young woman in her late 20's was arrested and charged with second degree murder in the shooting death of her husband. She had a 7-month-old baby and was pregnant with her second child. During the initial psychological evaluation, she admitted to having been battered by her now deceased husband. The psychological testing supported her having been a victim of trauma as well as demonstrated that she would be a good risk to be released from jail on bond to await her trial. If she stayed in jail, she would be less likely to be able to take care of herself during the pregnancy, nor could she take care of her baby at home. The Judge used the information provided by the supervising psychologist during her expert witness testimony at the bond hearing to decide to set a reasonable bond that this woman was able to meet over the husband's family's objections. The practicum student was present throughout all phases of this part of the case. He assisted in collecting interview data, formulating the case plan, administering some psychological tests, scoring and integrating interpretations with the supervising psychologist, and discussing the results with the attorney. He also was able to sit in on the attorney's meetings with other witnesses and became a part of the defense strategy team. This woman and her child have now been united, certainly a more positive result for both of them, and the client will be able to await her trial in her own home. (This case had a happy ending for the woman. After expert witness testimony by both the student who administered some of the psychological tests under the psychologist's supervision and the psychologist, the woman was found not guilty by a jury in September 1998.)

ANALYSIS OF THE PROCESS

The process of developing a practicum site in the community is usually a long and cumbersome one, particularly when issues of confidentiality and trust are as important as they must be when a criminal defendant's legal rights in addition to his or her health and mental health are at stake. However, in this case, Drs. Walker and Levant had a long history of working together in American Psychological Association governance activities and had been co-leaders for the past six years in an "intergender dialogue" presented at midwinter psychotherapy meetings. Each, individually, came with support from their bosses—Levant with the support of the new Nova Southeastern University president, an attorney, and Walker with the support of the elected Broward County Public Defender himself. Both the university president and the elected public defender also knew each other and were supportive of the collaborative program. By being able to work within the customary and usual rules governing practicums at Nova and at Broward Public Defender's Office internships (the practicum students were called "interns" in the courthouse), we did not disrupt either program by requiring an intolerable number of exceptions. This may well have helped maintain its success as there was less room for error or sabotage.

It is often difficult to get criminal defense attorneys to work with outsiders, including students, given their demand for confidentiality, especially while developing strategies to defend clients who have been charged with crimes. In this case, the students were all assigned to work on at least one major crime (murder) case that received high publicity because of the nature of the violence or the situation. Getting used to the idea that they would be interviewing a "murderer" was difficult for the students until they went in with the supervising psychologist the first time and realized that each defendant needed to be evaluated without those stereotypes. They learned to take specific precautions for their own and the client's safety. They also learned how to work as psychologists within a very rigid criminal justice system.

The supervisors liked working with the students; they provided good challenges and helped update their own knowledge when discussing new information being learned by students in their classes and readings. Forensic psychologists must continuously be able to back-up their findings with data; students learned how important knowing the psychological literature and research can be in helping these clients. During this semester, everyone began using the new WAIS-III cognitive test which was a bonding experience for students and supervisors alike. They also learned how to work together with criminal defense attorneys, some of whom may try to manipulate the data to say what they want it to say on behalf of their clients. Staying neutral during the evaluation phase became much more of a challenge especially when they then worked as part of a defense team once the data were collected.

ACHIEVEMENTS RELATED TO GOALS

The initial goals were to provide good services to clients (in this case, defendants) who probably would not have received services otherwise, and to train students to work as clinical forensic psychologists. In addition, we helped partner 10 forensic psychologists (Walker and 9 others) in the community with the major private university in Broward County. All involved in this project believe that we were certainly able to achieve these goals. The practicum will continue next year with double the number of students, and all the psychology supervisors have volunteered to be involved again. In addition, the university has decided to expand the forensic program to offer a specialization to students.

PROSPECTS FOR LONG-TERM SUSTAINABILITY

There is every indication that the courts and the Public Defender's Office want the students to continue working there. The new academic year has started off with students being assigned to two new courts; juvenile and involuntary hospitalization hearings. With the new clinical forensic specialization program that Nova is developing, there is every reason to believe that students will continue to want to choose this practicum.

LEARNINGS FROM THIS PARTNERSHIP

There were many different areas in which we learned some lessons from this partnership but perhaps some of the most important ones had to do with the conflict between the need for confidentiality and the need for good supervision of students.

Those students who were supervised by Nova core faculty were at a disadvantage if they were in a group setting, or if they had a faculty supervisor or other students in their practicum who were in other settings that might conflict with the need to keep information confidential. For example, one faculty member had a research and training program with one of the local police departments. This necessitated that the student he supervised take any cases she worked on from that police department to another supervisor to avoid conflict. Another faculty supervisor had someone in the group who worked on a private basis for a forensic psychologist who was frequently called in as a expert for the state attorney's office. Obviously, no identifiable cases could be presented when this person was present. In addition, the lawyers at the Public Defender's office were concerned about inadvertently breaking confidentiality when presenting to others in a group rather than just one faculty supervisor. Since students and psychologists need to work under the protection of the attorney, because psychology privilege unlike privilege from attorneys is insufficient to cover a defendant's rights to remain silent and not incriminate him- or herself, it became important to pay attention to these details. The faculty supervisor in this case agreed to hear the students cases individually and she was helped to present issues from her work that would not violate any confidentiality by not using any identifying information. The seminars with the other practicum students also served as a good discussion place for issues that came up in working with this particular population.

WHY WAS THIS A SUCCESSFUL PARTNERSHIP?

We believe that this partnership succeeded for many different reasons but particularly because of the good will of those involved. The lines of authority and communication were clear and did not get in the way. Furthermore, it was structured as a win-win situation for everyone. There was little room for petty problems to build up and become overwhelming because any issue that came up was dealt with immediately by Levant and Walker working together. The trust that had been established in prior relations helped us both to not get caught up in irrelevant system problems and everyone's concern for our clients and our students carried the day!

13 THE FAMILY SOLUTIONS PROGRAM: A COLLABORATION OF THE UNIVERSITY OF GEORGIA AND THE ATHENS/CLARKE COUNTY JUVENILE COURT

William H. Quinn
University of Georgia

'*You are the experts on this—tell me what I can do to help you make it happen*'— The juvenile court judge talking in 1991 to the author and associates about how a family intervention program might effectively address juvenile crime problems in the county.

The words of the judge were uplifting and challenging. We hoped they would be prophetic. He was conveying the opportunity to develop an innovative program; yet the statement challenged the team to be bold because the number of at-risk youth in the community was great. His message to the team was important because collaboration must include legitimate support expressed by representatives of institutions involved in collaboration. At the same time, an institution which has been in operation for many years, even decades, can be challenged by new ideas, and slow to change programs and procedures. In this early stage, we decided to accept this encouragement from the judge at face value and begin formulating an operational plan.

In 1991, Athens/Clarke County, Georgia was struggling with the increasing juvenile crime rate that was affecting perceptions of community safety, downtown business, and juvenile court resources available to process and intervene with youth. The community, home to The University of Georgia making it a center of culture, has a strong business community, and a professional work force. It is also an increasingly poor, minority, and urban community with high levels of poverty, high school dropout and teen pregnancy rates. For example, the percent of children living in poverty in Clarke County is 46.3% of the African American youth, and 10.5% of white youth, compared to state rates of 40% and 9.9%, respectively (Georgia Policy Council for Children and Families, 1998). The percent of juveniles arrested in 1996 in Clarke County was 14.1%, while the state average was 5.2%.

These concerns, among others related to at-risk youth, prompted increasing discussions among community professionals. These included the juvenile court judge, a staff member of the youth services state agency, a doctoral student in social work specializing in treatment of juvenile offenders, and faculty of the University's Marriage and Family Therapy Program.

Family intervention is a widely accepted modality of intervention in the Athens/Clarke County community. The Department of Child and Family Development has offered marriage and family therapy courses for several decades, and includes a doctoral program accredited by the American Association for Marriage and Family Therapy. The local mental health community includes many family therapy practitioners, including the spouse of the juvenile court judge. The State of Georgia has a licensure law in Marriage and Family Therapy. In the context of these local family intervention programs and emphases, a small group of professionals began a collaboration in which the community had opportunity to translate these resources into practice.

THE FIRST MEETING

The foundation of collaboration was laid at the first meeting among the professionals mentioned above. First, agreement was reached on the shared goal to address juvenile crime problems utilizing a preventive/interventive model that included the family. Second, there was agreement on the theoretical congruence among the professional team that families needed to experience a sense of possibility that their lives could be changed for the better. Thus, a solution/resource based program would be emphasized instead of a deficit/pathology based model. Third, there was consensus that new funding would be needed to initiate an intervention model that would have a reasonable chance of succeeding.

Following the meeting with the juvenile court judge, a proposal was written by the University members of the team utilizing their experience in grant writing. The proposal outlined a collaborative effort between the Juvenile Court and the University's Marriage and Family Therapy Program that would test an innovative multiple family group intervention program for juvenile first offenders. This proposal was funded by the Georgia Children and Youth Coordinating Council with the intent that three years of funding would be provided to test the feasibility of the program. The expectation by the funding source was that after three years, if the evaluation produced positive results, local and/or alternative funds would be secured to maintain the program. This initiative highlights two components of a successful partnership—development of a shared vision, and the willingness of the partners to share resources toward a common goal.

FAMILY AS A KEY CONCEPT IN INNOVATION

Family approaches to adolescent problem behavior have been demonstrated to be more effective than individual approaches. Family risk factors for juvenile delinquency have become well established (Forgatch, 1991; Larzalere & Patterson, 1990; Quinn, Michaels, Sutphen, & Gale, 1994). A multi-systemic approach in treating juvenile offenders in which the family is the unit of intervention has been empirically demonstrated as significantly curbing recidivism rates (Henggeler,

1992). Treating the family system of adolescent drug abusers has been shown to be effective (Joanning, Quinn, Thomas, & Mullen, 1992; Liddle & Dakof, 1995). Summarizing studies of family approaches to treat conduct disorders of adolescents, Chamberlain and Rosicky (1995) have provided further support for family inclusion in treatment of adolescents. Finally, the outcome evaluation of the program described here demonstrates a 21% lower recidivism rate for youth who have completed the Family Solutions Program vs. youth who do not participate in the program (Quinn, Bell, & Ward, 1997).

The intent of the innovative intervention program was to reach first offender youth in hopes that effective intervention might catch youth before they develop a delinquent identity, attach themselves intractably to a negatively influential peer group, and drop out of school. National data suggest that re-offense rates for first offenders are between 60-80%; thus, an effective first offender program that would decrease these rates would reduce demands of case management by the court, increase public safety in the community, and retain youth in viable educational institutions.

One aspect that set this program apart from others in the Juvenile Court which provided services to youth was that a clear expectation of parent involvement was established. The parents would be required to attend and siblings would be encouraged to participate as well. The result of this common view was that families in the community who were isolated, despondent, and possibly distrustful of professional systems needed to be invited to come together to form a critical mass that would draw on each other's experiences and create a sense of hope.

One of the longest and most important meetings held by staff was one in which the name of the program was determined. The selection of a name of an intervention program was considered important as it conveys a public perception that can either mobilize or repulse people and potential resources. Or, a name may not resonate at all with those in strategic positions of influence which leads to inaction. Given that delinquent youth were the target of intervention, a name that did not provide a stigma was important. After avoiding the trap of conjuring up an acronym, the name—The Family Solutions Program—was adopted. It has been retained since its inception over seven years ago. The FSP has remained intact because it provides the community with an identifiable name that conveys legitimacy.

SUMMARY OF THE PLANNED INTERVENTION MODEL

Juvenile court agreed to refer first offenders to the FSP. The court staff had many motives to do so, including to relieve the court staff of an overload of cases, provide intervention that was not readily available to many youth, and examine whether family involvement would make a difference.

First offender youth would be referred to the FSP intake coordinator who would conduct a risk assessment and inform the family of its obligation. The intervention program would explain details of the time and location of the program. The FSP was designed as a 10-week program. The content of the program was constructed from known research in two domains: (a) the risks and protective factors of juvenile delinquency, and (b) the properties of group process that promote behavior change. A curriculum has now been written and made available after 40 cycles of experience gleaning the most effective topics, discussions, and activities as reported by group leaders and families (Quinn, 1998). These topics include: group trust and cohesion, family cooperation, positive parenting skill enhancement, family contracting, conflict-resolution, educational success, decision-making and consequences, peer relationships, and a ritualized closure—called 'graduation.'

CHALLENGES IN UNIVERSITY-COMMUNITY PARTNERSHIPS IMPLEMENTING AN INNOVATIVE PROGRAM

There are a number of challenges when partnership initiatives are undertaken.

Ideology: Punitive/Benevolent. Initially first offenders were referred to a site for risk assessment some distance from the juvenile court. The purpose was to strategically posture the program as separate from the court, and foster the perception to the families of a benevolent program interested in reaching families under stress. While the idea seemed salient, in effect the plan was faulty in that families often did not appear for their risk assessment appointment and, thus, did not receive instructions related to program details. While some effort was invested in locating and funding a site separate from the Juvenile Court, a 50% no-show rate required the program staff to re-evaluate and return to the court as the intake site.

This change resulted in a stronger linkage between program officials and the families, since the adjudication process led immediately to a conference including the FSP liaison and the family. This was an example of FSP staff willingness to depart from the ideal preference for program operation. A concession was made in order to more adequately meet the needs of the court—to not allow court referred juvenile offenders to remain in limbo that would result in an increased workload for the court staff who would be required to review the case.

Flexibility while Adhering to Principles. One of the tenets of university-community collaboration offered by Fitzgerald and Abrams (1998) is that 'you can't always get what you want.' There must be a preparedness to remain flexible while simultaneously holding one's convictions to principles undergirding the program. The decision by the FSP leaders to abandoned the site separate from the court, originally intended to convey benevolence to families rather than punishment, was made in order to remain true to the principle of family involvement. If families for whatever reasons (e.g., transportation problems, poor coordination in scheduling, refusal to agree to the court's referral) were not making appointments to complete a risk assessment and receive details of the FSP, then a return to the court by the FSP was necessary for two reasons: (1) reach the families, and (2) demonstrate to the court that the program was committed to reaching families.

RECONCILING INSTITUTIONAL CULTURES

One of the inherent obstacles in partnerships that must be overcome is the differences in mission, goals, or procedures of various institutions. A reconciliation of differences in cultures must occur. Integrating a family-oriented prevention/ intervention model into a juvenile court system that is inherently punitive and remedial required changes in perception and acceptance that intervention was necessary. The traditional legal institution of court practices typically does not consider the family to share in the responsibility for youth behavior as it pertains to illegal acts. The challenge of integration was attempted by promoting a coordinated belief among the program staff and juvenile court staff that parents are significant contributors to program success. Professionals in the partnership have come together as the following steps were enacted. Such a cohesive approach required negotiations.

Parents would remark: 'I didn't do the crime, so why should I do the time?'; 'I don't have time to come, I have small children to watch'; 'I work at the time you offer the program'; or 'I don't have a way to get there.' To overcome this reluctance, the following actions were agreed upon among the partnership participants. The FSP intake coordinator would be present in the court when adjudications of first offenders occurred in order to explain the purpose and details of the program. Juvenile court staff, in their eagerness to meet the needs of youth and to remove youth from their caseloads, would advocate for youth to participate even if parents could not. The FSP staff remained true to the program requirement that parents must attend, and if they did not, the cases were referred back to the court for further review. The court workers have increased their participation in recruitment over time by making follow-up telephone calls to absent families requiring their presence back in court to reiterate the court's decision and expectations of the family. Communication and negotiation are ongoing characteristics of this collaboration.

RESOURCES AND STAFF

The management of resources requires regular monitoring, a reasonable sharing of resources, and a sense of fairness. The Department of Child and Family Development and College of Family and Consumer Sciences provided support for the program in several ways: release time for faculty to coordinate the program, facilities to conduct family intervention activities, office space for records, telephones and utilities, and secretarial support. The court, following the termination of grant funds, has secured funding locally or from the State Department of Juvenile Justice as recidivism data and family anecdotal data on successful program experiences have demonstrated its effectiveness. Furthermore, foundation support has been garnered to develop group leader training and program implementation in other communities in Georgia.

Staffing the program required recruitment and organizational management so that the responsibility for the program did not fall to one person or site. The linch-pin in the partnership is the FSP intake coordinator. This person is present in the court to receive referrals and personally meets with families referred to the FSP. The person is also an FSP group leader who understands the theoretical perspective (family inclusion with a solution-based program orientation) and limitations of the University's resources. University-community partnerships need personnel who can 'travel in both worlds,' and communicate the needs and circumstances of both groups.

Community coordination of the program is facilitated by the program leader who receives notification of all referrals to the program from the judge or juvenile court staff. The program leader is present at all adjudications of these referrals to administer a risk assessment (used to plan the upcoming program and evaluate the program) and to convey in person to the family the requirements of parent involvement, and the details of the logistics of the program such as where and when to be present. A personal contact with a FSP representative at this point helps put some families at ease and builds trust.

PROGRAM STABILIZATION

A vital part of the community-university partnership in the project has been the continuity of staff and the opportunity for students to mentor other students who follow. The program leader must receive compensation since major responsibility for implementing the program is expected. The initial program coordinator was paid for by a grant focused on innovative programs to address the rise in juvenile crime. This coordinator was a doctoral candidate with extensive background as a youth worker and family interventionist. After three years the grant ended. The initial coordinator received his doctoral degree and accepted a position at another university.

Since the program had demonstrated results pertaining to a reduction in recidivism and substantial anecdotal data from families and court workers, the Juvenile Court accepted responsibility for hiring the program leader. This event serves to reflect the confidence that can be built among partners when outcome results demonstrate benefits. Another graduate student who had done an internship as part of course requirements took over. As an intern, this person had helped the FSP program coordinator by charting cases and recruiting families. Therefore, she had a positive view of the FSP and was familiar with program implementation.

Currently a third person in the lineage of program coordinators has been in the position for almost three years. Her first contact with the FSP was as a student in the first author's undergraduate family intervention class where she as a class requirement had become familiar with an intervention program, and had observed and written about the FSP. This student also did an internship at the court under the tutelage of the previous coordinator. In this way the student learned about the referral process from the court to the FSP. The third coordinator proved her readiness for the role when she remarked one day about a family she was struggling to recruit into the program, "I am not giving up on this family, Dr. Quinn, because we all know that without the family very little will change for this child."

Locating the FSP Coordinator in the court for assessments and referrals provides a linkage between the university and community agency that reflects a role as program ambassador. This person as ambassador clarifies the mission of the program and confirms the united goals of those involved. Yet, the university's program director and the juvenile court judge and staff must directly communicate to more fully appreciate the mission and procedures of the two organizations. (The FSP Director attends court staffings and has lunch periodically with the Judge and Associate Judge to visit face-to-face with court personnel and confirm the commitment to first offenders and families.) The Judge has invited the program director to speak at the State of Georgia Juvenile Judges Conference to help promote the model in other communities. This event contributes to the university's mission as a land-grant institution that is expected to transfer original products developed within the institution to the constituents or communities who can benefit from these products—in this case, the potential decrease of juvenile crime and strengthening of family life in Georgia communities.

The network of those involved in FSP was expanded through undergraduate and graduate students who are majors in Child and Family Development. They provide assistance to FSP group leaders, co-leading discussion groups, directing group activities, serving as a source of feedback about family experiences heard informally before and after the program, and preparing program materials. These students receive academic credit through an 'independent study' course offered in the department. Since 1992, 88 students have participated. Their required papers at the end of the program suggest that this experience served as a capstone experience that provided an opportunity to apply their classroom study to 'real life.' The requirements for the paper are that they should avoid summarizing the events of the program, but rather describe their observations of the program's effects. Questions to which they respond include the following:

- 'What did the families gain from the program?'
- 'What occurred in the program that fostered the change?'
- 'What could have been done differently, and why?'
- 'Why were some families benefitted more than others?'

These questions require students to analyze the conditions under which beneficial intervention occurs, threats to program success, and how families with large differences can come together as a group in ways that are conducive to their success. The experience allowed them to discover that concepts and theories can be useful in providing a context for behavior change through intervention programming. Concurrently, the students were provided greater awareness of the challenges faced by families and interventionists regarding the resolution of problems embedded in life circumstances. As a result, the FSP experience allowed students the opportunity to evaluate whether such work was compatible with their career plans.

SOURCES OF FUNDING

In addition to the initial three year grant, the College of Family and Consumer Sciences provided funds through its outreach grants initiative to develop a curriculum for group leaders so that the program can be adopted in other communities within and outside the state.[1] Partial funding for the program has come from the local court allocation of 'services funding' which can be utilized for individual counseling, drug and alcohol screenings, psychological testing, and the like. The court made a committed decision to utilize some of these funds to support the continuation of the program. In addition, the regional administrator for the Department of Juvenile Justice lobbied for additional funds from the Georgia Council of Juvenile Court Judges to offer the program in other counties.

AN EARLY VICTORY

The impetus for continued collaboration between a university and community can sometimes require a successful short-term outcome, termed 'an early victory' by Fitzgerald and Abrams (1998). Progress in collaboration early-on provides sustaining energy and commitment by staff who are strategically located in the partnership organization. In addition, the early success breeds confidence in the plan thereby providing motivation for continued involvement and a shared vision.

In the FSP, the last session is 'graduation night,' which includes a pot luck supper in which families bring food, an inspirational speaker, and the presentation of cards and certificates. The Juvenile Court Judge was frequently invited to give the inspiration talk at graduation. The early victory came in the form of comments by parents in the program related to their successful involvement in the FSP which were shared with the judge during testimonials at graduation.

While there were difficulties early on with convening parents of some families for the FSP, those parents that did attend experienced a shift in their attitude that contributed to goal attainment in increased family cohesion and cooperation. Many parents bring an attitude of either ambivalence or disdain for the program and/or court intrusion. They may be embarrassed about being there and having friends from the neighborhood or community connect them to a juvenile delinquent child. Parents also may feel offended as they make an interpretation that somehow the child's delinquency is 'caused by' them or their relationships with their children.

The judge is aware of these attitudes when the adjudication process occurs and the referral to the FSP is made. Over the course of the FSP, however, parents begin to get comfortable, recognize the enjoyment of their own experience, and begin making alliances with other families. At FSP graduation, one parent remarked, 'You know, I didn't think I could afford the time to come to this program, now I realize I can't afford not to spend time with my child.' Another parent remarked, 'I have to thank you for all you have done (the leaders), it has made a big difference to our family.' A youth said, 'Thank you for being my friend during this program, I hope I never see you back here again!' (laughter) As the judge hears these remarks, he builds confidence that the program is worthwhile and deserving of support. Simply examining statistics on recidivism does not achieve full appreciation of the FSP, but hearing individuals and families express heartfelt gratitude and depict the changes that have occurred in their lives incrementally builds value even more. The judge's presence in hearing these family testimonials became the 'early victory' for the FSP.

ELEMENTS OF SUCCESSFUL COLLABORATION

Seven years of program development and implementation have provided a number of 'lessons' useful in guiding university-community partnerships that focus on youth intervention. The lessons learned in the FSP are outlined in this section.

1) *Alternative intervention programs advocated for by university representatives require conviction and continual oversight*. Family programs developed within traditional institutional service agencies face the challenge of rubbing against belief systems and practices that focus solely on the individual. The

individual focus is thought to be a more practical approach because societal expectations dictate individual accountability (in Eastern cultures historically the family and even the teacher were accountable for youth behavior even to the point that prosecution for illegal behavior could require punishment to the parents and even teachers). In addition, it is easier for an agency to target intervention for a youth rather than a family. Families may carry the belief system that the child alone is responsible for his/her behavioral choices. Thus, the family may be reluctant to oblige the treatment provider who requests its participation in intervention.

In the FSP, the University personnel remained determined that the court support the program's mission by advocating for family involvement. This meant that court case workers had to be reminded that a youth could not attend the program without parents. This was a particularly sensitive issue when an attendance report from the program coordinator to the court indicated a family absence. While the court worker wanted the youth to continue, the FSP coordinator was required to remain adamant that the court worker would need to locate an alternative disposition to the case. Otherwise, the integrity of the program (family involvement) would be threatened (parents might tell other parents, 'Oh you don't have to go to the program you were referred to, nothing will happen to you if you don't'). Adherence to the program's theoretical tenets must be steadfast.

2) *Initiators of a new program or institutional practice must cultivate and tend to the collegial relationships that are necessary between those that represent the new program and those that represent the institution.* Communication difficulties leading to disruptions in program practices exist when there are too few telephone conversations and personal exchanges. We have found that regular telephone conversations with the judges and probation officers help clarify the program and the shared expectations that exist regarding the operation of the program. These conversations include issues pertaining to the budget, family attendance, the referral process, and programmatic details such as when the next cycle of the FSP should begin.

3) *It is important that commitments made by personnel either representing the university or the community institution(s) be met.* For instance, there was initial difficulty as the FSP began with how to handle cases in which families did not attend the program. Whose responsibility was it to follow-up with the absentee families? Was it the court's responsibility since they have the legal leverage to invoke and maintain obligations to the court, or was it the FSP leader's responsibility since the cases were assigned to the program offered by the University? An example of a collaborative plan can be offered by the following scenario: (1) a list of families both present and absent for each session was faxed to the court by the FSP leaders after each session so that court workers were kept abreast of a family's status, (2) The FSP leaders would telephone absent families sometime prior to the next session to remind them of their obligation and the rule that only one absence was acceptable to qualify for graduation; (3) A family that was absent more than one time was formerly referred back to the juvenile court for further case review; and (4) The court worker would telephone, and meet with, any family which had been absent more than once to implement another case disposition and obligation (such as a formal and lengthier probation) or a referral back to the FSP for the next cycle of the program if acceptable to the FSP program leaders. The success of this plan hinged on each professional adhering to the plan and maintaining communication on issues pertaining to the status of each family case.

FSP leaders must maintain records of attendance and provide weekly attendance reports to the court; court workers must check these reports and follow-up with any families who have lost their eligibility to complete the program. Adherence to the plan is important so that FSP leaders can avoid threatened absences of other families who might assume that missed sessions don't result in any consequence. In addition, the court can confidently assume that families referred to the program are receiving treatment unless they are informed of absences. In this way, the missions of the court and the FSP are preserved.

4) *Outcome assessment is vital in stabilizing a program to protect and promote funding of the program and to substantiate the valid mission shared by collaborators.* Procedures for evaluation of an innovative program must be built into the program from its inception, and be adopted and valued. Reports of outcomes must be in the language of institutional leaders. For instance, judges may be primarily interested in recidivism and cost effectiveness, even though the quality of the family environment is important. The partnership, then, must ask itself how the initiative will be evaluated so as to be deemed valuable and deserving of continuation by both the community institution and University.

5) *There must be a positive public perception of the program. Representatives from the university must represent the program well in public.* Differences not yet fully negotiated in the university-community partnership must be silenced in public so that the perception of blame or unbalanced responsibility is avoided. Such negative perceptions will contaminate the collaborative spirit necessary for successful partnership. One example would be parents, teachers, and certain community critics who criticize the court for their juvenile arrest practices. The FSP does not view its role as a sounding board or conduit for change as it pertains to arrest practices. To do so would be trespassing on court jurisdiction and legal thought, with the outcome being a division between the court and the FSP.

PROSPECTS FOR PROGRAM SUSTAINABILITY

A number of achievements suggest that the FSP is a viable program that has established itself as a mainstream service delivery component of the court. One, the FSP is in its seventh year and the Judge and Associate Judge along with probation officers continue to enthusiastically support it. Two, the recidivism data suggest that youth who complete the FSP are significantly less likely to repeat offend (34%; N=248) than youth who do not complete the program (55%; N=248). Furthermore, the FSP 'graduates' who do re-offend do so less often than the FSP 'non-graduates.' Three, the judge reports these data to community leaders and the State Department of Juvenile Justice which builds confidence in the program and sheds positive light on his court's achievements. Four, the University continues to support the existence and growth of the program. Five, the number of communities adopting the FSP continues to grow. Communities in proximity to the University are contracting with the University to operate the program as they petition the State Department of Juvenile Justice for FSP funds, and communities some distance from the University are requesting FSP training sessions by the University FSP staff so that the local human service providers can deliver the program. Six, the Governors Task Force on Juvenile Crime has included the FSP as a recommended service to address juvenile crime in communities across the state, and the FSP was listed in a recent state report on crime prevention submitted to Attorney General Janet Reno.

CONCLUSION

The community-university partnership in operating the FSP has been successful for several reasons. In general success can be attributed to goal attainment as specified mutually by the University and the Juvenile Court. *First,* there was a shared view that the idea of including the family in addressing youth crime and behavior problems was viable. This shared belief system had to withstand threats such as parent refusal to accept case disposition to the FSP, ineligibility of youth who attended without parents, communication problems in contacting parents, and space problems in accommodating large groups comprising multiple families. *Second*, the evaluation design chosen included criteria important to the judges as well as University family researchers, such as recidivism rates, re-offense patterns, family reports of program experiences, and number of families who completed the program. In this way the Judge could communicate important information to his constituency of colleagues, civic leaders and politicians, and the State Department of Juvenile Justice. In addition, the students' participation from the University, as well as the provision of facilities, secretarial help, and utilities, lowered the budget costs expended by the Juvenile Court. A graduate research assistant provided by the College of Family and Consumer Sciences allowed for the establishment of a data gathering procedure to track recidivism that allowed outcome evaluation. *Third,* the university expanded its service learning mission of combining coursework on child and family development and family systems intervention with application to real family life struggles and dilemmas.

ENDNOTE

1. A complete written FSP Curriculum, The Family Solutions Program: A Group Program for Youth Offenders and Their Families, including videos and FSP brochures, is now available for adoption to any interested professionals.

The author wishes to gratefully acknowledge Dr. Christine Todd, Associate Dean for Outreach and Extension, College of Family and Consumer Sciences, and Associate Professor, Department of Child & Family Development; and Dean Sharon Y. Nickols, College of Family and Consumer Sciences, and Professor in the Department of Housing and Consumer Economics, who provided support to the Family Solutions Program, and reviewed an earlier draft of this chapter. The author also wishes to acknowledge the unswerving support of Judge James McDonald and Associate Judge Robin Shearer.

REFERENCES

Fitzgerald, H. E. & Abrams, L. A. (1998). Applied developmental science: A scholarship based approach to university-community collaborations. Presented at the Biennial Meeting of the Society for Research on Adolescence, San Diego, CA: February 26.

Forgatch, M. (1991). Parent practices: Mediators of risk for antisocial behavior. In J. B. Reid (Chair), *A social interactional model of the development and prevention of antisocial behavior and conduct disorder*. Symposium conducted at the Third Biennial Conference on Community Research and Action, Tempe, AZ.

Georgia Policy Council for Children and Families. Family Connection: Athens, GA (connection@athens.net), 1998.

Henggeler, S., Melton, G. B., & Smith, L. A. (1992). Family preservation using multisystemic therapy: An effective alternative to incarcerating serious juvenile offenders. *Journal of Consulting and Clinical Psychology*, *60*, 953-961.

Joanning, H., Quinn, W. H., Thomas, F. N, & Mullen, R. (1992). Treating adolescent drug abuse: A comparison of family systems therapy group therapy, and family drug education. *Journal of Marital and Family Therapy*, *18*, 4, 345-356.

Larzelere, R. & Patterson, G. R. (1990). Parental management: Mediator of the effect of socioeconomic status on early delinquency. *Criminology*, *28*(2), 301-324.

Quinn, W. H., Michaels, M., Sutphen, R., & Gale, J. (1994). Juvenile first offenders: Characteristics of at-risk families and strategies for intervention. *Journal of Addictions and Offender Counseling*, *15*(1), 2-23.

Quinn, W. H., Bell, K., & Ward, J. (1997). The Family Solutions Program. *Prevention Researcher*, *4*(2), 10-12.

Quinn, W. H. (1998). The Family Solutions Program: A Group Program for Juvenile Offenders and Their Families. The University of Georgia: Athens, GA.

14 AN OUNCE OF PREVENTION IS WORTH A POUND OF CURE

J. Jay Ney
University of Idaho

NATURE OF PARTNERSHIP

The Lewis-Clark Coalition for Families and Youth evolved from the "Making the Grade" town summit meeting held in Lewiston, Idaho, November 3, 1989. The goals of this meeting were: 1) To explore the current dimensions of at-risk youth problems in our community, assess the effectiveness of current programs, and identify possible new, broad-based efforts to meet the needs of all youth in the community; 2) To provide an opportunity for committed people to explore new program ideas and improve communication networks to meet the needs of at-risk youth more effectively; and 3) To encourage all members of our community to make or renew a commitment to do everything they can to help solve the problems confronting young people.

PURPOSES AND GOALS

"Making the Grade" was an innovative project of the National Collaboration for Youth designed to raise public awareness and stimulate action on behalf of youth at local, state, and national levels. Another purpose centered on educating the public about the critical problems that affect a significant number of America's young people and on providing opportunities for citizens to come together at the community level to develop and implement viable solutions to these problems.

ANALYSIS OF THE PROCESS

The unique focus of this project emphasized the interrelated nature of six trends that threaten to foreclose the future of at-risk youth—Functional Illiteracy, Juvenile Crime, School Dropouts, Substance Abuse, Teen Pregnancy, and Youth Unemployment.

ABC network television featured the "Making the Grade" project during a prime time special on September 14, 1989. The Lewiston town summit meeting was a follow-up to that program.

Twenty-six organizations, including the Lewiston Chamber of Commerce, publicized and distributed participant handbooks. One hundred seventy-five people attended the four-hour town meeting. Six point-of-view presenters (a high school student, the regional director of Head Start, a school teacher, the manager of an electrical company [also representing the Chamber of Commerce], a district judge, and a parent) discussed their perceptions of our community as related to functional illiteracy, juvenile crime, school dropouts, substance abuse, teen pregnancy, and youth unemployment.

A local report card for national, state, and local data for these risk factors was also distributed. The report card data was one of the motivating factors that brought people together. A summary of the data in report card format had not been done before. School personnel and other agencies were nervous that it was a reflection on them. Private industry representatives were implying something needed to be done. Spirited small group discussions magnified the concerns of parents, students, businesses, agencies, schools, law enforcement, and elected officials.

Following the meeting, 105 people signed commitment forms. Thirty individuals (including the president of Lewis-Clark State College, an attorney, school counselors, and representatives from area agencies and private industry) volunteered to develop a mission statement and goals for the formation of the Lewis-Clark Coalition for At-Risk Youth. (In 1997, the coalition changed the name to Lewis-Clark Coalition for Families and Youth.)

A video of the meeting and a blueprint for action were used to summarize the town summit meeting. Additional sub-committees were identified to address the following topics: Catalogue for youth services, crisis management, educational enhancement, parenting skills, and transportation activities.

Drafting the mission and goals statements, plus planning sub-committee activities and the at-risk data for the local report card, kept many people interested and active following the town summit meeting.

We meet on the first Monday of each month and have continued meeting each month, except for July and August, for the past nine years.

This was the first, and largest, youth and family collaborative effort to be initiated and sustained in this community in the past thirty years.

PROSPECTS FOR LONG-TERM SUSTAINABILITY

Developing letterhead stationery for the coalition helped to unify the group. Identifying organizations and specific individuals helped deepen commitments.

Annual election of officers has also enhanced the energy and expanded the vision for the coalition and, most importantly, for the community. I served as chair for the first five years. The chief of police was elected in 1994 to the position, followed by an executive of the Idaho Education Association, the superintendent of schools, the county juvenile probation officer, and currently, the comptroller for the *Lewiston Morning Tribune*.

Prior to formalizing the collaboration, the coalition was advisory, primarily because of the activities we sponsored. At one of our meetings, there was a debate about whether or not we should remain advisory or formally adopt articles of incorporation and non-profit status. The chief of police made a point by slapping his hand on the table and saying, "I get advice every day from lots of people. We need to get formally organized or dissolve." We voted to become an official 501-C3 non-profit organization. By-laws and articles of incorporation for a non-profit organization status were adopted in 1994.

This coalition has become a leader and primary voice for family and youth issues in Nez Perce County, Idaho, and Asotin County, Washington.

ACHIEVEMENTS RELATED TO GOALS

The coalition evolved from no budget—literally passing the hat for postage to mail meeting notices—to a $73,842 budget. Funding sources include the ES-USDA 4-H Program, Juvenile Justice System, United Way, Kiwanis Club, and the Idaho Department of Health and Welfare. A 1997 Adolescent Family Life grant provided funding for several abstinence programs which were implemented in cooperation with the Valley Family Resource Center, the Valley Boys and Girls Club, and the Lewis-Clark Coalition.

In 1994, the coalition became partners with the Valley Boys and Girls Club to establish a Valley Family Resource Center located in the Valley Boys and Girls Club building. The primary purpose of this entity is to provide counseling for families who cannot afford it. In 1998, 70 hours of counseling were provided to 18 families. The center also serves as a library for parenting resource material.

The Valley Family Resource Center was a stretch for the coalition and the Valley Boys and Girls Club. We have created a small business and need to clarify roles for decision making (such as hiring personnel, planning, budgeting, adoption of a counseling policy, time involved, and whose responsibility). All have made a deep commitment to this agreement.

The coalition was instrumental in developing and sponsoring an annual event called "Celebrate the Family Month." This event began in 1992 with the following goals: 1) To create the awareness that all families are important to society and communities within Nez Perce and Asotin counties; 2) To inform families of the resources available to them through employers, churches, agencies, schools, and law enforcement; 3) To provide an opportunity for family education providers to identify resources and present information to parents throughout Nez Perce and Asotin counties; and 4) To encourage families to participate in the educational and social events offered during the month of February and throughout the year.

Annually, there are over 50 events planned by schools, churches, and businesses that focus specifically on families and parenting. In addition, a two-page tabloid on parenting and family issues is published in the newspaper (26,000 daily circulation) each Friday for four consecutive weeks during "Celebrate the Family Month." Since 1997, six banners (3 ft x 20 ft) have been hung over major streets for the entire month of February. The banners read: "CELEBRATE THE FAMILY IN THE LEWIS-CLARK VALLEY."

Two thousand parents attend the "First Day of School," an annual event organized under the umbrella of the coalition. Members of the business community go to each school and talk about the important partnership among parents, schools, and the business community. They also talk about ways parents can assist their children to succeed in school.

Another sub-committee within the coalition organizes "Red Ribbon Week," an annual event that creates awareness to reduce the amount of alcohol and drugs consumed in this area.

In November of 1993, the Lewiston City Council adopted a resolution identifying the Lewis-Clark Coalition for At-Risk Youth as the organization to assist them and area law enforcement agencies to reduce criminal gang activity within the city via a community action team (CAT).

The Business/Education Alliance committee of the Lewiston Chamber of Commerce also evolved out of the town summit meeting, and that group has continued to meet regularly for the past nine years. Prior to the evolution of this committee, the Chamber of Commerce education committee was nearly defunct. Changing the name to Business/Education Alliance and attracting new leadership for this group has provided valuable communication among the schools and the business community.

LEARNINGS FROM THIS PARTNERSHIP

One of the biggest obstacles is to maintain and expand a shared vision and leadership. There is a continued rotation of new members in the coalition. We need a concise outline of who we are and a list of our accomplishments, otherwise membership interest drops.

Understandably, with the many community entities represented in the coalition, maintaining communication and keeping members informed of the goals and activities of all stake holders in the community and area is ongoing. The commitment as a community-building coalition helps to reduce token membership that uses the coalition for personal gain rather than community gain.

By identifying issues affecting families and youth, the coalition has helped reduce duplication of services. However, annual retreats are necessary to identify community needs and efficient methods of addressing them. This is a sensitive issue because of the competitive nature for funding which sometimes may not include all organizations.

WHY WAS THIS A SUCCESSFUL PARTNERSHIP?

We have found that by working together (collaborating—pooling resources, energy, ideas, and personnel) we can make a significantly greater difference than any single group or individual organization working independently. This partnership is successful because a core group of individuals are deeply committed to making it successful. These individuals are willing to meet, identify needs, share vision, and work together on a regular basis. Activities originally drove the program, and will continue to do so in the future. However, mission, goals, and needs of the community must be continually addressed by way of a strategic plan. Sharing leadership and experiencing the impact of wide visibility of activated programs has excited others to become involved.

15 FACILITATING PEACEABLE SCHOOLS

Deborah B. Gentry
Illinois State University

NATURE OF PARTNERSHIP

The peer mediation program described here was implemented in an elementary school in Normal, Illinois. Programs similar to it had previously been carried out in several other elementary schools in the same community. These efforts were a result of the collaborative thinking of community leaders. They realized the town's recent growth and progress was accompanied by stressful living and conflict among its increasingly diverse population. Educators were noticing that interpersonal conflicts, whether they originated during school hours or were prompted by difficulties at home or in the neighborhood, interrupted instruction and distracted students from engaging in sustained learning. A group of school administrators, educators, and parents determined a peer mediation program would be one of several strategies that could be carried out in an effort to teach the town's younger citizens to manage their conflict in positive and constructive ways. University faculty with alternative dispute resolution knowledge and skills agreed to consult with a given elementary school principal; train six elementary school teachers and selected 4th, 5th, and 6th graders in conflict resolution approaches; and assess parents' perspectives regarding student/child conflict management approaches. With continued mentoring on part of the university faculty, the initially trained teachers and students would subsequently train other teachers and students in their own and other schools in the district. In return, the principal and school district would approve the university faculty members' research related to program outcomes.

PURPOSES AND GOALS

First and foremost, the primary goal of this partnership was to bring about an improved classroom/school climate. It was hoped teachers would be able to spend more time providing instruction as a result of fewer disruptions for purposes of attending to student conflicts. Students would, in turn, benefit from this, resulting in increased learning. Another goal was to have students benefit from new knowledge and skills related to conflict resolution. It was hoped they would use such knowledge not only at school but also at home, thus improving their relationships with peers and family members, particularly siblings. A third goal was to determine just how salient this transfer of conflict knowledge and skill from the school setting to the home setting was. It was hoped the research study focusing upon such transfer would yield results worthy of dissemination to a wider audience. A final goal was to strengthen the community-university relationship that already existed.

ANALYSIS OF THE PROCESS

Though peer mediation programming which began at the high school level and eventually "trickled down" to primary grades had been shown to be successful in other locales, it was decided that creating a cadre of competent elementary-age student mediators who could help expand the program as they progressed through the school system was a worthy approach in this community. Implementation involved three phases: school sensitization, training, and practice.

PROCEDURES

Phase 1: School Sensitization

The author and a colleague, both faculty associated with Illinois State University (ISU), provided a two-hour seminar describing the theory and application of conflict management education in school settings for all of the teachers and administrators of the selected elementary school. All of the teachers, with special attention given to the fourth-, fifth-, and sixth-grade teachers, were asked to incorporate a series of conflict-awareness exercises into their language arts, social studies, science, and fine arts curricula over a four-week period of time. The ISU facilitators were available to assist the teachers in carrying out some of these exercises, many of which were taken or adapted from those designed for the Conflict Manager Program by the Community Board Program.[1] Members of the school's parent-teacher organization were informed of the proposed peer-mediation program and their support was solicited.

Phase 2: Mediator Selection and Training

After the conflict-awareness exercises were completed, the principles and procedures of the proposed peer-mediation program were explained to all of the fourth-, fifth-, and sixth-grade students in the school in a classroom-by-classroom fashion. This explanation included videotaped demonstrations of a "conflict manager" program in action. During classroom discussions that followed, the children were asked to identify qualities that would be beneficial in a competent mediator. The children said a "good" peer mediator would be honest and responsible, yet not shy or reserved. Next, the students were invited to nominate classmates to be schoolyard mediators for their school based on these criteria. Teachers made the final selections from those nominated, remaining cognizant of gender balance and racial representation. The teachers also considered the interest level of the student nominees as well as the degree to which they might already be committed to leadership roles within the school. After parental permission to participate was secured, the process of training the selected student "conflict managers" was begun.

All 27 of the selected students participated in a six-hour training, divided into three two-hour long sessions, that was both informative and experiential in nature. The content focused on these concepts: Cooperation, elements of positive communication, affirmation, and problem solving strategies. Skills included specifying the groundrules of the mediation process for disputants (agreeing to solve the problem, not to interrupt each other, to tell the truth, and to avoid name-calling and insults), helping disputants to identify the problem, probing for underlying tensions, and framing a durable solution. Some instruction was provided through large-group lecture/discussion and demonstration. Many learning activities and practice exercises called for the children to work in pairs or small groups of four. On these occasions, the two university faculty trainers and other adult volunteers (willing teachers and parents) shared the supervision of these activities. For greater detail about some of the instructional activities used, the reader should contact the author or consult a publication distributed by Family Information Services (Gentry, 1992).[2]

Phase 3: Mediator Practice

The final phase consisted of providing the trained students, on a rotating basis, with plenty of opportunities to perfect and utilize their new found abilities. When disputes between peers arose during recesses or lunch breaks, an assigned pair of mediators, typically a boy and a girl from different grade levels, would seek to assist the disputants in managing their conflict. Adult playground or lunchroom supervisors as well as teachers understood that they were not to intervene unless the conflict was a highly volatile one, the disputants could not find a satisfactory solution, or one or more of the parties requested adult involvement. The mediators were told to stop the mediation process if the disputants consistently broke procedural rules or if the conflict escalated to physical fighting. Each mediator was given the opportunity to serve as a mediator at least once every two weeks. The student "conflict managers" met with a faculty advisor on a regular basis to discuss any difficulties they experienced and to reinforce their previous training. The university faculty facilitators provided continued consultation. Other publications by Gentry and Benenson (1992; 1993) provide more detailed explanation about how the student mediators refined their skills.

ACHIEVEMENTS RELATED TO GOALS

When this peer mediation program was designed and implemented, evidence of the positive impact of similar programs had been reasonably well documented in the literature. While reconfirmation of such findings was desired, the university faculty facilitators of this endeavor primarily set out to determine the degree to and manner in which the elementary peer mediators involved in the program transferred the conflict management information and skills learned and practiced at school to the home setting for use in resolving conflicts with and between siblings. Each peer mediator and at least one of his or her parents were asked to participate in a structured interview just prior to and then again ten weeks after the training. This interview consisted of approximately 15 questions. Data collected during the interviews pertained to: 1) demographic information; 2) perceptions of the frequency, intensity, and duration of sibling conflicts; 3) the necessity and kind of parent intervention; and 4) the level of positive conflict management skills demonstrated by the children. Findings indicated that children perceived a significant decline in the frequency and intensity of conflicts with siblings. Parents perceived a similar decline in the frequency of such conflicts and in their need to intervene. Parents additionally perceived a significant improvement in their child's use of productive talk during conflicts. For further details about this study's results, consult Gentry and Benenson (1992; 1993).

This project would be suitable for replication or expansion, as its pretest-posttest, structured interview design is relatively uncomplicated. The educational activities used to train the student mediators could be adapted or substituted with others depending upon the cultural or age-related composition of the student body. Evaluative efforts have been undertaken for similar programs in other locations (Lam, 1989; Carter, 1995). Perhaps features of several previously implemented projects could be innovatively combined to create new applications. Developing parent education programs aimed at helping parents to understand how they can best facilitate their children's abilities to constructively manage their anger and impulsivity would be a logical next step as well (Colorado School Mediation Project, 1997).

ABILITY TO SUSTAIN EFFORTS

When this project was undertaken, few monetary resources were available to support it. Written materials to augment the classroom teachers' abilities to infuse peacemaking concepts into their regular curricula were purchased by the school. Written materials prepared by the university faculty trainers for use during mediation training were duplicated by the school's secretarial staff. The school provided cafeteria facilities as the location for the training as well as the special t-shirts worn by the peer mediators, identifying them as such, while they were on duty. Due to institutional valuing of faculty research pursuits as well as community service efforts, the time and expertise provided by the university faculty facilitators to this project were sponsored by their university.

This partnership has resulted in the formation of new partnerships. Other schools in this same district have asked for assistance in starting peer mediation programs, as have several community organizations. For example, the Boys and Girls Club has instituted a conflict resolution component into its after-school program for youth. The university has developed a peer mediation program for its own clientele. Once trained, college-age peer mediators have gained practice by volunteering their services at a local high school. Further, a community organization (called the Conflict Resolution Team) with diverse representation, including those from the public schools and university, has been formed and is planning a two-day event to focus community attention on alternative dispute resolutions programs and services.

Since this project was undertaken, the issue of youth violence has received increased attention. Local businesses may find a conflict manager program worthy of funding. Local and state government along with local and state social service agencies may be able to provide some financial and other kinds of assistance. It is recommended that persons interested in securing substantial funding to support peer mediation programming of their own design conduct a computer search for private foundation or federal government sources of funding with such interests. For example, the author has used the Illinois Researcher Information Service (IRIS). A recent IRIS search related to youth violence indicated Brach Foundation, Warner-Lambert Company, American Express, Metropolitan Life Foundation, and Mead Corporation Foundation as possible sources of private funds. As to federal government sources of funding, the IRIS search pointed to the National Institute of Mental Health within the Department of Health and Human Services, National Institute of Justice within the Department of Justice, and the Department of Education as possibilities.

LEARNINGS FROM THIS PARTNERSHIP

Not surprisingly, this partnership taught those involved that conflict among humans is inevitable, even when the focus of people's efforts is constructive conflict resolution. To varying degrees, as this project was carried out, conflicts about resources (printed materials, funding, time, space, etc.), goals, and methods arose. However, these conflicts were satisfactorily worked out leading to the best learned lesson of all: Community-university partnerships can be rewarding and beneficial to both entities.

WHY THIS PARTNERSHIP WAS SUCCESSFUL

This partnership was successful for two reasons. First, the mutual respect and commitment that was maintained by all the parties involved in the effort. Public school partners were enthusiastic about what they could learn from and share with the university partners. The reverse was also true. Second, tapping into the growing collection of resource materials on peer mediation programming helped to ensure success as well. Among the most valuable of resources were those accessed through an organization entitled "Conflict Resolution Education Network" (CREnet). In existence since 1984, CREnet (formerly called the National Association for Mediation Education or NAME) has promoted and continues to promote the development, implementation, and evaluation of school and university-based conflict resolution programs and curricula. Currently located in Washington, D. C., this organization has grown from a small, informal network of people interested in teaching students peacemaking skills to a primary national and international clearinghouse for information and resources, provider of technical assistance for program development, and source of training in the field of conflict resolution. Because conflict is an inevitable aspect of human interaction at all levels, available resources meet the needs of a variety of ages of students: Preschool, elementary, secondary, and post-secondary/college. A growing number of curricular resources which CREnet makes available for purchase attend to the needs of Hispanic, Chicano, and/or Latino audiences and are frequently printed in Spanish.

The organization sponsors a annual conference and sends its members a monthly newsletter filled with interesting articles entitled "The Fourth R." Among other noteworthy publications printed and distributed by CREnet is an annotated bibliography prepared by Bodine and Crawford (1998) which addresses rationales for conflict resolution programs in schools, various ways to design a program, and recommendations for implementing and evaluating a program. Also of value is a review and synthesis of evaluations of conflict resolution programs across the United States compiled by Jenkins and Smith (1996) and Blakeway and Kmitta (1998). Mastellone (1993) provides a theoretical and philosophical framework for persons interested in peacemaking. Practical information about setting-up peer mediation programs can be found in a publication by Community Boards (1992) and Cohen (1995). CREnet also recently published a resource guide for selecting professional trainers (Staff, 1996). This guide also provides a checklist of qualities to look for when selecting a trainer and an overview of the three most common conflict resolution models implemented in schools today.[3]

ENDNOTES

1. 1540 Market Street, Suite 490, San Francisco, California 94102; telephone: 415-552-1250; fax: 415-626-0595.
2. Family Information Services can be contacted at 12565 Jefferson Street NE, Suite 102, Minneapolis, Minnesota 55434-2102, telephone: 800-852-8112, and fax: 612-755-7355.
3. These and other resources can be obtained at reasonable cost by contacting CREnet at 1726 M Street NW, Suite 500, Washington, DC 20036-4502, telephone: 202-466-4764, Fax: 202-466-4769, web site: http://www.crenet.org.

REFERENCES

Blakeway, M. S., & Kmitta, D. M. (1998). *Conflict resolution in education research and evaluation synopsis and bibliography.* Washington, DC: National Institute for Dispute Resolution.

Bodine, R., & Crawford, D. (1998). *Handbook of conflict resolution education.* San Francisco, CA: Jossey-Bass.

Carter, S. L. (1995). *School mediation evaluation report: Project evaluation report 1993-1994.* Albuquerque, NM: New Mexico Center for Dispute Resolution.

Cohen, R. (1995). *Students resolving conflict: Peer mediation in schools.* Glenview, IL: Good Year Books.

Colorado School Mediation Project. (1997). *Handouts for parents.* Boulder, CO: Colorado School Mediation Project.

Community Boards. (1992). *Starting a Conflict Manager Program.* San Francisco, CA: Community Boards.

Gentry, D. (1992, May). Conflict management training for school and for home. In J. K. Comeau (Ed.), *Family information services professional materials* (pp. 29-42). Minneapolis, MN: Family Information Services.

Gentry, D., & Benenson, A. (1992). School-age peer mediators transfer knowledge and skills to home setting. *Mediation Quarterly, 10(1),* 101-109.

Gentry, D., & Benenson, A. (1993). School-to-home transfer of conflict management skills among school-age children. *Families in Society: The Journal of Contemporary Human Services, 74*(2), 67-73.

Jenkins, J., & Smith, M. (1995). *School mediation evaluation materials: Evaluation plan and instruments.* Albuquerque, NM: New Mexico Center for Dispute Resolution.

Lam, J. A. (1989). *The impact of conflict resolution programs on schools: A review and synthesis of the evidence* (2nd. ed.). Amherst, MA: National Association for Mediation Education.

Mastellone, F. R. (1993). *Finding peace through conflict: Teaching skills for resolving conflicts and building peace*. Amherst, MA: National Association for Mediation Education.

Staff. (1996). *Recommended standards for school-based peer mediation programs—1996.* Washington, D. C.: Conflict Resolution Education Network (CREnet).

16 CERTIFICATION BY LEARNING ON AN ALTERNATIVE SCHEDULE (CLAS)

Loretta P. Prater
Eastern Illinois University

NATURE OF PARTNERSHIP

It is becoming increasingly evident that academic institutions are challenged to meet the needs of contemporary populations and communities. The profile of the unmarried, 18-year-old, unemployed, full-time residential college student does not fit the profile of undergraduate students today. The CLAS program is a partnership initiative developed to broaden recruitment strategies and enhance opportunities for persons who might, otherwise, experience difficulty in completing requirements of an undergraduate degree in Child and Family Studies, especially in early childhood teacher certification. According to Love and Greer (1996), nontraditional programs can aid in supplying our nation's schools with well-trained educators who want to work with children and who could not acquire certification by traditional means. It was this kind of thinking that prompted the emergence of the CLAS program, an example of a partnership involving a university, a community college, and other community agencies.

PURPOSES AND GOALS

The five primary purposes and goals of CLAS are as follows:

1) Increase the number of certified teachers in Early Childhood Education and persons specifically prepared to work in community agencies serving families and children.
2) Remove barriers to enrolling in college by offering classes on an alternative schedule.
3) Provide quality higher educational opportunities to a diverse and changing population of non-traditional students.
4) Demonstrate proactive efforts to build and strengthen partnerships between the university and other community agencies/institutions.
5) Increase the number of students participating in a 2+2 articulation agreement with a community college.

ANALYSIS OF THE PROCESS

CLAS was designed at the University of Tennessee at Chattanooga by the author. The creation of CLAS allowed non-traditional students to complete a bachelor's degree in Child and Family Studies. One unique feature of CLAS is that students could enroll full-time while continuing current employment. The Child and Family Studies Program, within the Department of Human Ecology, offers two degree concentrations, Early Childhood Teacher Certification, and Child and Family Services. Most CLAS participants seek early childhood teacher certification.

The CLAS program was initiated in the Fall of 1995. The first challenge in the process was the selection of participants. Criteria for selection included fulfillment of all requirements for admission to the university, submission of a completed CLAS application, submission of a transcript to document at least 60 hours of transferable college credit with a minimum 2.5 GPA, and documentation of circumstances to qualify as a non-traditional student. After a vigorous summer recruitment effort, 19 students, ranging in ages 25-65 were enrolled. Participants represented diverse groups, including 17 females and 2 males, and 13 white students and 6 African-Americans. Among the cohort group were 6 persons with a bachelor's degree and 10 with an associate's degree (Prater, 1996).

Although there has been some concern regarding alternative teacher education programs expressed by some groups, the CLAS program was designed to embrace established curriculum. According to Dial and Stevens (1993), the Association of Teacher Educators has all but denounced alternative certification, proposing 22 minimum standards that should be followed by states using alternative routes. CLAS students follow the same curriculum as other students progressing through the Pre K-3 program. The major difference is that the classes are offered at a time convenient for these students. CLAS is the answer for students who have been employed for years at the associate's degree level, but felt that their jobs prohibited their returning to school.

A major strength of the CLAS program is that required classes are offered on Saturdays within two 8-week sessions of extended class times. This format allows one to complete 12 semester hours within a calendar semester by attending classes only on Saturdays. Other selected required classes are offered during two evenings on a rotational basis. The format described above operated during the fall and spring semesters, with a modified Saturday structure for summer school.

ACHIEVEMENTS RELATED TO GOALS

The University of Tennessee at Chattanooga and Chattanooga State Community College have a 2+2 articulation agreement in Early Childhood Education. This arrangement has been strengthened. Although many community college students become employed immediately after receiving their associate's degree, CLAS enrollment allows them to continue working toward the bachelor's degree. Therefore, there are fewer instances in which the associate's degree becomes the terminal degree. Thus, the number of certified teachers in Early Childhood Education increases, as opposed to the number of paraprofessionals working in child care centers increasing. Some participants select the non-certification major option of Child and Family Services, which prepares them to work in various community agencies serving children and families. Another worthwhile achievement is that these graduates are not only prepared to work with families in the community, but are better prepared for their existing roles as parents, spouses and other family members.

Many of the CLAS participants are employed with the Head Start program. Through a Head Start grant initiative, each of their participating employees received a grant to cover the tuition cost for 6 hours each semester. In addition, administrators of Head Start allowed employees to use accumulated leave days to be away from the facility to complete student teaching requirements. Some of the students depend on this financial assistance to continue their education. This support from Head Start is significant in removing a financial barrier to some participants completing the program. In addition, while studying for the bachelor's degree, Head Start employees are gaining valuable knowledge and skills which can be applied in their Head Start classrooms.

There was also a significant partnership achieved with the local public school system. In the instance of one CLAS student, who had a bachelor's degree but was working on Early Childhood Certification, employment was offered in an early childhood position through a waiver agreement while completing certification. The university allowed her year in that position to serve as a supervised internship to meet student teaching requirements. She completed all requirements to become a licensed teacher. In another instance, a teacher assistant participated in the program. Her school principal allowed her to work a semester of flex-time in order to take a course unique to her situation. She has completed her requirements and is now a full-time teacher in an elementary school setting. In both instances, these teachers are working in urban school settings. This is an important fact to note. Because of the maturity of CLAS participants, a wealth of life experiences were brought into the classroom. This is a critical factor, considering the demographics of urban schools. Interestingly, older students tend to favor working in urban settings and are more likely to remain at those schools, in comparison to younger students completing teacher education programs (Haberman, 1994).

Internal barriers within the university were removed for CLAS participants. Partnerships between university departments have been created and nurtured. Some of the required classes offered in the alternative format are available through other departments because of the needs of CLAS students. For example, there are classes which were never offered in the evening or on Saturday, which are now available during those alternative times.

PROSPECTS FOR LONG-TERM SUSTAINABILITY

The goals of CLAS have been met. CLAS has been successful, beginning with the first year of initiation. Since the beginning of CLAS, four Saturday classes have been offered each semester during the academic year. During the first year of CLAS, these classes produced 147 and 285 credit hours, respectively. These numbers certainly suggest the prospects for long-term sustainability. Through collaboration with the College of Arts and Sciences, selected required evening classes have been offered. In some instances, classes now have the maximum allowable enrollment, which is proof that there was a need for this option. CLAS has now been institutionalized and other departments are viewing the structure as a way to meet some of their needs, especially those areas in which community college graduates are immediately employed without considering transferring to a four year institution.

Because program enrollment requires at least 60 hours of completed college credit, it does not take students 4 years to complete CLAS. Therefore, CLAS has alumni who have already completed the program and are now teaching in early childhood education settings. These alumni are also helping to sustain the program through informal recruiting. They are telling others about their experience and the process through which they received their bachelor's degrees. One such supportive former student was the very first CLAS graduate, a 40-year-old wife and mother who had received an associate's degree in early childhood 15 years before enrolling in the program. She had been working in Head Start while trying to "figure out" how she could complete her schooling. Because of the manner in which CLAS is packaged, she was finally able to get the classes she needed to graduate with her bachelor's degree in Early Childhood Education.

For years the term life long learning seemed to hold little meaning. Today, it is definitely a reality. Another prospect for long-term sustainability is that CLAS is focused on the older student. Although classified as non-traditional, the presence of a growing number of mature students on college campuses is redefining the concept of the traditional student. CLAS is uniquely positioned to serve this growing population of older students desiring to complete their education, but who are fiscally responsible for supporting families. For this population, CLAS and comparable prototypes, are solutions.

LEARNINGS FROM THIS PARTNERSHIP

A significant accomplishment of CLAS is that it represents an excellent example of creating synergy among previously competing entities. The program illustrates the advantages of letting go of "turfs" in order to serve those in need. Establishing networks to utilize the resources of other groups results in a successful venture in which all benefit. CLAS is an example of identifying a need, using parts of various resources, and creating a visible product to enrich lives. CLAS and the successful results are possible because of this partnership. As the creator of CLAS, I liken the process to one of putting together a puzzle in which none of the pieces seem very useful until the whole is completed. It is only then that one is able to look at the beauty of the whole picture and feel a sense of accomplishment.

WHY WAS THIS A SUCCESSFUL PARTNERSHIP?

The success of this partnership is not a mystery. The goals were embraced by all involved. The students, the university and community college and their internal partners, Head Start, the public school system, and family members of participants all had a vested interest in the success of CLAS. The nature of the benefits varied, but all benefited. The success hinged on the cooperation of all entities working in concert for a common cause.

REFERENCES

Dial, M., & Stevens, C. J. (1993). The context of alternative teacher certification. *Education and Urban Society*, *26*(1), 4-17.

Haberman, M. (1994, Winter). Preparing teachers for the real world of urban schools. In R. A. Edelfelt (Ed.), *Educational Forum*, *58*(2), 162-168.

Love, F. E., & Greer, R. G. (1996). Recruiting minorities into teaching. *Education Digest*, *61*(6), 52-55.

Prater, L. P. (1996, July). *Higher ground, each one reach one, and CLAS*. Paper presented at the American Association of Family and Consumer Sciences Annual Conference, Nashville, TN.

17 IMPROVING CHILD CARE SYSTEMS IN ILLINOIS AND GEORGIA: PARTNERSHIPS BETWEEN THE LAND-GRANT UNIVERSITIES AND STATE AGENCIES

Jo Cato
Deborah Wilkes
Georgia Department of Human Resources

Susan Maxwell
Georgia Child Care Council

J. Lee Kreader
Anne Wharff
Illinois Department of Human Services

Christine M. Todd
The University of Georgia

This chapter outlines a journey—a journey involving one faculty member, five state agency professionals, and many local collaborators on a quest to help working families care for their children; a journey that has spanned 14 years, two states, and affected the lives of children, parents, and child care professionals in 261 counties; a journey that has changed the culture of state agencies, two land-grant universities, and local communities; a journey that is not yet over.

As the lone faculty member, I (CMT) provide the only link between the two state child care collaborations outlined in this article. As a result, I have been elected narrator for the two groups. I accept this role reluctantly; to be singled out from the group is an unusual role for me. I have learned over the past years that collaborations persist, in part, because individuals are willing to put aside their personal identities to promote the accomplishments of the group. But without a single narrator, this story would be uninterpretable. So, I reluctantly have agreed to serve as the "voice" for the two collaborations. However, all partners listed in this chapter serve as authors.

NATURE OF THE PARTNERSHIP, GOALS, AND OUTCOMES

In the 1980s, America was in crisis. Mothers were flooding into the work place to sustain their families' incomes in response to economic downturns and the shift from a manufacturing society to a service economy and the information age. At the same time, our child care delivery system barely existed. Care was hard to find, often of low quality, and, for many families, inaccessible because of high cost or lack of transportation. Training for child care professionals was sporadic, of varied quality, and for some subgroups of child care professionals—such as family child care providers and school age care providers—virtually non-existent in most communities.

In response to this situation state departments of human resources, land-grant universities, and non-profit organizations in many states began work to improve the availability, accessibility, and quality of child care in local communities. This chapter outlines my involvement in two university-community collaborations to improve state child care systems: 1) a 12-year collaboration between the University of Illinois and Illinois child care organizations; and 2) following my move to Georgia in 1996, my integration into a pre-existing collaboration between the University of Georgia and Georgia child care agencies.

The overall goal to be achieved in both the Illinois and Georgia collaborations was to develop an infrastructure that would improve the quality of child care available to families and increase the ability of those families to locate, recognize, and access high quality care. Although the university-community collaborations in each state developed totally independently of each other, there were some similar outcomes. For example, the collaborations in both Georgia and Illinois resulted in the creation of state-wide child care resource and referral (CCR&R) systems, integrated state-wide training systems for child care providers, and the development of school-age care professional organizations in each state. There were also unique outcomes as the collaborations in each state addressed state-specific issues. The collaboration in Georgia, a state which only recently developed a monitoring system for regulated family child care providers, focused some of its energy on the creation of a family child care inspection system and training supports for home providers. In Illinois, the need to integrate separate child welfare and child care systems facilitated the creation of a technological infrastructure linking the CCR&Rs, state agencies, and the University via the Internet as well as collaborative efforts to analyze state-wide child care supply and demand data for use by local communities and policy makers in decision-making.

The nature of the collaboration in each state is best described as a collection of individuals who, by virtue of the compatible missions of their institutions and their common passions in life, have found each other and have chosen to work together and share their respective resources to achieve a common goal: Accessible, affordable, quality child care. As has been found in the research literature on collaborations (Bergstrom, Clark, Hogue, Perkins, & Slinski, 1995), compatible missions and common goals are the cornerstone on which successful partnerships are built. At an institutional level, common missions and goals give members "permission" to be part of the collaborative and provide the rewards for their efforts. But personal commitment is essential as well. All collaborations have their ups and downs. It is the "fire in the belly," as Debbie Wilkes describes it, that keeps each person committed when the going gets tough. Therefore, both shared institutional missions and individual commitments have been cornerstones of both the Illinois and Georgia child care partnerships.

It is also important to recognize that even though we have billed each state's effort as a university-community partnership, in fact, the university has been only one of many partners in the collaboration in each state. This is not to say that the university was unimportant. At various points in time, what the university had to offer was unique. At that time, the university came forward and provided leadership for that project or activity. This is a second characteristic of sustained, successful university-community partnerships—members are willing to lead when needed but are comfortable in a supportive role at other times.

What is needed for successful university-community outreach collaborations is fundamentally different from how success is defined in the research arena (McCall, Groark, Strauss, & Johnson, 1998). For researchers, first authorships, continued and ever increasing grants, and constant leadership roles in professional societies are required to be viewed as a successful faculty member. This mode does not work in many outreach collaborations, however, because faculty members are unable to control real life the way they can their research agendas. In the real world conditions change. Your area of expertise may not be needed at the moment. To push for its inclusion would mean one of two things: Either the progress toward goals will be sidetracked because what you have to offer is not the best way to address the issue at that time; or, as a faculty member you will be stretched beyond your area of expertise. In the research world, this would be akin to asking an outstanding researcher in the area of personality development to suddenly provide leadership in a major research initiative in neuroscience.

Like a good member of a football team, the university must always be there on the bench, but only come onto the field when what the university has to offer is what is needed to win that particular play. In some years, the university started a lot. In others, the university mostly warmed the bench. This approach represents a new form of leadership that is emerging, one that focuses on leadership as a group-level function rather than a trait of a single individual (Sandmann & Vandenberg, 1995). To be good collaborators, university faculty must recognize when it is time to play and when it is time to sit on the bench.

ANALYSIS OF THE PROCESS

Several researchers have suggested that collaborations represent the interplay between systems (Lerner & Simon, 1998; Todd, Ebata, and Hughes, 1998). Characteristics of the individuals, the agencies and institutions involved, and society will all affect the nature of the collaboration. Analysis of how the Georgia and Illinois child care collaborations developed support this view. In this section we describe the formation of the two state collaborations and illustrate how these influences affected the development of the partnerships.

Finding Collaborators. My advent into the Illinois child care collaboration came because, as a new Extension faculty member, I was required to provide training to child care providers. To help me better understand the child care system, the director of our child development lab school put me in touch with the local child care licensing office and I soon became integrated into that network. As chance would have it, one of the licensing representatives was promoted to the state office that was responsible for overseeing the federal Dependent Care grants. Because of working with me at the local level, she knew about the resources of the University and asked us to take on a small project—the development of a videotape and newsletter for school-aged child care providers. The visibility of this initial project opened doors for the University with many child care groups. We had demonstrated that the University had something useful to offer—a very necessary condition for being invited into a collaboration.

My integration into the Georgia child care system was equally serendipitous. Three weeks after arriving in Georgia, a faculty member asked if I would like to accompany him to a child care conference in south Georgia. One of the people I met that day was an Extension agent who ran the local child care resource and referral. I shared with her my interest in resource and referral and we discussed some of the common challenges faced by R&Rs in Georgia and Illinois. When I left the conference the agent made several phone calls to let others in the child care network know about this new person who had come to Georgia. By the time I returned to the office, I had a message waiting on my desk from Susan Maxwell, one of the co-authors of this chapter, who further facilitated my integration into the Georgia child care collaborative.

Two observations can be derived from these examples. First, collaborations typically form through personal connections. The second lesson is that having credibility at the local level is critical to being invited into a collaboration. Too often, universities want to lead without demonstrating first that they understand the issues and have something to offer. It is critical that faculty spend time "in the trenches" with local communities to gain insights, form networks, and build credibility. Faculty who do this will have little problem gaining entry into successful partnerships.

Societal influences. The development of the Illinois and Georgia child care collaboratives also illustrate how societal forces can affect both the direction and outcomes of the collaboration. It is not coincidence, for example, that both Illinois and Georgia developed state-wide resource and referral systems, integrated training systems for providers, and professional associations for school-age providers. The federal Dependent Care and Child Care and Development Block Grant funds provided to states during the 1980s and 1990s were specifically designed to promote the development of these child care structures. Much of the early success of both the Illinois and Georgia collaborations can be attributed to the availability of federal funding to promote the work of the collaborations. Currently, welfare reform, the explosion of child care related research, and the increasing focus on accountability are affecting both collaborations. These recent societal influences have furthered collaboration between the University of Georgia and the child care collaborative. For example, the Office of Regulatory Services and the University of Georgia are planning a research study to identify the characteristics and training needs of "informal" caregivers—often relatives and friends—who care for children in families moving from welfare to work. This information will be used to develop training materials for use with this audience and will also add to the research literature in this area.

Institutional and Community Climate. Like societal influences, the resources and cultures of the University and the state child care agencies in Georgia and Illinois have influenced the collaboration. Successful collaborations occur when each partner has resources that are needed by the collaboration. For example, the university-based Cooperative Extension Service in both Illinois and Georgia could rapidly get information and training down to the local level because the county Extension offices were linked electronically. The University also could provide access to distance education technology for training child care professionals and had expertise in data management, analysis and evaluation. In contrast, state agency professionals were experts in understanding the child care profession in its many forms and settings. State agencies provided sites for university students to expand their classroom learning through internships and service learning projects. The state agencies also were a source of funding for many projects and were in a position to develop policies and procedures that would facilitate the work of other partners. By learning about each other's resources we were able to easily determine which partner was in the best position to provide what was needed at the moment. This reduced competition and also allowed each organization to specialize in what they did best.

University and agency cultures can also create impediments to be overcome. For example, early in the development of the Illinois collaboration a university administrator wanted to eliminate the university-based resource and referral agency because it was simply a service unit. Fortunately this did not occur. Future administrators did, however, insist that the resource and referral agency tie into all three missions of the university—teaching, research, and service. In retrospect, this was one of the key actions that led to the sustainability of both the university resource and referral and the larger child care collaboration. Getting students and other faculty involved in the child care initiative moved the collaboration from the status of a stand-alone outreach project to that of an integral part of the university.

Another constant struggle facing the collaborations in both Georgia and Illinois was the incompatibility between the university and state agency fiscal procedures. Anne Wharff and I spent many hours helping each of our respective fiscal offices understand the accounting system of the "other side." As the partnerships evolved, we were able to help the fiscal units of our respective organizations find ways to work together more efficiently. This same process is now occurring in Georgia.

One component of the culture at the University of Georgia that places a stress on the collaboration is the indirect cost rate for outreach grants. As McCall et al. (1998) have mentioned, state agencies and non-profit organizations have a very difficult time accepting the concept of indirect costs. It would be far better for the collaboration if the university allowed costs for space, phone, accounting and administration to be carried as direct rather than indirect costs. Our collaborators accept these types of expenses as legitimate. They simply have a difficult time seeing how these translate into a standard percent of each contract.

Clearly, universities and agencies each have cultures that can facilitate or impede university-community collaborations. Both Georgia and Illinois represent diverse states with a major city, several smaller cities, and large rural areas. Early in the Illinois collaboration this presented an impediment. There was continual competition between urban and rural areas for scarce resources. Moreover, the vast distances separating urban and rural professionals made it difficult for each group to learn more about the needs of the "other."

Within the Illinois state child care agencies there was a strong commitment to help all children and families—no matter where they lived. As a result of this climate, substantial time and resources were directed at encouraging a collaborative, rather than a competitive climate between urban and rural communities. This was done by paying for representatives from the diverse areas to come together for planning meetings and giving careful attention to where and when the meetings were held. The University of Illinois also made available at cost its teleconferencing system which would allow up to 50 people to participate at one time on a conference call. The state agencies further promoted a collaborative climate by insuring that state and federal dollars were distributed equitably between urban and rural areas. Although it took many years to develop trust and understanding between urban and rural groups, this approach has been highly successful. Instead of competing, child care organizations from throughout the state now pull together to address common needs.

The role of the individual. Like societal and organizational influences, the way individuals act within partnerships affects the collaboration. One characteristic of individuals evident in both Georgia and Illinois was and is a commitment to work collaboratively. This commitment expressed itself in many ways. Trust emerged from our successes—that is when members fulfilled their commitments to the partnership and the outcomes moved us closer to our collective goal. Trust also emerged when we insured that all partners shared in the credit for successes (and, occasionally, responsibility for our failures). When turf issues or problems arose within the collaboration, various members would attempt to mediate the situation. As trust developed between members of the group it became easier and easier not to "take offense" at some statement or action of another partner.

In summary, the characteristics of individuals, the culture of institutions and communities, societal influences, and serendipity all affect collaborations. Understanding each others' culture and learning to put the goals of the collaboration ahead of your own goals and those of your organization are essential to developing effective partnerships.

INDICATORS OF SUCCESS

In identifying the indicators of success for the Illinois and Georgia university-community collaborations many dimensions could be considered. From the perspective of the university, the opportunity to work collaboratively with state agencies has greatly enriched our research and teaching programs. Students have gained valuable research and evaluation skills as they worked on projects such as determining impediments to using child care supply and demand data at the local level, creating a procedure for geomapping supply and demand data to better identify the child care needs of low income families, and identifying whether various types of child care providers have different training needs. The close working relationships that have developed among collaborators in each state have also been rewarding. But we count as our greatest achievement the improvements in the child care delivery system that have come about in Georgia and Illinois due, at least in part, to our university-community partnerships. When we began this journey a decade and a half ago there was no coordinated training system for child care providers in Georgia or Illinois. Families could not contact a resource and referral to find a care arrangement because CCR&Rs did not exist. There was no systematic way to identify where additional child care was needed or to foster its creation. There were few child care subsidies for low income families. Last year 50,000 Illinois and Georgia parents were able to contact a resource and referral to locate care, 35,000 new child care slots were added, 45,800 child care providers received training through a coordinated system, and 120,900 low-income children received child care subsidies. We have a long way to go to achieve the dream of accessible, affordable, quality child care for all children. But we have come a long way. The journey continues.

REFERENCES

Bergstrom, A., Clark, R., Hogue, T., Perkins, D., & Slinski, M. (1995). *Collaboration framework: Addressing community capacity*. Columbus, OH: USDA Cooperative State Research, Education, and Extension National Network for Collaboration.

Lerner, R. M., & Simon, L. A. K. (1998). Directions for the American Outreach University in the twenty-first century. In R. M. Lerner & L. A. K. Simon (Eds.), *University-community collaborations for the twenty-first century: Outreach scholarship for youth and families* (pp. 463-482). New York: Garland Publishing.

McCall, R. B., Groark, C. J., Strauss, M.S., & Johnson, C. N. (1998). Challenges of university-community outreach to traditional research universities. In R. M. Lerner & L.A.K. Simon (Eds.), *University-community collaborations for the twenty-first century: Outreach scholarship for youth and families* (pp. 203-230). New York: Garland Publishing.

Todd, C. M., Ebata, A. T., & Hughes, R. H. (1998). Making university and community partnerships work. In R. M. Lerner & L.A.K. Simon (Eds.), *University-community collaborations for the twenty-first century: Outreach scholarship for youth and families* (pp. 231-254). New York: Garland Publishing.

Sandmann, L. R., & Vandenberg, L. (1995). A framework for 21st century leadership. *Journal of Extension, 6*. Available from www.joe-ed@joe.org.

18 PROJECT FAMILY: A PARTNERSHIP INTEGRATING RESEARCH WITH THE PRACTICE OF PROMOTING FAMILY AND YOUTH COMPETENCIES

Richard Spoth
Virginia Molgaard
Iowa State University

INTRODUCTION

Project Family involves a community-university partnership directed toward "action-oriented research" (e.g., Small, 1995). As such, it aims to achieve two goals: To generate knowledge that will advance the science of family-focused competency building and to enhance the well-being of participating families and children. The project's ultimate purpose is to strengthen the competencies of general population families and children on a broad scale—to ensure that a larger number of children develop into healthy and adaptive adults in the project's targeted general populations.

PARTNERSHIP AND PROJECT BACKGROUND

Lerner and Simon (1998) suggest that America may be wasting its most precious resource, the human capital represented by its youth. They report epidemiologic data indicating historically unprecedented problems confronted by contemporary families and youth, including the high prevalence of risk behaviors among youth, many of whom are growing up in poverty. Project Family aims to address the problem of the prevalence of high-risk behaviors among youth through collaborative approaches to problem-focused scholarship and action-oriented research. In the Project Family case, this entails a collaborative, stepwise progression through the problem-oriented phases and tasks of preventive intervention research articulated by the Institute of Medicine (Mrazek & Haggerty, 1994). These tasks include problem definition and needs assessments, intervention design, intervention outcome study, and dissemination of empirically-supported interventions.

The Project Family partnership began with collaboration between the authors of this chapter, a preventive intervention researcher, and a state Extension Specialist at a land-grant university.[1] The collaboration between the prevention researcher and this specialist initiated a three-way partnership among university-based prevention researchers, university-affiliated Extension personnel at the state and county-levels, and local community-level participants.

The first author joined the university as part of an effort to develop an applied research center (subsequently titled the Social and Behavioral Research Center for Rural Health).[2] In an initial meeting with the second author, her description of the Extension Service suggested its potential for contributing to the development of the center. This conversation also inspired an early joint effort in the form of a prevention-oriented workshop conducted as part of a larger Extension program. Subsequently, the first author and research colleagues secured funding from the National Institute on Drug Abuse to conduct a research project including preventive intervention outcome studies. Collaboration on the Extension workshop, the dialogue on the applied research center development, and the receipt of an intervention research grant set the stage for a series of meetings of the authors with other Extension personnel.

The object of the meetings on the intervention research project funded by the National Institute on Drug Abuse (NIDA) was to explore a number of specific activities for collaboration. These included, for example, planned contacts with Extension personnel working in the communities where the project was to be implemented. As part of this process, the authors solicited input from the Extension personnel on intervention implementation tasks (e.g., recruiting schools for the project, finding local people who could be hired as group leaders).

Initial Extension involvements were very productive and, consequently, the authors and their colleagues decided to propose another large-scale longitudinal intervention outcome study, employing a similar approach to collaboration among prevention researchers, state and county-level Extension personnel, and community participants. The introduction to the proposal cited the potential for the Extension System in project implementation and, ultimately, large-scale dissemination. It was funded by the National Institute of Mental Health (NIMH) and provided further opportunities for refining the collaborative process. Continued success of the collaboration provided impetus to write other proposals designed to extend the work of the collaboration (see section on project contributions).

It is important to note key characteristics of the Project Family partnership associated with its maturation in the context of multiple, grant-funded preventive intervention research studies. As a result of this developmental process, the structure and function of the partnership has varied to some degree across Project studies and activities. In some activities, such as needs assessment surveys, Extension personnel were involved, although partners outside of the Extension system (e.g., from other state agencies and universities) played the major role. In other activities, state- and county-level Extension personnel assisted primarily with local setting implementation activities. There are yet other project tasks (e.g., dissemination) in which Extension personnel took the lead and researchers had relatively less involvement. This chapter focuses primarily on Project Family partnership activities in which Extension personnel at the state and community level collaborated extensively with university researchers in order to facilitate linkages between university researchers and local community residents.

RATIONALE FOR THE FOCUS ON COMPETENCY BUILDING

A commonly accepted definition of competence is a pattern of effective adaptation in the environment (Masten et al., 1995, Masten & Coatsworth, 1998). For children, competence is indicated by success with major developmental tasks (e.g., attachment to caregivers, self-control, school adjustment) and with specific domains of achievement (e.g., academics). For parents and guardians, competence involves the ability to set appropriate standards, monitor and effectively discipline youth, and provide nurturance and support. Project Family interventions are designed to teach skills and behaviors that enhance competencies, along with the reduction of risk factors originating in the family (e.g., a pattern of coercive parent-child interactions).

The Project Family partnership focus on family and youth competency training was suggested by an emerging literature on child resiliency (see review by Grover, 1998; also, Kumpfer, Molgaard, & Spoth, 1996) as well as on the adaptive functioning of families in the development of child problem behaviors. Masten and Coatsworth (1998), for example, describe child relationships with competent, caring adults as a "powerful adaptive system" that protects child development in both favorable and unfavorable environments.

There are a number of strategies for strengthening family and youth competencies and adaptive functioning in general populations. One of them is the widespread dissemination of empirically-supported family competency-building programs through community-university collaborations. Although there appears to be widespread application of family-focused interventions, currently disseminated interventions are rarely proven or evaluated, particularly through randomized controlled studies, especially as implemented in special populations (Kumpfer, 1992; Spoth, 1997; Spoth, Redmond, & Lepper, in press).

In order for dissemination to be truly effective, two things should happen. First, dissemination should be preceded by programmatic outcome research and, second, effective partnerships involving program developers, researchers, and local communities should be organized. Under optimal circumstances, initial development of partnerships can occur through programmatic outcome research. In this way, research can be carefully integrated with practice across the major tasks of the preventive intervention research process (Mrazek & Haggerty, 1994). In Project Family, the integration of research with practice has been greatly facilitated through its three-way partnership of project researchers, Cooperative Extension personnel affiliated with a land-grant university, and communities participating in the project. Following an overview of Project Family goals and objectives addressing each of the major tasks of preventive intervention research, the partnership contributions will be described in more detail.

PROJECT FAMILY PARTNERSHIP GOALS AND OBJECTIVES

The primary goal of Project Family is to study the efficacy of universal family and youth competency training interventions, through randomized, controlled investigations. The findings of these studies are used not only to determine whether tested interventions are effective, but also to examine models of interrelationships of variables that determine how the intervention affects targeted outcomes, in order to guide intervention refinement (Spoth et al., 1998; Spoth, Redmond, Hockaday, & Yoo, 1996; Spoth, Redmond, & Shin, 1998). For example, one model has examined the extent to which a family-focused intervention directly influenced young adolescent tendency to use alcohol and the extent to which its effect on young adolescents was an indirect result of positive influences on parenting (Redmond, Spoth, & Shin, 1998). These models are central to the integration of intervention research with practice (e.g., Mrazek & Haggerty, 1994). The other goals of Project Family include: (a) intervention needs assessments, using probability sample surveys of risk and protective factors in state populations targeted for prevention programming; (b) consumer research investigating factors that influence family and youth participation in intervention and intervention research activities, in order to develop improved methods for engaging youth and families; and (c) the development of effective strategies for the dissemination of empirically-supported family and youth-focused preventive interventions through the assistance of the national Extension Service.

PARTNERSHIP OUTCOMES IN PRACTICE AND RESEARCH ARENAS

The Project Family Partnership has been successful in securing funding from several National Institutes of Health (NIH) institutes and other federal agencies[3]—for work directed toward the refinement and enhancement of family and youth competency-building in general populations. In addition to successfully securing competitive grant dollars, several key contributions of the Project can be identified in both the practice and research arenas.

Contributions to Competency-Building Programming and Practices

Positive Intervention Outcomes

As noted previously, Project Family is an action-oriented research project and, as such, its purpose is not only to generate knowledge through research, but also to directly enhance the well-being of participating youth and parents. An example of the direct contribution to families, one of the tested interventions, the Iowa Strengthening Families Program, has shown positive results for both parents and youth with a sample of 422 families. Intervention and control group comparisons showed significantly improved parenting behaviors directly targeted by the intervention (e.g., clarification of substance use rules and consequences, increased level of positive parent-child involvements) which, in turn, were strongly associated with general child management (e.g., general standard setting, monitoring, effective discipline) and parent-child affective quality (e.g., expressions of positive affect) (Redmond, Spoth, Shin, & Lepper, 1998; Spoth, Redmond, & Shin, 1998). Outcome data for youth show significant intervention-control differences in gateway substance use, conduct problems (physical aggression, minor theft, property damage), school-related problem behaviors (e.g. truancy, cheating), peer resistance, and affiliation with antisocial peers at the one- and two-year follow-ups. As an example, of the two-year follow-up there was a 56% relative reduction in first-time use of alcohol without parental permission in the intervention group

(Spoth, Redmond, & Lepper, in press). Importantly, there was evidence of an increasing divergence of outcomes for the intervention and control groups through the second year follow-up.

The published results of this research have bolstered dissemination efforts by the second author and other Cooperative Extension personnel. As an example, published findings have generated interest in program implementation and group leader trainings. In Iowa the Extension Service has trained over 600 group leaders and the program has been offered in 91 communities. It is also being implemented in 26 states; in four of these cases, proposals have been submitted to seek funding for intervention outcome evaluation projects.

Family Engagement Strategies

Project Family investigations employing consumer research methods have helped to clarify the factors that influence families to engage in competency-building interventions and in related research activities. Although studies have been conducted with relatively homogeneous general populations of rural families, they have shown important variations in family engagement factors, such as attitudes, beliefs, and preferences concerning interventions (e.g., Spoth & Redmond, 1993; Spoth & Molgaard, 1993; Spoth & Redmond, 1994). At the same time, a small number of stable family characteristics (e.g., education) are often related to participation decisions (e.g., Spoth, Goldberg, & Redmond, in press).

Family engagement findings have guided the development of practical strategies for recruitment and retention for program services. Project reports have described recruitment strategies and other implications of findings for addressing variations in parent beliefs and preferences (Spoth, Ball, Klose, & Redmond, 1996) and for accommodating families' educational background (Spoth, Redmond, Kahn, & Shin, 1997). As another example, project studies have suggested that a primary consideration in recruitment strategies is the practical constraints imposed by time and scheduling realties among parents. Using a combination of consumer study data, information on local community events (e.g., ball games, church night), and individual family preferences, optimal scheduling plans have been derived. Overall, project research has underscored the need to devote substantial project time and resources toward efforts to gain family attendance in and cooperation with project activities.

Needs Assessments

Community needs assessments are commonly employed by the Extension System to guide program efforts. In addition, Project Family has conducted needs assessment studies at the regional and state level, in cooperation with state universities, state agencies, and state regional planning committees that include regional stakeholders (representatives from various sectors of several communities in the region) and Extension System representatives (see Spoth, Ramisetty-Mikler, & Goldberg, 1995a, 1995b). Regional stakeholders have provided input on the development of survey instruments used to collect data on empirically-based risks and protective factors indicating a need for specific types of prevention services. For example, a recent household survey showed that among the domains of risk and protective factors (community, family, and individual), those originating in the family were the most predictive of substance onset and other conduct problems among children (Lutz et al., 1998). These findings will help guide resource allocation and program planning in various regions of the state.

Dissemination Strategies

As previously noted, family- and school-based universal competency building interventions are widely disseminated, but they are only rarely evaluated (Spoth, 1997; Spoth, Redmond, & Lepper, in press). When interventions with no evaluation data or theory-base are implemented, chances are great that time, energy and money will be spent with little to show for the effort. At the same time, programs proven to be effective are more likely to address well-documented needs for competency-building and the reduction of risk behaviors among youth and their families in general populations. Perhaps the most noteworthy contributions of the Extension-assisted Project Family partnership with Iowa communities are the strategies and procedures it is developing for the dissemination of empirically-supported interventions to improve competencies of family and youth in general populations. Because the partnership has involved collaboration with personnel from within the system that will ultimately disseminate the interventions on a broad scale—through needs assessment, participant engagement and outcome study phases—intervention implementation procedures are already tailor-fit to the dissemination system. This has set the stage for a large-scale, multi-site dissemination project currently in the planning phase.

Family and Youth Program Policy

Because of the practice and research-related achievements of the Project Family partnership, the authors have been in a position to provide policy input to various federal and state agencies. Funding agencies are increasingly recognizing the need for accountability in program delivery. In addition, they are increasingly encouraging groups who receive funding for local programs take the time and effort to evaluate program outcomes. In the past, many funding agencies were satisfied with "head counts" of participating individuals, but now there appears to be movement towards making program funding contingent on the local group's use of programs proven to be effective.

One example is the set of guidelines (Principles of Effectiveness) issued to recipients of funding from the Safe and Drug Free Schools Program. The first author is on an expert panel whose charge is to develop criteria to guide identification of programs consistent with the principles of effectiveness.

Contributions to Practice-Oriented Competency-Building Research

Because of its orientation toward action research, the Project Family partnership has attempted to contribute to the advancement of competency-building intervention outcome evaluation research. Although Extension personnel have played less direct roles in this arena, those roles have been critically important to what has been accomplished. For example, the successful Extension-assisted implementation of the controlled Project Family outcome studies was necessary to contributions that have been reported in the scientific literature and presented at numerous conferences. This literature includes, for instance, previously mentioned reports directed toward clarification of how interventions achieve their effects and with what population segments they are most effective. Such work is intended to guide the refinement and application of competency training interventions.

The refinement of the methodology for family-focused preventive intervention evaluation is, ultimately, of great benefit to the implementation of the interventions themselves (see Mrazek & Haggerty, 1994; Russell, Kahn, Spoth, & Altmaier, 1998; Spoth, in press). In addition, there are a number of methodological problems to be solved and deficits to be addressed that are important to the practical goal of the advancement of research-based family and youth competency-building interventions. These include the need for randomized controlled evaluation designs with adequate sample sizes; long-term follow-up assessments of outcomes; evaluations of intervention fidelity; and adequate attention to missing data and participant attrition, among a number of others (see Russell et al., 1997; Redmond, Spoth, Shin, & Lepper, 1998; Spoth, in press; Spoth, Redmond, & Shin, 1998; Spoth, Yoo, Kosterman, & Shin, 1997; Spoth, Reyes, Redmond, & Shin, in press).

In part, based on the project's attention to these methodological issues, as well as its success in building partnerships in program research and practice, one of the recently-funded Project Family studies, the Capable Families and Youth (CaFaY) Project, has received a prestigious MERIT Award from the National Institute on Drug Abuse. Also, the project has been selected one of ten research-based projects recognized in the National Institute on Drug Abuse publication on preventing drug use among children and adolescents (National Institute on Drug Abuse, 1997).

PROSPECTS FOR LONG-TERM SUSTAINABILITY

An important reason for creating community-university partnerships is to ensure that, following acceptable demonstration of intervention effectiveness, an effective mechanism for dissemination within communities is available. Extension's presence in nearly every county in each of the 50 states provides a network of youth- and family-serving professionals who are committed to providing interventions designed to build competencies and reduce risks, in order to encourage healthy development among young people. Extension prides itself on being one of the few "research-based" organizations within communities, with the charge of applying the latest research from land-grant universities. Further, Extension has highly trained professionals housed at land-grant universities, typically with Ph.Ds, who are in a position to promote the research-practice linkage.

Thus, Extension's widespread local presence, its mission, and its staff expertise make it an ideal organization for promoting long-term sustainability of proven interventions. In the Project Family case, early and continued involvement of Extension System personnel has resulted in intervention implementation that is sensitive to the local community context. The history of collaboration has set the stage for longer-term promotion of family and youth competency-building programs. As previously noted, a large-scale multi-site dissemination research project is currently in the planning stage.

CHALLENGES AND LEARNINGS FROM THIS PARTNERSHIP

There are a number of challenges in creating meaningful and long-term working partnerships between university researchers and the extension service, along with the communities served by Extension. Over its history, Extension's most important characteristic is its presence and ongoing relationship within the local community. As mentioned above, Extension is involved in local needs assessments and is active in responding in a timely fashion to expressed needs. The Extension commitment to "early responding" creates problems in working with a research project which moves through the multiple phases of the Institute of Medicine's preventive intervention research model (Mrazek & Haggerty, 1994), typically over a period of years. Also, a partnership with a research project involves a significant allocation of time and energy from Extension specialists—resources that are, consequently, not available to meet immediate needs for consultation and development of new teaching materials for use within the state's Extension System. Several people within the system must make major adjustments to Extension's normal way of doing things. First and foremost, state Extension administrators must see the value of the extension-research partnership and make modifications in expectations for the specialist's involvement in Extension's ongoing programming. Next, the specialist must relinquish large areas of responsibilities in order to devote the needed time and energy to the partnership and the work involved therein. At the same time, field staff within Extension must accept a change in the specialist's responsibilities and be willing to accept a new definition of her or his role.

A second set of challenges concerns differing vocabularies and intervention evaluation concepts among Extension personnel and researchers. In reference to the project described in this chapter, federal funding agencies in the National Institutes of Health (NIH) use phrases such as "mental health problems," "prevention of substance abuse," and "epidemiological trends"—phrases that are not often used by Extension personnel. Even though much of Extension's work with youth and families involves problems, issues, and concerns suggested by those phrases, Extension staff are not likely to be accustomed to such phraseology. In a recent study of Extension's work in the area of prevention of mental health problems, it was discovered that university-level Extension specialists did not report doing work in this arena, even though they were currently dealing with prevention of depression and suicide, stress management, preventive parenting practices and lowering risks of adolescent substance abuse (Molgaard, 1997). Another example of differing usages of phases and concepts is highlighted by considering the term "research-based." Extension personnel are proud to say that their interventions are research-based but that may not mean that the interventions have been scientifically studied and found to be effective. Rather, in the Extension context, the term "research-based" refers to an intervention design informed by research on risk and protective factors. This difference in meanings imputed to the phrase "research-based" reflects significant variations in researcher and Extension personnel concepts and models of intervention evaluation. Both sides in the partnership need to learn and appreciate each other's meanings and intent.

Despite these and other challenges, the partnership described here has created opportunities for the both the partners and the organizations or projects they represent. The research project itself has benefited immensely from the assistance of both the specialists involved and the contributions of Extension field staff who have provided local contacts, information and support. Communities participating in the research have responded positively, in large part because of its support by local extension personnel. At the same time, Extension has benefited in many ways. The specialist primarily involved in the partnership has had the opportunity to concentrate her efforts on the adaptation and testing of a major curriculum. Because of positive research findings, the curriculum has received national recognition and widespread application. Extension as a whole has benefited by direct connections to the research community, in-service trainings by research staff, the opportunity to be trained in and use a nationally recognized curriculum, and the knowledge of their support in contributing directly to a much-needed field of research on reducing adolescent problems and developing more competent youth and caregivers.

CONCLUDING COMMENTS: WHY THIS PARTNERSHIP HAS WORKED

There are several important reasons why the partnership among university researchers, Extension Service personnel, and local community residents has been successful. First and foremost is the commitment of the researchers and Extension personnel to be open-minded about their respective differences in approaches to the challenging tasks at hand. In this connection, the first author has had an enduring commitment to the value of working through the Extension Service, as a local partner in assisting with the evaluation and dissemination of prevention programs. In addition, the specialist who was the primary Extension partner was willing to manage the competing demands of Extension and the research project.

Second, the necessary administrative support has been provided. The state Extension specialist's administrator has seen the value of the partnership and given the needed support to make the research project a significant part of Extension's mission in the state. This person encouraged staff throughout the state to become involved as needed. In addition, the director of the center housing Project Family research has been supportive of the partnership. Third, Extension field staff have demonstrated willingness to provide significant assistance in several phases of the project, including: consultation on project design, help in recruitment of research families, and service as local liaisons between community and university. Finally, the respect local community residents have for Extension field staff has been instrumental in their motivation to cooperate with Project efforts.

It is fitting to conclude with a statement synthesizing key points made in the chapter. The most important factor in the success of the Project Family partnership has been the partners' common cause of family and youth competency building, pursued with an open-minded, problem-oriented approach, and with respectful responsiveness to differences of partner opinions about problems and solutions.

ENDNOTES

1. The official title of the Extension service is the Cooperative State Research, Extension and Education Service (CSREES) but throughout the paper it is referred to as the Extension Service. The state specialist involved in the partnership described in this chapter is a Family Life Specialist and serves both Youth and Families staff. The role of a state Extension specialist involves taking findings from relevant research and disseminating them to the public within the state. In that role, the state specialist reviews and interprets research literature, writes articles for local newspapers and newsletters, trains staff and, in general, serves as a consultant for field staff across the state.
2. Seed funding for center development was provided by Iowa Methodist Medical Center, Des Moines, Iowa.
3. Project Family studies are currently funded by the National Institute on Drug Abuse, the National Institute of Mental Health, the National Institute of Alcoholism and Alcohol Abuse, and the Center for Substance Abuse Prevention. Past funding has included support from the Center for Substance Treatment.

REFERENCES

Grover, P. L. (Ed.). (1998). *Preventing substance abuse among children and adolescents: Family-centered approaches* (Reference Guide) (2nd in the Prevention Enhancement Protocols System [PEPS] Series, Center for Substance Abuse Prevention). Washington, DC: U.S. Government Printing Office.

Kumpfer, K. (1992). *Strengthening America's families: Promising parenting and family strategies for delinquency prevention.* Washington, DC: U.S. Department of Justice, Office of Juvenile and Delinquency Prevention.

Kumpfer, K. L., Molgaard, V., & Spoth, R. (1996). The Strengthening Families Program for the prevention of delinquency and drug use. In R. D. Peters & R. J. McMahon (Eds.), *Preventing childhood disorders, substance abuse, and delinquency* (pp. 241-267). Thousand Oaks, CA: Sage.

Lerner, R. M., & Simon, L. A. K. (1998). The new American outreach university: Challenges and options. In R. M. Lerner & L. A. K. Simon (Eds.), *University-community collaborations for the twenty-first century* (pp. 3-24). New York: Garland.

Lutz, G. M., Spoth, R., Crew, B. K., Neppl, T., Fahrney, K., Ramisetty-Mikler, S., & Roth, K. (1998). *Iowa Substance Abuse Prevention Needs Assessment: Public Survey Findings.* Research Monograph Report to the Center for Substance Abuse Prevention for the Iowa Department of Public Health. Cedar Falls, IA: University of Northern Iowa, Center for Social and Behavioral Research.

Masten, A. S., Coatsworth, J. D., Neemann, J., Gest, S. D., Tellegen, A., & Garmezy, N. (1995). The structure and coherence of competence from childhood through adolescence. *Child Development, 66*, 1635-1659.

Masten, A. S., & Coatsworth, J. D. (1998). The development of competence in favorable and unfavorable environments: Lessons from research on successful children. *American Psychologist, 53*(2), 205-220.

Molgaard, V. (1997). The Cooperative Extension Service as a key mechanism for research and services delivery for prevention of mental health disorders in rural areas. *American Journal of Community Psychology, 25*, 515-544.

Mrazek, P., & Haggerty, R. (Eds.). (1994). *Reducing risks for mental disorders: Frontiers for preventive intervention research.* Washington, DC: National Academy Press.

National Institute on Drug Abuse. (1997, March). *Preventing drug use among children and adolescents: A researched-based guide* (NIH Publication No. 97-4212). Rockville, MD: Author.

Redmond, C., Spoth, R., & Shin, C. (1998, June). *Adolescent propensity to use alcohol: Long-term outcomes of a universal family-focused preventive intervention.* Symposium paper presented at the Society for Prevention Research Sixth Annual Meeting, Park City, UT.

Redmond, C., Spoth, R., Shin, C., & Lepper, H. (1998). *Modeling long-term parent outcomes of two universal family-focused preventive interventions: One year follow-up results.* Manuscript in review process.

Russell, D. W., Kahn, J., Spoth, R., & Altmaier, E. M. (1998). Analyzing data from experimental studies: A latent variable structural equation modeling approach. *Journal of Counseling Psychology, 45*(1), 18-29.

Small, S. A. (1995). Action-oriented research: Models and methods. *Journal of Marriage and the Family, 57*, 941-955.

Spoth, R. (1997). Challenges in defining and developing the field of rural mental disorder preventive intervention research. *American Journal of Community Psychology, 25*(4), 425-448.

Spoth, R. (in press). Family-focused preventive intervention research: A pragmatic perspective on issues and future directions. In R. Ashery (Ed.), *NIDA Research Monograph on drug abuse prevention through family interventions.* Rockville, MD: National Institute on Drug Abuse.

Spoth, R., Ball, A. B., Klose, A., & Redmond, C. (1996). Illustration of a market segmentation technique using family-focused prevention program preference data. *Health Education Research, 11*(2), 259-267.

Spoth, R., Goldberg, C., & Redmond, C. (in press). Engaging families in longitudinal preventive intervention research: Discrete-time survival analysis of socioeconomic and social-emotional risk influences. *Journal of Consulting and Clinical Psychology.*

Spoth, R., & Molgaard, V. (1993). Consumer-focused data collection in prevention program evaluation: Rationale and illustrations. *Evaluation and the Health Professions, 16*(3), 278-294.

Spoth, R., Ramisetty-Mikler, S., & Goldberg, C. J. (1995a). *Parent reported risk and protective factors for substance use among Iowa elementary and middle school children.* Research Monograph Report to the Center for Substance Abuse Prevention and the Center for Substance Abuse Treatment by the Iowa Department of Public Health. Ames, IA: Iowa State University, Social and Behavioral Research Center for Rural Health.

Spoth, R., Ramisetty-Mikler, S., & Goldberg, C. J. (1995b). *Teacher perceptions of risk and protective factors for substance use among Iowa K-8 school children.* Research Monograph Report to the Center for Substance Abuse Prevention and the Center for Substance Abuse Treatment by the Iowa Department of Public Health. Ames, IA: Iowa State University, Social and Behavioral Research Center for Rural Health.

Spoth, R., & Redmond, C. (1993). Identifying program preferences through conjoint analysis: Illustrative results from a parent sample. *American Journal of Health Promotion, 8(2)*, 124-133.

Spoth, R., & Redmond, C. (1994). Effective recruitment of parents into family-focused prevention research: A comparison of two strategies. *Psychology and Health: An International Journal, 9*, 353-370.

Spoth, R., Redmond, C., Hockaday, C., & Yoo, S. (1996). Protective factors and young adolescent tendency to abstain from alcohol use: A model using two waves of intervention study data. *American Journal of Community Psychology, 24*(6), 749-770.

Spoth, R., Redmond, C., Kahn, J., & Shin, C. (1997). A prospective validation study of inclination, belief, and context predictors of family-focused prevention involvement. *Family Process, 36*, 403-429.

Spoth, R., Redmond, C., & Lepper, H. (in press). Alcohol initiation outcomes of universal family-focused preventive interventions: One- and two-year follow-ups of a controlled study. *Journal of Studies on Alcohol* (invited article for special issue on alcohol and the family).

Spoth, R., Redmond, C., & Shin, C. (1998). Direct and indirect latent-variable parenting outcomes of two universal family-focused preventive interventions: Extending a public health-oriented research base. *Journal of Consulting and Clinical Psychology, 66*(2), 385-399.

Spoth, R., Redmond, C., Shin, C., Lepper, H., Haggerty, K., & Wall, M. (1998). Risk moderation of proximal parent and child outcomes of a universal family-focused preventive intervention: A test and replication. *American Journal of Orthopsychiatry, 68(4)*, 565-579 (invited article for special section on preventive intervention research).

Spoth, R., Reyes, M. L., & Redmond, C. (in press). Assessing a public health approach to delay onset and progression of adolescent substance use: Latent transition analyses of longitudinal family preventive intervention outcomes. *Journal of Consulting and Clinical Psychology.*

Spoth, R., Yoo, S., Kosterman, R., & Shin, C. (1997). Applying readily accessible graphical techniques to assess curvilinear relationships and detect outliers: The case of protective family processes. *Evaluation and the Health Professions, 20*(3), 353-364.

19 ESTABLISHMENT OF AN INTERDISCIPLINARY COLLABORATIVE DEGREE PROGRAM IN EARLY CHILDHOOD STUDIES

Shirley Hymon-Parker
University of Maryland Eastern Shore

NATURE OF THE PARTNERSHIP

In 1992 the Department of Human Ecology received a grant from the U.S. Department of Education-Title III program to develop an interdisciplinary degree program in Early Childhood Studies. The purpose of the grant was to bring together several disciplines at the University of Maryland Eastern Shore (UMES) for the development of an undergraduate degree program. *The Maryland Plan for Post-Secondary Education* (1992) challenged higher education institutions in the state to improve the quality of elementary and secondary education by educating effective teachers for the state's school systems. This program lays the foundation for quality education by training caretakers as well as educators who will work with children from birth through grade three. *The Maryland Plan* also addresses the regional needs of the Eastern Shore, noting that teachers in the area need more continuing education opportunities. There are no other degree programs on the Eastern Shore of Maryland that lead to initial early childhood certification (Maryland State Department of Education, 1996). This program will increase educational accessibility and attainment of all Maryland citizens by overcoming the disparities in educational opportunities and will allow for access and choice for residents of the Eastern Shore.

PURPOSE

In addition to establishing the degree program, the grant provided funding for the establishment of an Early Childhood Laboratory. The laboratory would offer early educational stimulation to children ages 3-5 of faculty, staff, and students at UMES, and to children from the local community. The laboratory would also provide school involvement activities for parents and grandparents through parenting workshops and transition counseling for new parents. The community would benefit from the lab because it is the only childcare program in the three county area

(Somerset, Wicomoco, Worcester) that has an educational component and will be linked to a baccalaureate degree. The primary focus of other child/day care centers located in the area is the provision of caregiving services. University-degree-seeking students will benefit as they apply knowledge learned in class to situations experienced in the lab school during the completion of practicums and internships.

Initially the program was to be developed and implemented by the departments of human ecology and education at UMES. The chairs of these departments were later notified by the chair of the Department of Education at Salisbury State University (SSU), located just fourteen miles north of UMES, that SSU, too, was interested in developing an Early Childhood degree program. New state guidelines established under the University System of Maryland Vision I and II Plans presented a strong mandate for collaboration between institutions for new programs. Furthermore, the mandate prohibited duplication of degree programs for the two campuses located on the Eastern Shore of Maryland (Action Plan for Reinvesting the System's Resources, 1994). It became clear at this point that collaboration between the Department of Education at SSU and the Departments of Education and Human Ecology at UMES was inevitable and salutary.

Implementation of the collaborative Early Childhood Studies program between SSU and UMES will enable the two institutions to meld their historical antecedents of teacher preparation into a cohesive program of teaching excellence. Both approved mission statements identify teaching as an institutional focus. Teacher preparation is a shared responsibility for both.

A 10-member committee was formed to develop the degree program. The committee comprised six faculty (two from each of the three departments), the three department chairs, and the director of UMES-SSU collaborative programs. SSU and UMES faculty were involved in conceptualizing and creating the Early Childhood Studies program from the beginning. Equal partnerships and ownership are in operation.

ACHIEVEMENTS

Four years after grant notification, our accomplishments have been significant and include:

1) Development of a memorandum of understanding that addresses issues pertaining to admission, tuition, registration, graduation, curriculum, class size, faculty assignment, internships, program implementation, and the establishment of a steering committee to monitor and evaluate the program.
2) Development of a teaching major in Early Childhood Education and a non-teaching major in Child Development.
3) Completion of the degree prospectus and proposal detailing the recommended four-year course sequence for each major including course descriptions. Both documents have been approved by the University System of Maryland and the proposal has been forwarded to the Maryland Higher Education Commission (MHEC) for state program approval.
4) Establishment of an Early Childhood Lab School housed at UMES and managed by the Department of Human Ecology. Twenty-four cheerful and enthusiastic little boys and girls are currently enrolled in the lab. The ethnic

mix of roughly 50/50 Black-White ratio makes for a very diverse, positive, and ecologically valid learning environment. The Department of Human Ecology received Title III funding to support two university faculty positions, and to furnish and equip the lab. Cooperative Extension Service facility funds were set aside to renovate an existing facility at UMES for the lab school.

LEARNINGS FROM THE PARTNERSHIP

Developing this program was not without its share of challenges as the two universities worked through sensitive but relevant issues. The core issues included: courses needed for the program; who would develop/teach new courses; need for new faculty lines and availability of funds to support additional faculty; where the new faculty would be housed (SSU/UMES); who would supervise new faculty; program cohort size; and supervision of interns. The appointment of a new chair in the Department of Education at SSU set the committee's progress back as the new chair became acquainted with the proposed program and learned to navigate through the various layers of institutional review necessary for the development of a new program. The appointment of a new university president and a new vice president for academic affairs at UMES slowed the development too. Again, the committee experienced delays due to these individuals' desire to be clear on all aspects of the proposed program and Systems requirements before forwarding the proposal to the next step.

During the four-year developmental period, we learned that nothing is as simple as first believed. We discovered that patience is a prerequisite to collaboration and that successful collaboration requires shared decision-making, wherein all parties assume mutual and equitable responsibility for planning and managing the program. Administrative support was also found to be crucial because administrators have the authority to reallocate and redistribute resources necessary to implement the program. In addition, administrators' support and involvement symbolically and operationally signal the importance of the collaborative effort as well as the need for others to cooperate and participate.

WHY THIS WAS A SUCCESSFUL PARTNERSHIP

This partnership has been successful for several reasons: the program meets a curricular need for the region; there are perceived educational benefits for all parties; the close proximity of both institutions tends to encourage open and regular communication; it eliminates program duplication; it enables the universities to share resources and facilities as appropriate; and the support of strong and competent leaders who are devoting energy and time to make the partnership work. The memorandum of understanding signed by the department chairs, deans, and provost/vice president of academic affairs expresses both universities' commitment to the partnership and their interest in having long-term sustainability for the program.

REFERENCES

Action Plan for Reinvesting the System's Resources. (1994). University of Maryland Eastern Shore/Salisbury State University (UMES/SSU). Princess Anne: Author.

Maryland Higher Education Commission. (1992). *The Maryland Plan for post-secondary education.* Annapolis: Author.

Maryland State Department of Education. (1996). *Maryland teacher staffing report 1996-98.* Baltimore: Author.

20 EXTENDING HEAD START TO HOMELESS FAMILIES: A UNIVERSITY-COMMUNITY PARTNERSHIP

Sally A. Koblinsky
Elaine A. Anderson
University of Maryland

> "...and I be dreamin' that I would get my mama a house... and she would have her own bed, and a curtain... and we would have a lot of food, food all the time and sometimes candy... and my sister and me, we be going to school every day, just like some other kids..." (Martin, age four)

Martin, his sister, and mother represent one of the increasing number of homeless families in the United States. Families with children are the fastest growing segment of the homeless population, accounting for 43% of the homeless in 1993 (U.S. Conference of Mayors, 1993). Most of these families are headed by single mothers (Kondratas, 1991). In addition to the "official homeless" in shelter or on the streets, thousands of poor families find temporary residence in overcrowded dwellings where they "double up" with relatives or friends.

The many stressors experienced by homeless families may adversely affect young children's health and development. Noisy, overcrowded shelters may contribute to higher rates of infectious illnesses and limit opportunities for children to develop new cognitive and social skills. Homelessness may also strain parent-child relationships, as parents expend all their physical and emotional resources to meet basic needs, leaving little time to nurture their children.

To examine the influence of homelessness on parenting and young children's development, the authors initiated a collaborative research partnership between the University of Maryland/College Park and the United Planning Organization Head Start Program in Washington, D.C. Funded by the Administration for Children, Youth and Families (ACYF) in 1991, this three-year study involved more than 300 Head Start families. The goal of the research partnership was to determine if there are differences in the developmental status of homeless and housed Head Start children, and to examine the relationship between family variables (e.g., social support, coping strategies) and child outcomes. Of particular interest was the relationship between family factors and changes in homeless children's skills and self-concept during the Head Start year.

On the basis of early research findings revealing potential benefits of Head Start exposure and the desire to serve the nation's neediest children, ACYF increased its commitment to homeless families. In 1993, the agency funded 16 three-year demonstration programs to increase homeless children's participation in Head Start. The authors then established a second university-community partnership with Baltimore City Head Start to increase the enrollment of homeless families in Baltimore's Head Start centers. The authors and other faculty in the Family Studies Department also conducted evaluations of the Baltimore City program as well as a second homeless demonstration program sponsored by the United Planning Organization, "Bright Beginnings," in Washington, D.C.

The collaboration between university faculty and community Head Start programs in research and program development resulted in a number of creative strategies to address the complex needs of homeless families. These strategies enabled the partnership to overcome serious barriers to serving homeless children and their parents. Major lessons learned from the partnership are summarized below.

GIVING A VOICE TO THE STAKEHOLDERS

One of the most important strategies in our partnerships has been the early inclusion of homeless families and Head Start representatives in project planning and decision-making. Preliminary meetings with these stakeholder groups enabled us to incorporate their voices and recommendations in the grant proposals. After the projects were funded, homeless families and Head Start personnel were active participants on advisory committees and smaller project work groups (e.g., parent outreach, classroom curriculum). Head Start parents and family service coordinators on the research advisory board assisted in recruiting homeless parents and selecting measures that were sensitive to the racial/cultural characteristics of the sample. Both the Baltimore City Head Start and Bright Beginnings demonstration programs hired homeless parents to serve in project staff positions. To further expand the input of homeless families, the authors conducted focus groups at shelters with homeless parents whose children were not attending preschool. Many of these parents went on to enroll their children in Head Start and to become beneficiaries of the project. These strategies gave Head Start personnel and homeless families a sense of project "ownership" and mobilized them to achieve project objectives.

UNDERSTANDING THE CULTURE OF THE TARGET POPULATION

Although homeless families are often treated as a homogenous group, they differ along many dimensions, including racial/cultural background, family structure, geographic location, and pathways to homelessness (e.g., job loss, domestic violence, substance abuse). The majority (90%) of homeless families involved in our projects were African American, headed by women, and residents of inner-city neighborhoods. Thus, it was important for all university students involved in our research project to develop knowledge of the cultural values, family strengths, language styles, needs, and coping strategies of lower income African American families. Training sessions, readings, and homeless shelter visits helped student researchers develop an understanding of the culture of the target population. Half of the students participating in data collection were African American, increasing parents' comfort with the research process. Insuring that all project staff demonstrated respect for cultural diversity enhanced the researchers' ability to establish rapport with parents and to obtain accurate information.

INVOLVING THE LARGER TARGET COMMUNITY

The authors discovered that many homeless families were in need of services that went beyond the mission and resources of the university-Head Start partnership. Therefore, the original partnership took steps to involve the larger community in the demonstration programs for homeless families. Linkages were established with many community agencies that provided services to homeless families, including federal entitlement programs, health agencies, social service programs, food and clothing banks, churches, public schools, and the business community. Volunteer service groups, such as the Junior League (the original sponsor of the "Bright Beginnings" program) were especially effective in marshaling educational, employment and legal resources for homeless families. Through representation on project advisory committees, community organizations learned about Head Start and an array of local services for homeless families, minimizing duplication of effort and enriching service delivery. By working with Head Start to establish resource and referral networks for homeless families, the researchers demonstrated their commitment to improving family well-being and earned the trust of collaborating community agencies.

EVALUATING OUTCOMES IN THE SPIRIT OF STRENGTHENING PROGRAMS

Partnerships initiating new programs need to compare the outcomes of their activities to their original program goals. One effective strategy of our university-community collaboration was to frequently evaluate project objectives, use a variety of process and outcome measures, and maintain a climate of openness and interest in improving program effectiveness. The authors helped both Head Start staff and families understand the importance of program evaluation and involved these constituents in defining indicators or benchmarks of program success. Parents participated in focus groups and interviews assessing program outcomes, receiving small incentives for their involvement. Both the project advisory committees and Head Start staff then used evaluation results to review and refine program operations, taking such actions as lengthening the Head Start day and hiring a homeless mother as a parent outreach coordinator. This process enabled constituents to think strategically about project goals, prioritize their objectives, celebrate program achievements, and mobilize community support for their programs. Thus, program evaluation helped to engage and empower homeless parents, as well as maintain project momentum.

DISSEMINATING INFORMATION TO KEY AGENCIES

Often the results of research/demonstration projects are not available until multi-year projects are completed. However, sharing the results of early data collection and early program evaluation may help to improve delivery of services to that target population before the conclusion of the grant period. The authors disseminated preliminary findings of their study to the National Head Start Bureau, and made presentations summarizing project findings at local, regional, and national Head Start conferences. As a result, many Head Start programs requested in-service training about the unique needs of homeless families and asked for clarification of Head Start policy on enrollment and attendance of homeless children. Programs also used initial feedback from homeless parents to develop parenting interventions and strategies for supporting homeless families. Early sharing of project data strengthened the university-community partnership and increased the quality of service to homeless families. By disseminating results at other professional meetings (e.g., National Association for the Education of Young Children, National Council on Family Relations), the authors also benefited from the insights of other researchers, early childhood educators, and service providers working with homeless families.

SUSTAINING PROGRAMS

Maintaining or institutionalizing innovative programs requires a major commitment of time, resources, and leadership. To insure the continuation of innovative projects, it is important that partnerships consciously develop strategies for continuing program services from the beginning. In our partnerships, members made ongoing efforts to build public and private support for the homeless family programs through reports to the National Head Start Bureau, community agencies, and homeless service providers. Celebrations of the opening of new Head Start centers serving homeless families included community officials, volunteer groups, local media, and homeless parents. Using data from evaluations of the demonstration programs, an attorney who served as president of the "Bright Beginnings" advisory board prepared legislation that would continue Head Start funding for all 16 homeless family demonstration projects. Introduced and passed by the U.S. Congress in 1996-1997 session, this Head Start Authorization Bill insures that there will be permanent resources for model Head Start programs serving homeless children and families.

CONCLUSION

The partnership between the University of Maryland Family Studies Department, the United Planning Organization, and Baltimore City Head Start has fostered applied research, program development and evaluation, and policy formation to serve the needs of homeless families. The success of this partnership appears largely due to: Establishing a sense of "ownership" of project goals and activities by key stakeholders (homeless families, Head Start personnel); building a trusting, respectful relationship among partners; establishing a working alliance with the larger community; and assessing and reporting project outcomes in a timely manner. As a result of these strategies, in six short years, we have seen applied research translated into creative programs and permanent policy that will improve the lives of homeless young children and their families.

REFERENCES

U.S. Conference of Mayors. (1993). *A status report on hunger and homelessness in America's cities: A 26-city survey*. Washington, DC: Author.

Kodratas, S. A. (1991). Ending homelessness: Policy challenges. *American Psychologist*, *46*, 1226-1231.

21 THE GOUCHER COLLEGE-CHOICE MIDDLE SCHOOLS PROGRAM PARTNERSHIP

Judy Jolley Mohraz
Carol Weinberg
Goucher College

Leigh Curtis Higgins
Choice Middle Schools Program

Commencement was still two weeks away as the president, dressed in full academic regalia, headed across the Goucher campus for another commencement ceremony. Processing to "Pomp and Circumstance," ten eighth graders were graduating from the Choice Middle Schools Program, and the college wanted to honor the moment. The ceremony, a mixture of formality and high jinx, marked the end of the students' participation in the Goucher component of their program—a program of tutoring, recreation, and mentoring for high risk adolescents from two middle schools in a low income area of Baltimore County. Every week during the academic year they had traveled to the idyllic suburban campus to work—and play—with Goucher student volunteers. Many of these adolescents had never ventured very far beyond their neighborhoods before entering the Choice Middle Schools Program. The college might as well have been on Mars. One of the goals, therefore, of the program had been to make a college campus as familiar and inviting to them as their local school yard.

"I expect several of you," the president told the graduates, "to return as entering freshmen at Goucher four years from now." As each student came forward to receive a certificate or card and a Goucher Alumni t-shirt from his or her tutor, applause and cheers erupted from the assembled group of Goucher volunteers and Choice Middle Schools and Goucher professional staff. Not by accident was this afternoon laced with the symbolism of a college graduation. The message was clear: Those at-risk students had stuck with an after-school program for three years and the college had faith in them and their futures. Another message underlay the event as well: Diverse constituencies could work together in an effective partnership.

NATURE, PURPOSE AND GOALS OF THE PARTNERSHIP

The Choice Middle Schools is a community-based intervention for middle school students at risk of school drop out. The Shriver Center at the University of Maryland Baltimore County provides administrative oversight to the program. Choice Middle Schools is funded by the Maryland State Department of Education and is part of the Maryland's Tomorrow Middle School Initiative. The goals of the program are as follows:

- To improve school attendance
- To decrease disciplinary referrals
- To decrease out of school suspensions
- To improve grade point average in core subjects

Although problems in these areas manifest themselves at school, they are often reflections of negative influences at home and/or in the community. To counteract these influences, Choice Middle Schools provides services for students and their families using casework teams consisting of highly energetic and committed bachelor's level individuals. Through individualized case management, these casework teams provide 24 hour a day, 7 days a week support to students and their families. These services include: Daily home visits to communicate student progress to parent(s); parental support and crisis intervention, and curfew monitoring; and advocacy and support services in areas such as mental and physical health. In an effort to increase communication and accountability regarding the child's educational progress, these activities are combined with a strong presence in the schools by casework teams. Daily attendance monitoring and follow up, intervening in disciplinary situations, and communicating with teachers and administrators about student academic and behavioral progress is the main focus of these casework teams during the school day.

The program is designed to boost these middle school students' academic skills while providing them with a wide range of experiences and activities to increase their engagement in school and the learning process. The tutorial program at Goucher College was designed with this goal in mind.

A major goal of this partnership, from Goucher's perspective, is to channel the college students' desire to work with young people into a program where their efforts could be put to best use. Goucher also wanted to expand students' awareness of, and involvement in, the lives of children from different backgrounds and circumstances—seeking to open up their worlds just as Choice Middle Schools looks to broaden their students' lives in a complementary direction. The college volunteers are able to develop their own tutoring and mentoring skills through this program and they also experience the gratification that comes with committing themselves to a semester-long relationship with a middle schooler.

ANALYSIS OF THE PROCESS

The Choice Middle Schools-Goucher partnership has developed over the course of the last four years. In the summer of 1994, Goucher's coordinator of community service, Carol Weinberg, first met with Leigh Higgins, the assistant director of the

Choice Middle Schools Program to discuss working together on a big brother/big sister type program. Goucher's previous effort to create such a program with a grassroots group in Baltimore City had not been successful, primarily because of limited staff in both groups to structure and supervise the program.

At this initial meeting, we discovered that while Goucher was looking for a structure to be a part of, Choice Middle Schools was seeking additional college tutoring centers for their program which had just begun. One of the Choice Middle Schools' satellites was located in a low-income area of Baltimore County about a half hour from Goucher. The collaboration began during fall semester, 1994 and the program has evolved each subsequent semester based on regular feedback from the Choice Middle Schools staff and students and from the Goucher volunteers and coordinator of community service.

The tutor was upset. She felt as though Gayle, one of the Choice Middle Schools caseworkers, had spoken with her student too harshly and publicly. The tutor, Mary, approached one of the Goucher team leaders, in tears, to talk about what had taken place. The team leader brought her to Goucher's coordinator of community service. Together they talked about the situation and then brought Randy, the Choice Middle Schools educational coordinator into the discussion. Randy set up an immediate impromptu meeting for all Goucher and Choice Middle Schools' staff involved.

This was an opportunity for the caseworker to hear the tutor's reactions and for the tutor to learn about the context of the caseworker's comments. The student's problematic behavior over the last few weeks at home, at school, and in the community had led to an agreement between Choice Middle Schools and the student's parents about what steps would be taken if the student continued to misbehave. Gayle, the caseworker, was acting on that agreement. The Goucher tutor and team leader began to understand that their experience with the students—for less than two hours a week—was only a small part of the on-going contact that the caseworkers had with them. They realized that in Gayle's actions they were seeing a later stage of an escalating process that could be misunderstood and perceived as unreasonable. Gayle became aware that the misunderstanding could have been avoided if there had been more communication with Mary, the tutor, about what had been going on with the student.

A corner was turned in the partnership that Monday afternoon in March. In part it was because each side gained a new awareness and respect for the role the other played in the process. On a larger level, it was because the discussion was carried on without defensiveness and because it became clear that the children were everyone's number one priority.

Sufficient staffing and clearly defined responsibilities contribute to the success of this partnership. These roles and responsibilities have become more effectively focused as a result of our early experiences working together. The list that follows notes specific responsibilities of each role in the Goucher tutoring component.

- Choice Middle Schools:
    - educational coordinator—oversees educational programs at several sites; helps train Goucher tutors
    - team manager—supervises caseworkers; comes regularly to sessions at Goucher; trains tutors

  - caseworkers—transport students to Goucher; serve as resource for tutors; reinforce school-home-Goucher connections
- Goucher:
  - coordinator of community service—oversees logistics and arrangements on campus; comes regularly to sessions; serves as resource for team leaders
  - team leaders (students)—recruit tutors and serve as resource for them; plan and run all activities
  - tutors—work with Choice Middle Schools students one-on-one for a full semester (each session involves one hour of tutoring and 1/2 hour of group activity)
  - chair of the education department—trains tutors

ACHIEVEMENTS RELATED TO GOALS

John began his involvement with Choice Middle Schools as a sixth grader. He was a new student to the area, was repeating the sixth grade, and was having a difficult time adjusting to his new surroundings. Over the next three years, during his involvement with the program, John became more comfortable in his surroundings and developed into a very good student. However, there was still something lacking—John had no interest in his own academic future. John was solely interested in playing basketball at the NBA level, completely overlooking a college education, and when asked if he wanted to attend college, he would often reply, "yes, only if I can play basketball for them."

As a seventh and eighth grader, John was enrolled in the tutorial program at Goucher College. In an atmosphere conducive to studying, and with the help of the one-on-one attention he received from his tutor, John was able to make up the missing assignments he couldn't complete at home. But besides being able to complete school assignments, the Goucher tutorial program allowed John the opportunity to speak with the tutors about the many different fields of study and reasons for coming to college. Today, John is still interested in going to college and playing basketball, but first and foremost, he is interested in going to college to study in the hopes of one day becoming an architect. Choice Middle Schools, in conjunction with the Goucher tutorial program, provided John with a valuable lesson: Life is more than just playing basketball, and a college education is the key to opening many doors in his life.

All of the students who participate in the Goucher tutorial program are at risk for school drop out. The factors that place them at risk are numerous, and the remedies to their situations are varied. That is why Choice Middle Schools seeks to explore all the possible avenues to reach a child until something "clicks." For some students, it is the Goucher tutorial program that "clicks." It may be the one-on-one attention they receive from caring adults that bolsters their self-esteem, it may be the exposure to the college setting that encourages students to achieve in school in the hopes of one day attending college, it may simply be the fun they have while at tutoring that motivates students to attend school on those days. Whatever it is, Goucher tutoring reaches some of these students in a very special way. Students with chronic attendance problems began attending school every day. Students with below average grades improved their GPA almost a full point during the semester of their Goucher tutoring.

The Choice Middle Schools Program at Goucher has grown in both numbers and strength since 1994. We began with sixteen tutor/student pairs and now have twenty-four pairs each week. Tutor applications have consistently increased each year. In any semester, approximately half of the tutors have tutored in the program before, and a number of Goucher students have participated throughout their entire four years of undergraduate study. Some of the students who tutor in Choice Middle Schools have gone on to work in similar programs elsewhere after they have graduated. The impact of the program on the volunteers can, perhaps, best be described in their own words:

> "I simply felt good about myself being able to help the kids and have a positive influence on them."
>
> "I found this to be an incredible experience, thoroughly rewarding and worth every minute of my time."
>
> "I was able to observe a lifestyle different from my own and in the process I was able to analyze myself."
>
> "This got me back into working with youth, helped me to realize how much I enjoy teaching, and helped me realize how special each individual is and how much middle schoolers can teach college students!"
>
> "This program made me feel really optimistic for the world because the kids were so great, and it made me feel like I could really make a difference."

WHY THE PARTNERSHIP HAS SUCCEEDED AND WHAT WE HAVE LEARNED

When we first met to plan the program, it was understood that the middle schoolers would have snacks each day as soon as they arrived at Goucher. The community service program at Goucher had a limited budget, and Carol met with the director of dining services who agreed that they could provide these snacks at a very reasonable cost. You get what you pay for! The straw that broke the camels back, so to speak, were the celery stalks filled with peanut butter. The Choice Middle Schools students provided feedback through the expected channels. They complained to the caseworkers in the cars going home, and their concerns made it back through the team manager to the assistant director of the program. Leigh called Carol at Goucher and Carol had to tell her that "with the budget we've got available to us, this is the best we can do." Leigh was quick to respond: "Our funding can cover it. For some of our kids this food after school is really important; they may not get much dinner at home." Carol spoke with Goucher's director of dining services again and discovered that what we needed were "mini-meals"—submarine sandwiches, fruit, and juice. With the Choice Middle Schools Program underwriting the cost of the mini-meals, we've been able to provide more substantive snacks for the kids ever since.

In the third year of the program, Goucher added a new activity to help expand the Choice Middle Schools students' exposure to college life. CAUSE, Goucher's student community service organization, offered to fund "dinner in the dining hall" one night each semester for all the Choice Middle School students. Tutors use their own meal tickets and we all crowd around several large tables in the Goucher dining hall. This has turned out to be a wonderful opportunity for the seventh and eighth graders to enjoy the "all you can eat" world of college dining, to meet their tutors' friends and classmates, and to see more of what college life is all about. The experience also gives the Goucher tutors an opportunity to see their own world through the eyes of their young friends.

The success of this partnership is a result of mutual commitment, complementary skills and strengths, and a willingness on all sides to be open to improvement and expansion. For example, although the Choice Middle Schools Program at Goucher started out as an effort within the volunteer community service program, during the last two years Goucher's education department and Choice Middle Schools have ventured into new levels of the partnership. Goucher has begun to use the tutoring program as a field work assignment for some students in several different classes. Choice Middle Schools staff have also been willing to share their expertise beyond the confines of the tutoring program. The Choice Middle Schools educational coordinator, for example, has taught a session on classroom management in Goucher's student teaching seminar.

In addition, as the education department explores the possibility of establishing professional development schools, departmental members have focused their attention on the area of the county that includes the two middle schools from which the Choice Middle Schools Program draws their students. This step could allow Goucher to become involved with the Choice Middle Schools students' educational environment in new ways.

There is a tremendous trust felt by both partners. We came together at the very start of the Choice Middle Schools Program and have, in essence, grown together. There has never been a feeling of one partner trying to fit into the other's already well-established program. We started small and grew as we got a handle on any problems. This was able to happen because we quickly communicated any concerns—from first year confusion about roles and responsibilities to early lacks of communication between tutors and caseworkers to student complaints about the kind of meat in the sandwiches served for snacks. We found that there was a sincere willingness on both parts to creatively solve any and all problems together.

The bottom line as to why this Choice Middle Schools-Goucher partnership works may sound simplistic, but it is nonetheless true—we like one another. We enjoy working together and we marvel at how much more we can accomplish together than separately. And both partners have never lost sight of who the program is designed to benefit—the students!

22 THE BENEFITS OF A PHILANTHROPIC-UNIVERSITY-SCHOOL COMMUNITY PARTNERSHIP: THE CAMBRIDGE "SAY YES TO EDUCATION" STORY

Tracey L. Hurd
Anne Larkin
Lesley College

Jose Ribeiro
Cambridge Public Schools and Lesley College

This chapter describes a philanthropic-university-school partnership, Cambridge "Say Yes to Education" (SYTE), that was established with a goal of supporting a group of students developing towards educational success. While the charter of the partnership was (and is) to support a group of disadvantaged students developing towards the attainment of a post-high school education, the collaboration, and the program, has become much more. It has been a conduit for positive, sustainable, systemic change.

In order to contextualize the story of the successful partnership, we first briefly chronologue the genesis of the collaboration as well as the nature and logistics of the unique partnership. Next, we discuss the explicit and implicit goals of the partnership. Third, we analyze the unique processes, manifestations, and benefits of the collaboration. Finally, we close by examining achievements, goals, and lessons learned about the nurturing of long term sustainable partnerships.

The data for this chapter are derived from a series of in-depth interviews with four of the "key players" of the partnership, two of whom were involved (the two elementary school administrators) and two of whom are involved (the SYTE Director and the SYTE Coordinator) directly with the children and families. During these interviews, the participants were asked to reflect on the genesis, evolution, strengths and weaknesses of the project. Interviews were tape-recorded and analyzed for common themes and disparities.

INTRODUCTION

In 1990, Lesley College was approached by two philanthropists, one of whom was an alumna of the college. They hoped to start a collaboration between their foundation (The Weiss Foundation), Lesley College, and an urban school community to support a group of students. They wanted to provide for those students ongoing support towards obtaining a college education, and the guarantee of full tuition funding by the Foundation. They asked Lesley College to find a class—a grade full of students—who lived in an urban setting, that faced many challenges that accompany living in a low socio-economic area. The Foundation placed their trust in the personnel of Lesley College to determine a public school and class. In turn, the Foundation pledged financial support for personnel within Lesley College and the school system to implement their tuition guarantee program.

NATURE OF THE PARTNERSHIP

When Lesley College agreed to become partners with the philanthropic foundation for the SYTE partnership, the first step was to recommend to the Foundation an urban school site. The process of choosing was left primarily to the SYTE Project Director, who was a full professor in the School of Education. "I did a lot of homework," the Director explained. There were four criteria set forth by the foundation; the school had to be (1) multicultural, (2) low socio-economic, (3) inner city, and (4) a Kindergarten through 8th grade school. The Lesley College SYTE Director spoke with colleagues and explored the needs of Cambridge, the city in which the university is based. Research in the service of choosing the school was done without revealing the scope of the possible project. Only the Foundation and the university knew about the planned partnership. After the thorough process of review, when a truly challenged school was chosen, the principal was told of the plans. That was *one day* before the scheduled announcement. The principal was asked to gather all the families of the children in the second grade for an important announcement that would change their futures. The excitement was immense when the Lesley College personnel, Cambridge Public School administrators, and the philanthropists presented their promise of an augmented education and fully paid college tuition.

According to both university and public school administrators, the basis for trust was formulated in the selection process. The SYTE Director remarked, "A factor of choosing the school was finding a principal who was a leader—who said, 'I will support anything you do.'" The school Principal echoes, "I knew that the program would be good for the whole school—not just the children that were in that grade." Together a team of university and school-community representatives (parents, teachers, and administrators) searched for a Program Coordinator, who would work with the SYTE Director in the school as the liaison to Lesley College and SYTE children and families. A clinical psychologist, who had worked for years in the chosen elementary school before taking another position in the school system, was recruited. He accepted the position.

The Program Coordinator position was (and is considered) critical by all participants in the partnership: The philanthropic foundation, Lesley College and the school-community. Who would fund the position became a "turf" issue. The

Program Coordinator explained, "There was an issue of salary. The SYTE salary [as provided by the foundation] would not have compared to the salary of a psychologist in the Cambridge Public Schools (CPS). So I said that I cannot accept it. . . But there was tremendous excitement about the program. The Superintendent of the [Cambridge Public] Schools said that I could remain a member of the CPS staff for the duration of the SYTE project. Lesley College agreed to pay the money provided by the foundation to CPS and then the rest of the salary would be provided by CPS. It's a nice example of complete cooperation between a school system in a city and Lesley College." Within the first year of the program, the Program Coordinator was additionally appointed as Associate Professor in the College.

GOALS: EXPLICIT AND IMPLICIT

The explicit goals of the SYTE are to provide a college education (or alternative post-secondary opportunities) and ongoing support to the 69 children who were a part of the chosen class in the designated urban school. As a means of actualizing the gift of a college education, the SYTE program also seeks to provide or give access to the services (counseling, crisis intervention, academic tutoring, summer programs, drop-out prevention) necessary to truly support students. According to all reports, the needs of the particular cohort of children in the SYTE program are extensive: 80% were eligible for free lunch during Grade 3 and nearly 50% were referred for special needs interventions. In addition, the project was implemented at a time when state funding for student counseling interventions services had been cut. The challenge of supporting the students within the community was great for both school-community and university players.

The implicit goals of the SYTE project went beyond supporting the group of chosen students, to supporting and enriching the school. The SYTE Director explained, "My attitude was that we were a member of that community [the school community]. If we did not [reach out to the all school community members]—if we did not do that—they would not have accepted us a true members. If one alienates any of these people, that person would not receive support. Teachers, administrators, janitors—everyone. We knew that it was a community of individuals that cared about kids, even if they didn't always have all the expertise necessary. Any training we did, any program we offered, was open to everyone."

The SYTE project was interpreted by Lesley College personnel comprehensively: To enrich the school experiences of the program's children, the elementary school had to be enriched. The SYTE Director explained, "We understood that somehow we had to bring this group together. Teachers were isolated, hard work and no rewards. It was a school that needed to come together to say, "We are one school serving all children." The Program Coordinator affirmed, remarking, "To help a child adjust to circumstances and to succeed is to try to create a good fit between teacher and child. We made a tremendous effort to create a fit, from working with individual scheduling, school scheduling, curriculum planning, 'teaming' [facilitating teachers working in teams]." Enriching the school overall was an implicit (although at times explicit) goal of SYTE. The Principal commented, "They [the Director and the Program Coordinator] were *here*. They were part of the team. Other children who were not SYTE children would benefit. And that was very good."

Evaluation and Research

The conceptualization of SYTE goals afforded many natural points of evaluation. The daily assistance of children and families was evidence of achievements on the path of supporting SYTE children. Improvements in the school, including teachers' interest in training or support from Lesley College, were another source of informal evaluation. As SYTE players engaged in a hands-on manner in the program, evaluation became secondary. Record keeping (e.g. the chronologuing of program features including contact with children in the program, all printed materials, reports, etc.) was conducted with care. A skilled program assistant, who was also a trained teacher, was added to the SYTE Lesley College team to facilitate this effort.

At the start of the SYTE program, the university had enlisted the assistance of a researcher who formulated a program of research to examine the explicit goals of SYTE. A plan, to follow the SYTE program participants longitudinally, was proposed. However, the study was not funded by the Foundation, the College, or other sources. A study of the implicit goals of SYTE was never formally developed.

The absence of a research plan was lamented by all stakeholders in the partnerships. However, recently SYTE personnel developed a strategic plan of research to focus on both the implicit and explicit goals of the program. Lesley College and Foundation monies have been allocated for this research.

PROCESSES, MANIFESTATIONS AND BENEFITS

When reflecting on the process of beginning the SYTE program, the Program Director sighed and said, "It was *very* difficult. It [the school] was very fragmented, not together as a community. The notion of haves and have nots, needed to be dispelled." Reaching out to the children and families in the program and working within the school to create community were the large tasks of the SYTE program. Several factors emerge as key to both processes.

Creating Trust between the Lesley College SYTE and the School-Community

While a foundation of good will existed at the inception of the program, the building of trust was a critical factor in the SYTE program process. The Program Coordinator was known and respected in the school community. His presence and Lesley College's sanctioning of his role, facilitated trust. The Program Coordinator remarked, "I knew the atmosphere and the culture of the school, from administrators to janitors, and that facilitated our tasks tremendously—from getting an office, to being able to have teachers willing to talk with us, to having the authority to talk with teachers."

The SYTE Director talked about working hard to make herself known, familiar and trusted: "I was a city kid, too, and I let that be known. I got to know the [teaching] aides. I joined the School Improvement Council. Letting them [the school community] know that we were there for *all* of them made a difference." In addition, the SYTE team was supported by the administration of the elementary school and the central administration for the CPS. During the early years of the program, the SYTE staff met several times a month with both administrative teams.

Creating Shared Community

In addition to building trust, the goals of SYTE required the building of a shared sense of community. The unity of the SYTE team from Lesley College in pursuing their efforts to create community is cited by both school-community and university players. The Program Coordinator commented, "One of the reasons we succeeded is that the Director and I were totally together. It was a school in which people were *very* entrenched... The Director provided things to teachers to make them feel appreciated. And we extended that to the whole staff."

In order to work towards enriching the school and creating community, the Program Director and the Program Coordinator, worked with teachers directly on team curriculum planning. Funding from the SYTE project and additional teacher aides provided by the CPS system, made teacher planning meetings more possible. The idea was new to the teachers, who were used to isolated teaching. The goal of teaming was to create community and also influence the quality of teaching available to the students.

The Director explained, "Some teachers were entrenched. It was very difficult for some of them to accept change. I said to the Principal that we'll team third and fourth grades and talk about curriculum. The first year was just getting to respect each other and build camaraderie. Initially, I led the meetings and the Program Coordinator recorded the minutes. Then, I was unable to attend and the Program Coordinator took over leadership of the meetings. After a period of time, the teachers took over those roles. The Principal remarked, "It [teaming] was not easy. It was happening already in the upper grades. It was one of the better things [about the SYTE program]."

The Director and Coordinator used team meetings to create a shared substantive focus on providing quality education, together as one community, for all children. When teachers began to actually work together on thematic curriculum, SYTE provided money for materials, field trips, training and other resources. Since teams often worked in two grade level units, children from other classes gained equal access to the resources and teaching. Intervention with teaching teams followed the SYTE participants' grade level. "Every other year," the SYTE Director remarked, "we started over again [with a new team of teachers]."

When the SYTE children graduated from the elementary school, the SYTE Lesley College personnel had worked with teams from Grades 3 through 8. Teaming is now part of the school culture and community. The genesis of teaming with a focus on curriculum arose from the work with SYTE personnel; now, however, the process has been sustained by the teams of teachers on their own.

Attending To Individual Needs

While the SYTE project worked hard to create institutional cohesion, community and trust, it also focused on meeting the individual needs of SYTE children. The Program Coordinator provided counseling to SYTE students. Interns from the university worked under the Coordinator's supervision to provide counseling. The Program Coordinator intervened with individual children, monitoring all aspects of their academic progress, their schedules (including afterschool and summer), and their plans. He became a member of the School Support Team, that comprised teachers, parents, and psychologists, who met weekly to work towards considering the needs of students. Since the Program Coordinator has a sense of the "pulse" of the SYTE students, he is also an important conduit to the Foundation. At times during the SYTE program, the philanthropists have asked to learn about the progress of students. The Coordinator plays a critical role in that effort.

GOALS AND ACHIEVEMENT

The goal of providing support for SYTE towards the achievement of a college education for the designated group of children, is difficult to document. The story is still unfolding. More than half of the program participants no longer attend CPS. All participants are still in contact with the Program Coordinator; all are still eligible for the tuition benefit. Anecdotal evidence, and eight years of weekly if not daily crisis intervention, attest to the achievement of support for the students. As the SYTE team ready the children for college or other post secondary opportunities, they have placed new demands on their program participation. For example, students who have unsatisfactory academic progress are eligible for summer camps of their choice only after they have completed summer academic tutoring. The Program Coordinator comments that some students have said that he is "on their case 24-7," and that is true. There is a sense of frustration in the ongoing need to support a small number of students, that leads to the question, 'Is it fair or cost effective for the Coordinator to spend 75% of his time with 25% of the students in the program?'

The Foundation does not place constraints on SYTE students' program participation. The Program Coordinator's role is to support students and guide them. Although it is only implied in the students' agreement with the Foundation, ultimately all SYTE students are entitled to the promised college tuition regardless of their participation in recommended courses of action. The Program Coordinator continues to monitor, intervene, and often be an advocate on behalf of SYTE students. During separate, open ended interviews, one school community administrator and the Program Coordinator suggested that there might have been some potential benefit to an agreement that set forth Foundation-mandated conditions for remaining in the program.

The implied goal of enriching the elementary school community in which the SYTE was located has been met, by all accounts. The image of the school has been changed dramatically. Team planning continues, as does the thematic curriculum introduced by the SYTE Director. In addition, the school's links to Lesley College have multiplied. Three of the Coordinator's interns came from the Lesley College Counseling division and provided therapy for the students. After the first year of the SYTE program, the elementary school was chosen by Lesley College as a professional development school. Training from Lesley College is widely available. Student teachers from the College are plentiful at the elementary school.

In addition, other research/intervention programs have been attracted to the elementary school. The SYTE Director encouraged university colleagues to consider partnerships with the school. At present, a comprehensive literacy program associated with Lesley College is being implemented in the school. In addition, the College has facilitated connection with other institutions around full inclusion and teacher training. Both the school community itself and the school community partnership with the university have been strengthened as a result of the SYTE program. Clearly, sustainable community change has evolved from the SYTE project involvement.

LESSONS LEARNED ABOUT CREATING SUSTAINABLE PARTNERSHIPS

The SYTE project demonstrates the utility and power of the combination of philanthropic, university and school community collaboration. Circles of collaboration are evident on many levels. The Foundation provided a vision and funding for the program, and also provided freedom and autonomy to the university to develop a plan to implement that program. The university created a partnership with the school community. The school community was respected by the university and the key position of Program Coordinator was filled by someone who was already trusted and respected by the community constituents. The university made becoming a part of the school community a high priority. The school community administrators pledged and provided support for the SYTE initiatives: They opened their doors to systemic intervention and change.

These are the largest and most visible circles of collaboration. Many other small examples occur during each day and week of the program. A systemic effect of the program aimed at supporting children was the development of positive, multi-layered circles of co-learning and action that transformed a school in need and enriched all partnership members. Each member of the partnership was and is critical to the success of the program. There are shared resources of personnel and funding. There is shared responsibility and care for both the SYTE children and the community in which they exist.

Often programs aimed at interventions for children and youth focus narrowly on those target populations. The conceptualization of the SYTE program by the university broadened the focus. The unfolding of the SYTE children's experiences is a critical part of the SYTE program. However, those explicit goals of the program are finite. Through the examination of this successful community partnership, that has spurred self-sustained and newly generated community change, an example of the potential benefit of limited partnership for broader change has emerged. Most importantly, the lives and work of all participants in the SYTE program, and its accompanying philanthropic, university, school community partnership, are enriched and transformed. Valuable lessons have been learned.

23 REVITALIZING THE COMMUNITY THROUGH NEIGHBORHOOD AND INSTITUTIONAL PARTNERSHIPS

Dale Lucy-Allen
Jennifer Seydel
Springfield College

> Urban America is where the nation's fabric is now experiencing its most serious strain. Violence, unemployment, poverty, poor housing, and pollution often occur at the very doorsteps of some of our most distinguished colleges and universities. How can the nation's campuses stay disengaged? Ira Harkavy, director of the University of Pennsylvania's Center for Community Partnerships, warns that 'universities cannot afford to remain shores of affluence, self-importance, and horticultural beauty at the edge of island seas of squalor, violence and despair' (Boyer, 1994, p. A48).

Over the past six years, Springfield College has been challenged to participate in addressing the needs of the urban neighborhood in which it resides. To answer this call, the College has had to wrestle with the many challenges necessary to change the attitude of the institutional culture toward the community, and to reestablish relationships within the neighborhood. The College and community partnerships that have resulted from facing these challenges are dynamic collaborations that involve participation at all levels. Undergraduate and graduate students, faculty members, administrators, neighbors, leaders of community based organizations, and the governmental agencies that impact the solutions have all worked together to create service and educational programs tailored to meet the needs of children and families in the community and participants on the campus.

In this chapter we provide the context for the development of two college-community collaborations in Springfield, Massachusetts. We share the developmental progression of the Partners Program, which formed the foundation of Colleges Serving the Community, and served as the incubator for the S.A.G.E. Project. A discussion of the two partnerships, one that was initiated by an individual from within the neighborhood and college and another that was initiated by institutions from within the community, is included. We discuss how the individuals and institutions involved in these collaborative programs have accepted ownership for the outcomes of the programs, and are working toward sustaining the programs. An overview of the salient lessons learned from the development of these collaborative programs and the key elements for their success conclude the discussion.

REVITALIZING THE COMMUNITY THROUGH PARTNERSHIPS

Springfield College's mission is to educate students—in spirit, mind, and body—for leadership in service to humanity. The College's commitment to academic excellence and the practical, service-oriented curriculum prepare its undergraduate and graduate students for careers in the human-helping professions, including education, physical education, recreation, allied health sciences, and human and social services. For more than 110 years, graduates have filled key positions in youth organizations and nonprofit agencies, and have been pioneers in such fields as recreation and municipal parks, sports and sports management, adaptive physical education for persons with disabilities, and rehabilitation services. Alumni represent a cross-section of highly successful professionals who are outstanding in their chosen fields, such as teachers, physicians, head coaches of U.S. Olympic Teams, elected officials, and other prominent leaders in the public and private sectors.

In 1992, the College renewed its institutional commitment to local community outreach under the strategic initiative named by College President Randolph W. Bromery as "The Hill Renaissance." Through this initiative, President Bromery challenged the College community to become more involved in revitalizing the local neighborhood. In response to this challenge, the College's Office of Student Volunteer Programs completed a study of the residential undergraduate students to determine if they were interested in becoming involved with the neighboring community through service programs. Over 75% of the residential population, of 1,800, responded, with the following results: a) 66% wanted to be involved in service programs in our community; b) 75% desired the opportunity to assist youth in either educational or recreational activities; and c) projected time commitments ranged from one time events to 10 hours per week. Focus groups were held with students who wanted to volunteer. At about this same time, a resident of the neighborhood and principal of one of the neighborhood elementary schools approached Dr. Bromery to explore the possibilities of meeting the needs of the children at the William N. DeBerry Elementary School. Students who had participated in the focus groups were challenged to develop a program that would address the responses of the study and this request from the community.

THE PARTNERS PROGRAM

During the Fall of 1993 recruitment began for an after-school service program, the Partners Program, that would match college students with children from the William N. DeBerry School. To determine the best way for the College to work with the school, a team of faculty, students and administrators from the College met with a team of teachers, parents and administrators from the DeBerry School to design the program. As the team identified the strengths and needs of the community and college, the following goals emerged:

- To provide unique educational and recreational opportunities for the DeBerry students by using campus and community resources .
- To provide urban educational opportunities for the largely suburban college students by using the community and neighborhood as the College's primary service-learning partner.
- To provide the students at the DeBerry School with weekly exposure to a college campus and discussion about obtaining a college degree.
- To include parents in the activities to enable them to connect with their child's school.
- To provide college student leadership opportunities and support to operate service programs.

The Partners Program has grown from the original 28 Springfield College students, matched with 28 DeBerry youth, to include 150 students from three local colleges and three neighborhood schools. American International College (AIC), Springfield Technical Community College (STCC), and Elias Brookings and Homer Street Schools joined the program in 1995. This program formed the foundation of a new collaborative effort entitled Colleges Serving Community (CSC).

During the first three years of the program, development and design was guided by a council of parents, teachers, college faculty, administrators, and college students. The program model includes matching a college student with a youth, between third and eighth grade, one day per week for three hour sessions over a 24-week period. Each week the pairs meet at the respective public school and spend one hour working on academic enrichment, then travel to either SC or AIC to participate in a recreational, educational or cultural activity for 1 hour. The final hour allows the partner pairs to dine together in the College dining hall. Youth are then transported home or are picked up by their parents. Monthly social events are held for parents and guardians, teachers, college students, and youth. These events have included outings to Stage West Theater and to the Basketball Hall of Fame, attending gymnastics exhibitions, hearing storytellers, and attending an Olympic Track and Field Clinic.

In the Fall of 1995, the CSC collaboration, was implemented further with support from Learn & Serve America. The goals of this program were:

- To expand the Partners Program to include sites at three elementary schools and one middle school;
- To increase the number of one day service events sponsored by three colleges;
- To alter the institutional infrastructure to include support for service-learning at three colleges; and
- To provide support for and increase the number of faculty members utilizing service-learning to meet educational and community needs.

Over the past three years, CSC has had a positive influence on faculty and administration in all three collaborating institutions. The professional network created by the CSC has provided the opportunity for faculty and administration to increase utilization of service-learning through training and technical assistance, mini-grants, and to support integration of service-learning and release time to develop the infrastructure needed at the institutions to sustain and support this program.

THE S.A.G.E. PROJECT

As the Partners Program and CSC progressed, the relationship between Springfield College and the Springfield Public Schools strengthened. In the spring of 1996, the Western Area Office of the Massachusetts Department of Youth Services (DYS) and Springfield Public Schools (SPS) approached the college to participate in addressing another crucial issue within the community. DYS, SPS, and the District Attorney's Office were involved in developing a comprehensive strategy to reduce juvenile crime and provide educational services for high-risk youth. In the summer of 1996, a task force comprising representatives of the DYS, SPS, and Springfield College began to work toward developing an educational strategy that would support school success for youth who are adjudicated or at high risk of criminal involvement in the community. The S.A.G.E. Project is the result of this collaboration. This ongoing project, the S.A.G.E. Project, maintains four programs:

- The S.A.G.E. Collaboration—to foster the collaborative efforts between the public and private sectors of the community, justice system, and educational institutions as they address the needs of high risk youth.
- The Springfield College Authentic Graduate Education (S.A.G.E.) M.Ed. Program in General Counseling and Education—a teacher and school adjustment counselor certification program designed to increase the number of secondary educators within the Springfield Public Schools with the expertise to meet the needs of high risk youth.
- The Springfield Adolescent Graduation Experience (S.A.G.E.) Secondary School—an alternative high school which includes a comprehensive prevention strategy to address the needs of high risk and adjudicated youth.
- S.A.G.E. AmeriCorps Program—a service program that provides up to twelve S.A.G.E. M.Ed. students the opportunity to gain a full year of experience working as mentors and tutors with the high-risk and adjudicated students that attend the S.A.G.E. Secondary School.

The S.A.G.E. Collaboration comprises scholars and practitioners representing a broad range of public institutions in education, corrections, and human services within Springfield. Individuals in this group have been involved at various levels of the planning and development of the S.A.G.E. M.Ed. Program, the S.A.G.E. Secondary School, and the S.A.G.E. AmeriCorps Program. Their expertise has been essential to implement the unique combination of best practices that continue to shape the S.A.G.E. Programs.

The purpose of the S.A.G.E. M.Ed. in General Counseling and Education Program is to prepare secondary educators with the skills and knowledge necessary to work with high risk students in traditional and nontraditional programs. Pre-service and in-service teachers are taught to integrate psycho-education, behavior management, and experiential education techniques and methods into the curriculum. Recruitment of students for this program is guided by the projected needs of the Springfield Public Schools over the next ten years. As an integral part of the S.A.G.E. M.Ed. program, ten to twelve graduate students participate in the S.A.G.E. AmeriCorps Program. Guided by the public school teachers, school adjustment counselors, and the Supervisor at the Springfield Adolescent Graduation Experience, (S.A.G.E.) Secondary School, M.Ed. students gain practical experience with high-risk students as they perform their year of service as tutors and mentors through the AmeriCorps Program. Springfield College provides limited tuition support to all S.A.G.E. AmeriCorps members.

The Springfield Adolescent Graduation Experience, (S.A.G.E.) Secondary School, a Springfield Public School, has been created through this collaboration to develop an effective educational model for high-risk and adjudicated youth. This program utilizes a comprehensive behavior management system and information exchange system that enhances cooperation between all agencies providing services and supervision to these youth. The curriculum at the school integrates community service learning, adventure education, and school-to-work programs to support the social and vocational development of the students while they work toward meeting the learning outcomes for SPS graduation. The faculty and staff at the school work closely with Springfield College faculty and S.A.G.E. Project Director to support the development of the AmeriCorps members serving in the school.

ANALYSIS OF PROCESS

The Partners Program, subsequently CSC, and the S.A.G.E. Project reflect four essential building blocks for successful college-community partnerships: a) administrative leadership; b) identification of real need within the community *and* the College; c) commitment by individuals at all levels of the College and community; and d) the development of a collaborative process that includes clearly identified roles and systems for shared responsibility, lateral accountability and program planning. As one might imagine, the impact of these collaborative programs have had a ripple effect on the whole community.

The influence of the support by Springfield College President, Dr. Bromery for community outreach has had a dramatic impact at all levels of the College community. With administrative leadership, the College community has participated in the development of a comprehensive strategic plan for the College. This revisioning process, known as Vision 2003, clearly projects the college's role in the community and includes service-learning and community outreach as part of the academic process. Since 1995, this plan has provided direction and a renewed vigor for outreach in the community.

As the Senior Management Team and the Deans of the five academic schools accept outreach as an important part of the academic preparation of Springfield College students, administrative systems have been created to support service-learning throughout the campus. A faculty governance committee, the Committee for the Advancement of Service Learning (CASL), has been created to explore and recommend ways that service-learning can be integrated into the academic curriculum. In addition, the Office of Institutional Advancement has increased its efforts to support the expanded community outreach. Over the past three years this has included filling two vacant positions including a grants officer to assist with proposal development, coordination, and reporting.

It has been our experience that projects that meet a need within both the College community and the local community have a higher degree of success and longevity. The need for after school programming for youth and the interest of Springfield College students in service were key factors in the creation of the Partners Program. Because the program was designed to meet these needs the commitment of all of the partners has been sustained. In the case of the S.A.G.E. Project, the need within the community had been clearly identified prior to contact with the College. The S.A.G.E. M.Ed. Program has been able to fill the need for a graduate level program in secondary education.

In both of these programs, much time and energy has been expended by all of the participating institutions during the development and implementation phases. As the idea for the Partners Program germinated, it was nurtured by a committee that included college administration, faculty, students, and public school administrators, teachers, and parents. The level of personal investment by these individuals sustained the idea before funding support was secured. While this method of development has led to a very special design, it created the added obstacles of obtaining new resources, each step of the way. Fortunately, this program and subsequently CSC has been successful in obtaining and leveraging resources from many collaborators to expand the outreach and community impact.

On the other hand, the S.A.G.E. Project was initiated from within the administrative structure of the Western Area Office of the Massachusetts DYS and the SPS. Because one of the main goals of this project was to enhance the collaborative efforts among the governmental agencies serving high-risk and adjudicated youth, this Project maintained an Advisory Board and Executive Committee that was purely administrative through the first eighteen months of planning and implementation. As the Project has progressed and the administrative issues have been resolved, it has become more important for faculty and staff at both the College and the S.A.G.E. Secondary School to work together.

As each program developed, it has become necessary to nurture the collaboration as well as the project. We have found that it has been important for all partners to have equal input into program planning to insure a sense of shared responsibility and lateral accountability. This level of cooperation has required each institution participating in the program to develop an increased level of ownership, involvement, and trust of the other partners.

Both projects have had key faculty and administrators that have been able to facilitate and manage the college-community collaboration. These College and community members have been able to identify four essential elements in their leadership roles: Respecting the traditions and structures of all partners; maintaining the integrity of the collaboration over loyalty to any one partner (including the employer); ensuring that all partners have a voice; and maintaining a visible and vocal role in the community.

ACHIEVEMENTS RELATED TO GOAL

The data provided for the achievements related to the goals of CSC are taken from the 1996-97 Evaluation Report authored by Dr. Arthur Bertrand and Associates. The Partners Program was evaluated by the public school youth, teachers and administrators, and parents, as well as, by the college participants and student leaders. The Partners Program has had a considerable impact upon both the College and the community. It has drawn them together in a partnership that has begun disintegrating the lines which have kept the two communities apart in the past. Public school students spend time at Springfield College and become acclimated to its culture. Thus, the two communities that had been separated over the years are drawn together with a goal of providing a better education to the public school and college students. The resulting community impacts are impressive:

- In the first five years of the Program, over 700 pairings have occurred for mutual learning experiences between college students, youth and families.
- SC's traditionally white, middle class students are placed in a multicultural setting that better prepares them to be educators for individuals that may have different learning styles and values than their own. Many of these students are now considering teaching in an urban school, something that was not considered previously.
- Youth who initially may not have included education as a life goal, are now including college and a specific major as a long term goal.
- Teachers and school staff have reported that the youth have increased their academic performance levels and are attending school with fewer absences throughout the year.
- Teachers and school staff have reported that the youth are less likely to be disruptive in the classroom and have an improved self esteem.
- Parent(s)/Guardian(s) have become more involved in their child's education by interacting with the public school staff and visiting the school more frequently.
- The utilization of service-learning by Springfield College faculty has increased from four during the 1993-94 academic year to 29 during the fall of 1997.

In the initial evaluation report of the S.A.G.E. Project, completed by Mr. Frank Llamas, in May 1998, all key stakeholders indicated that there was universal support and commitment to the S.A.G.E. collaboration. One hundred percent (100%) of those interviewed replied that the interagency case management system that has been created through the S.A.G.E. Project has improved the services provided to the students involved in the juvenile justice system. Respondents also consistently reported that the S.A.G.E. M.Ed. Program, in conjunction with the AmeriCorps Program provided a new approach to teacher training that greatly improves the old model. In addition, they felt the S.A.G.E. M.Ed. Program is laying the groundwork for effective strategies to train teachers to develop the expertise to meet the needs of urban at-risk students. One respondent commented, "The future of teacher preparation lies in these kinds of field-based programs."

Other results include:

- Fifty students attended the S.A.G.E. Secondary School in its first year of operation.
- Fourteen graduate students completed the first year of the S.A.G.E. M.Ed. Program.
- Thirty youth involved with the juvenile justice system, received improved supervision through the information management system created by the S.A.G.E. Project.
- Over 17,000 hours of service to the Springfield community was provided through the S.A.G.E. AmeriCorps Program.

Additional collaborative outreach efforts, by Springfield College, over the past four years include: a) Project S.P.I.R.I.T., an undergraduate program designed to increase the number of minority teachers in Springfield; b) Integration of service-learning in 56 undergraduate and graduate courses during the 1997-98 academic year; c) Increased numbers of athletic team members participating in youth clinics and as peer educators with the Time Out for Communities program; and d) The creation of an America Reads Program with the Springfield Public Schools and community-based organizations; and e) For the past four years the Summer Enrichment Program (SEP) provides Springfield College and high school students the training and support to lead educational, recreational, cultural, and community service related activities for over 3,000 youth and families each year at six urban parks that were traditionally vacant each summer.

LESSONS LEARNED FROM THESE PARTNERSHIPS

There have been many lessons learned from the development of these college-community collaborations and the rapid expansion of community outreach at Springfield College. The most salient of these include: The importance of open communication between the College and community; the importance of flexible program leadership that allows the college-community collaborations to evolve and change as the partnerships strengthen; and the necessity for centralized coordination and clear communication within the college community by the leadership of community outreach programs. By responding to these three lessons internally, Springfield College has become a more responsible partner in community revitalization.

Open communication between the College and the community has been a key to the success of each of the collaborative programs we have discussed in this chapter. Because of the college's mission of service to humanity and the selection of faculty and administrators for their excellence as teachers and/or practitioners in their fields; more so than for their record of research and publication, many of the individuals leading the college-community programs have been able to establish real authority with community partners rather than role authority. This factor has allowed them to work closely with the community and relationships are based on honesty, trust and genuine respect. As these peer relationships have developed, not only does commitment to the program become a value, but commitment to the healthy professional and personal development of each person involved becomes a value. Within this atmosphere of collaboration, open communication allows the partners to clarify roles, share resources more readily, and build on the strengths of the program and individuals while managing areas on concern. Students, faculty, community members, teachers, and principals involved are empowered to be the leaders who provide the formation and direction for the programs.

These working relationships have allowed each program to grow and change as the partnerships have strengthened. When this occurs, it has been important for the leadership at the college to be flexible and responsive to becoming an active community partner. It has also been important for the entire College community to be more aware of the impact of their decisions and actions on these partnerships. Although resignations and retirements of key figures within the College community may only seem important within the college community, as stronger and more effective partnerships are developed within the community these actions also create a ripple effect and can sometimes create stress within the community. Decisions by the Board of Trustees can also impact college-community collaborations. As community outreach increases, additional institutional, community based, and external support is also necessary. Leadership, from the College and community, must respond positively to these needs to enhance a trusting relationship within the community. We believe that securing this support is directly correlated with the degree of success in initiating and sustaining our outreach efforts.

As the College has become more involved with the community, it has become evident that it is important to develop an internal process to manage and coordinate the partnerships and resource needs that have developed between the College and community. At the current time the College is exploring a number of options to make this happen. It is not the goal of the College to take ownership of ongoing projects, but rather to serve as the bridge and incubation tank that shares all aspects of programming to meet shared needs. The development of a Center for Community Partnerships is being formalized and may provide the needed infrastructure to increase the success and opportunity for outreach to be sustained. We believe it is important that this effort be supported by the President and become an institutional priority.

The opening of the proverbial doors of the College by Dr. Bromery in 1993 has been the catalyst for five years of partnerships to revitalize the Springfield community. These partnerships continue to be successful because the needs of the community and the College remain the focus of program development. As the culture of the community and the College has changed we are able to see the impact within the community through improved relationships and through the increasing numbers of youth and families involved.

REFERENCES

Boyer, E. L. (1994, March 4). Creating the new American college. *Chronicle of Higher Education, 40*(27), p. A48.

Harkavy, I. (1992, Summer). Universities and inner cities. *Planning for Higher Education, 20*(40), 27-33. Summer 1992.

24 CAMEO FEATURE NEWS: UNIVERSITY AND COMMUNITY PARTNERSHIP DISSEMINATES CHILD DEVELOPMENT INFORMATION

Nancy Martland
Fred Rothbaum
Tufts University

NATURE OF THE PARTNERSHIP

How do grass-roots agencies and programs lacking the expertise and the budget to publicize their work get their message out to the communities they serve? How do scholars and researchers, who publish their work primarily in professional journals, make the latest in child development research accessible to the public? CAMEO Feature News (CFN), an internet-based project at the Eliot-Pearson Department of Child Development at Tufts University, brings together the community and the university in a novel partnership that addresses both of these questions.

CAMEO Feature News is a unique blend of Child Development and Journalism. This university-based news service works directly with community-based agencies and programs that deliver direct service to children and families, as well as the interested public, to disseminate solution-oriented stories to the mainstream news media. CAMEO Feature News, which is operated entirely by faculty and students, assigns staff to work with agency personnel to produce story materials for journalists, called Cameo Summaries. The summaries include a personal account about a client/participant, information about the program, contact information for story subjects, relevant expert comments and research, names and addresses of experts, references and web links. Cameo Summaries are released to journalists at the CAMEO web site (www.jumbohub.com/cameo) and by Email.

WHY CAMEO FEATURE NEWS?

It seems to be a truism in academia and among children's advocates that the press just doesn't get it right. In the case of coverage of children, research tends to support this conclusion. A study by Kunkel (1996) revealed that, while children and child-related topics are covered regularly in the print and broadcast media, the majority of stories focus on children either as victims or perpetrators of violent acts. Moreover, the reporting itself tends to be one-dimensional, focusing on the sensational and surface features of the story rather than presenting a fuller context that gives the story depth. According to Cathy Trost, Director of the Casey Journalism Center at the University of Maryland, "The bad news is that there are still plenty of barriers to good coverage, and too much of the reporting about children is still shallow or sensational." (Trost, 1996, p. 48)

The enormous power of the media both to educate and to influence public opinion on children's issues is well-documented (Bonk & Wiley, 1994; The Advertising Council, 1995). Poor reporting on children creates a double bind that CAMEO Feature News seeks to correct. First, such reporting has negative effects; second each superficial report wastes an opportunity to inform the public, practitioners, and policy-makers. Wexler (1993, p. 18) highlights the adverse effects of sensational reporting, using the example of child abuse. He writes, "Despite the best of intentions, the media are doing serious harm to the children caught up in the protective system. The media have contributed to the atmosphere of hysteria that surrounds child abuse." Wexler goes on to advocate reporting that goes beyond taking a story at face value. He suggests that journalists covering abuse stories find out what the relevant laws are, that they examine the cost structure and financial aspects of child protection, that they broaden their sources to move beyond the rolodex, and that they treat the next abuse "crisis" story with a measured reponse that will not encourage panic.

The Kidsbeat which has developed in the 1990s (Trost, 1996) includes reporters who specialize in covering children; these journalists have done much to improve the quality of coverage. According to Carole Simpson of ABC News, the Kidsbeat is an idea whose time has come: "The response to the 'American Agenda' and to the stories I have done about children has been phenomenal... the public seems to love them. And public officials have reacted most positively." (Columbia, 1992, p. 226). Simpson went on to describe effects of her reporting, including supplying clips for Representative Dan Rostenkowski to use to put forward a children's agenda in Congress, and the rescue of WIC funding. A study by the Casey Center found that "More than half of 62 newspapers and news services surveyed in 1995 had added children and/or family beats in the previous three years." (Casey, 1995, p. 2). Despite these recent inroads, much remains to be done. The Casey report goes on to say, "One of the most urgent issues is how the media can better convey depth and detail about the causes and consequences of children's problems." (Casey, 1995, p. 4).

The superficiality of coverage is the fault of experts as well as journalists. Just as the reporters fail to make themselves adequately informed about research, experts do not take responsibility for translating their work into terms comprehensible to the general public. Experts are "...trained to publish descriptions of knowledge generated by developmental science in language and journals inaccessible to parents, teachers, practitioners, policy-makers and others who could apply the knowledge to directly promote the welfare of children and families." (Fisher & Osofsky, 1997, p. 2; Sigel, 1990).

CAMEO Feature News attacks the double bind by providing journalists with the material they need to develop an in-depth feature that explores significant issues surrounding a news event. CFN collects personal accounts from community organizations, researches them, and prepares a Cameo Summary for journalists. Several related summaries along with supporting material such as references, background information, and lists of story leads and key issues are combined into a

Topic File. We notify journalists of our Topic Files that are relevant to breaking news events and emerging trends, thus providing easy access to material that supports the writing of high-quality related coverage and sidebars. Working together, the university and the community can have an impact on the way that children are covered in the mainstream media.

PURPOSES AND GOALS

CAMEO's main goals are: (a) to educate the public about child development by improving the quality of media coverage of children and families, and (b) to encourage more media attention to the many constructive community efforts on behalf of children and families. With regard to the media, CFN aims to promote solution-oriented coverage, coverage with depth and context that moves away from sensationalized accounts of children's lives, and coverage of under-represented populations. The contexts of greatest importance to CFN are:

- research findings about child development that are relevant to issues addressed in the Cameo Summary
- the methods and goals of agencies and programs which serve the persons described
- opinions of scholars and practitioners regarding the personal account, the program/agency, and the research addressed in the Summary.

This information is presented in an accessible manner to enhance its impact and usefulness to the public.

CAMEO Feature News has two goals in working with community organizations. First, to collaborate with grass-roots programs to highlight the stories of people who work with children every day and of the children and families they serve. While CFN is dedicated to "getting the word out" about community-based initiatives, it is not simply a public relations service; in the process of providing depth and context, CFN sometimes raises issues and concerns that these agencies would rather ignore. For example, research may be cited that fails to support the efforts of a similar community program or that questions their methods.

Second, CAMEO Feature News strives to provide access to a variety of resources plentiful in a university setting but typically unavailable to community programs. Of paramount importance is access to information technology. Most of the local agencies lack sophisticated information systems such as Email and world wide web access; CFN uses state-of-the-art technology available in a university setting to enhance its community partners' ability to take advantage of the power of the Internet to distribute information about their work. Faculty child development expertise, including both extensive practical knowledge and cutting-edge applied research, complements the information that agencies supply about their activities and enriches what they can offer to the press.

CFN capitalizes on the enthusiasm of students for the project by using their energy, their growing skills, and their generous contribution of labor to operate the service. At Tufts University, over 300 students give of their time through the campus service organization, the Leonard Carmichael Society. We believe this is representative of the abundance of student volunteer labor and energy available on campuses across the country. To date, over 30 students have participated in CFN for periods *in excess of* 100 hours each.

ANALYSIS OF THE PROCESS

While CAMEO Feature News was initiated within the university setting, community agency representatives played an important role in its planning and design. Early in the process, CAMEO leaders met with community leaders and local journalists to gather information about the needs of each group, as well as their ideas about how CAMEO could help to meet those needs. This collaboration continued and is ongoing. University faculty and students (the project director is a Ph.D. student) designed the prototype product—the Cameo Summary—and a process for collecting and producing summaries, but input from the community and the media shaped the work.

Journalists from across the country were surveyed early in the design phase to ascertain their general receptivity. In March 1998, journalists from the New England region provided feedback about the initial release of Cameo Summaries. Both surveys were invaluable in generating ideas and suggestions which were incorporated into the project plan, leading to a greatly improved product. For example, the more recent survey led to the decision to provide multiple personal accounts within each file and to focus on stories related to hot breaking news.

While the long-term plan is to use the web site to attract and gather stories, we realized that we needed to seek out community organizations actively during CFN's initial phase. Working with umbrella agencies such as the Children's Trust Fund, we were able to identify the most promising programs, which were then contacted personally by the director to enlist them as partners. We plan to continue to initiate collaboration with community organizations.

When the story collection stage began in 1997, the university contacted several direct-service agencies and programs. In most cases preliminary contact was made by the project director, who telephoned the program director. The reception to these calls was uniformly enthusiastic. When offered the opportunity to collaborate with CAMEO Feature News to produce stories about them, the only reservations involved the confidentiality of clients/participants. To address this concern, CFN designed a policy which allows story subjects to use pseudonyms in the posted Summary, and to designate a contact through which reporters can have access to them.

The university and community collaborate in all three major phases of the process leading to a Cameo Summary: Collection, analysis and research, and production.

In the collection phase, CFN staff and agency staff work together to acquaint each other more fully with the nature of Cameo Summaries and of the goals and operations of the agency. They then discuss possible subjects for the personal account. Agency personnel then put the CAMEO staffer in touch with the subject they believe can provide the most compelling personal account, and this subject is interviewed by a trained student member of the CAMEO staff.

In the analysis and research phase, agency personnel serve as expert contacts for the Cameo Summary, helping CFN staff to understand fully the salient aspects of the personal account and the surrounding circumstances. Agency personnel have also been willing to make themselves available to reporters. Agency administrators and staff are at times good sources of information about academic experts, research, and references that are particularly meaningful to their work. In general, agency personnel give generously of their time to support the analysis phase of the summary.

In the production phase, the dialogue between CAMEO and the local agency continues, but the parties are mindful of the need for increased reporter/subject boundaries. In light of the necessity for objective reporting, agencies cannot collaborate in the writing of the final version of the CAMEO Summary; however, in this alternative journalistic model, limited input is accepted. Agencies receive a copy of the final version. It is understood from the outset that factual inaccuracies will be corrected, but that the content and analysis included in the summary is otherwise non-negotiable. Both the subject of the story and the agency administrator retain the right to withdraw the summary at any time.

ACHIEVEMENTS RELATED TO GOALS

As a result of the Summary production process, CAMEO Feature News has made substantial progress toward realizing many of its initial goals. Outreach by CFN to community organizations created a network of community contacts that we expect to further cultivate, as well as to expand with new contacts. CFN's approach, which involves agency personnel in the identification and analysis of story material, has strengthened ties between these community organizations and the university partner; an atmosphere of mutual respect developed as the two groups cooperated to create a final product for distribution to journalists.

CAMEO Feature News has successfully engaged journalists by creating a group of "CAMEO Consultants" mainly from among prominent Boston-area reporters and editors (e.g., from several newspapers, local television stations, and National Public Radio). This included the recipients of the initial release of Cameo Summaries; they provided excellent feedback which was highly positive and encouraging, as well as several thoughtful suggestions for refinements that would make the summaries more useful and attractive to them. Several stories have appeared in the Boston media as a result of CFN, among them pieces aired by WHDH, the Boston NBC affiliate and WBUR, the Boston NPR outlet, and published in the Boston Parents' Paper.

Regarding the goal of educating the public about child development, CFN has addressed this primarily through the incorporation of expert information within the Cameo Summaries. Because the project is university-based, it has been relatively easy to accomplish this goal; the university faculty have embraced the work of CAMEO and have extended themselves to support it. Faculty in the Department of Child Development have been enlisted to serve in two ways. They consult with CAMEO staff to assist with identification of issues and research relevant to the personal accounts, thus providing valuable analytical support. Faculty have also been willing to call upon their personal network of colleagues as needed for particular Cameo Summaries. This allows CFN to work from a base which draws upon the most highly-respected scholars and researchers from across the country. CAMEO Feature News has begun to develop contacts with experts both through faculty assistance and through the creation of our own database. Using web sites such as ProfNet which locate academic experts in response to reporter's queries, as well as the more conventional databases such as PsychLit and Lexis-Nexis, CAMEO staff have created an expert database, which we will continue to expand. Materials have been developed that introduce experts to CAMEO Feature News and that invite them to continue to work with us. To date, the response from experts we have contacted has been very positive; these experts see the value of working with journalists to improve reporting, and they are willing to make the investment of time necessary.

PROSPECTS FOR LONG TERM SUSTAINABILITY

We believe that CAMEO Feature News is ahead of the technology curve in the way it addresses the needs of community organizations to inform the public about their activities. This is reflected in the enthusiastic response from such organizations. As more and more news outlets realize the public appetite for solution-oriented stories that address child and family issues, we believe that CFN is well-placed to serve as a much-needed resource for this kind of reporting. The development of sustained reciprocal relationships with many members of the media places CFN in an ideal position to take advantage of this emerging media trend.

The CAMEO projec t has developed a model for staffing and operating a news service from a university site that can continue successfully, and we believe, can be replicated at other university sites throughout the country. We envision the establishment of CAMEO Feature News "bureaus" on other campuses across the county. Materials to support the creation of a bureau and the training of staff have already been developed here at Tufts; CFN will make them available to others. Regional bureaus could gather stories locally, much as CFN presently does in the New England area; all Summaries would be posted on one web site with material indexed by both content and location. This would allow the production of the home-grown stories that are the bread and butter of the local reporter, as well as national distribution of stories that are of broader interest.

Student staffing is a tremendous advantage in many ways, particularly financially. Since CFN is a free service largely dependent on foundations, it is essential that costs be minimized. Students provide a very intelligent, highly motivated labor pool, whose efforts have been rewarded in part by the awarding of course credit. Since student involvement requires substantial supervision by well-trained professionals, it is fortunate that faculty, whose time is donated, and advanced graduate students, who receive course credit, are able to supervise their training. In addition, CAMEO Feature News has created a set of training materials and supporting materials to facilitate the development of a student-staff, with good results. The present director, who has extensive training and experience as an educator, has the primary responsibility for developing materials and training the staff.

With a well-designed web site, an attractive product, and the operational structure in place, CAMEO Feature News enters the next phase in its development, that of marketing itself to its several constituencies. CFN must make itself known to a wide network of journalists as a valuable source for stories and supporting material; it must also get the word out to the many community organizations that serve children and families. As those partners increase in number and take on a more active role in the compiling of Summaries, the number of Summaries CFN can produce will increase exponentially. Plans are currently underway to address this next phase of marketing.

Long term sustainability, of course, rests on adequate financial support. CAMEO Feature News is a novel approach to a familiar problem. It brings together the field of journalism/media and child development/academia in a new way that has enormous potential to improve the coverage of children. Funding poses a distinct challenge, in part due to the novelty and creativity of the approach we have taken; it is difficult to find funders who have defined their funding priorities flexibly enough to encompass such a hybrid. Foundations are accustomed to funding media efforts or child development efforts, but they rarely fund projects at the intersection of these disciplines. Other avenues of support, such as fee-for-service or sponsorship offer promising possibilities once the service is more fully developed.

LESSONS LEARNED FROM THE PARTNERSHIP

Bringing CAMEO Feature News from the idea stage into concrete reality was an eye-opening venture. One discovery was that the university needed to reach out aggressively to community groups in order to enlist their participation. Once the initial contact was made the response was uniformly receptive and enthusiastic. Another discovery was the variety of work going on that we didn't know about until we began to approach both umbrella organizations and local community groups. Yet another was the somewhat shocked discovery, from our perch in a sophisticated research institution, of the extent to which organizations lacked access to technology we considered routine, such as Email. We were even more surprised to find that many reporters were in the same predicament, and that journalists, especially those in TV, had few contacts in academia and no research funds or personnel devoted to research.

On the university end, we learned how rewarding and enlightening it can be for students to move into the field and work with practitioners to identify the important stories there, to visit programs and meet clients. They are eager to apply their knowledge from the classroom, especially the advanced undergraduates who view CFN involvement as a transition to the real world of work. The CAMEO experience is valuable as a hands-on application of knowledge. In addition, it stimulates thinking and motivates students to learn more. We also realized how valuable the support and participation of our colleagues was to the project; it is critical to marshal and nurture their involvement.

WHY WAS THIS A SUCCESSFUL PARTNERSHIP?

CAMEO Feature News is an unusual partnership. It was something that hadn't been tried before and that evolved out of input from several constituencies. Factors contributing to success included:

- mutual goals shared by university and community partners
- university initiation of contact with community partners and active solicitation of their ideas

- umbrella organizations and individual community agencies were eager to collaborate and willing to make a considerable effort to see that work was successful
- intense involvement of Tufts faculty and students
- support from Tufts administration in the form of resources (funds, space)
- support and interest from the end users of this service—journalists.

REFERENCES

The Advertising Council. (1995). *Summary of the Advertising Council's Strategic Task Force on Research*. Unpublished manuscript.

Bonk, K., & Wiley, M. (1994). *Communications strategies for policy agenda setting*. New Haven: *Quality 2000* Working Paper.

Casey Journalism Center for Children and Families. (1995). *Children and family journalism: Out from the shadows. Media coverage of children and family issues* (Research Report). College Park, Maryland: Casey Journalism Center.

Columbia University Graduate School of Journalism. (1992). *Report of the 1992 media conference, "Focus on Children: The Beat of the Future"*. New York, NY: Columbia University Graduate School of Journalism.

Fisher, C. B., & Osofsky, J. (1997). *Training the applied developmental scientist for prevention and practice: Two current examples*. Social Policy Report: SRCD, Vol. 21, p. 1-18.

Kunkel, D. (1996). How the news media "see" kids. In E. E. Dennis & E. C. Pease (Eds.), *Children and the media*. New Brunswick, NJ: Transaction Publishers, pp. 57-62.

Sigel, I. E. (1990). Ethical concerns for the use of research findings in applied settings. In C. B. Fisher & W. W. Tryon (Eds.), *Ethics in applied developmental psychology: Emerging issues in an emerging field*. Norwood, NJ: ABLEX, pp. 113-144.

Trost, C. (1996). From unseen and unheard to Kidsbeat. In E. E. Dennis & E. C. Pease (Eds.), *Children and the media*. New Brunswick, NJ: Transaction Publishers, pp. 47-56.

25 DEVELOPING AN EXTENDED SERVICES SCHOOL: A SCHOOL-COMMUNITY-UNIVERSITY PARTNERSHIP

Mary E. Walsh
Dita G. Andersson
Michael A. Smyer
Boston College

For the past several years, faculty and students from Boston College have been engaged in a school-community-university partnership committed to improving the life chances of children and families in the local community. The development of this partnership has a complex history involving many aspects of the both the university and the community. In this paper, we describe the nature of the partnership (i.e., its purposes and goals), the process through which this partnership developed, its goals and achievements, and some of its key learnings regarding what factors best facilitate the development of a successful partnership.

NATURE OF THE PARTNERSHIP: ITS PURPOSES AND GOALS

The partnership that has developed between Boston College, the Gardner Elementary School, and the local community has as its primary purpose the enhancement of the academic and social development of children by forging strong connections between family, school, and community. Located in a Boston neighborhood about four miles from campus, the Gardner Elementary School faces the complex issues typical of urban schools across the country (Wang & Kovach, 1996). Of the population of 500 students, 80% percent are students of color and 80% percent meet the federal poverty guidelines. For 78% of these children, English is a second language with more than 31 different languages spoken among their families. The more immediate goal of the partnership has been to transform this traditional, urban public school into an "extended services school" which would: 1) extend the school day to provide before and after school programs for children and evening programs for adults, and 2) extend the range and availability of services offered to both children and adults. Through this transformation, the partnership hopes to enable all children to become successful learners and productive citizens.

DEVELOPMENT OF THE EXTENDED SERVICES SCHOOL: AN ANALYSIS OF THE PROCESS

The development of the Extended Services School was the product of a complex series of interactions between the university and the Gardner Elementary School. The university faculty had first become involved with this school in a manner typical for academics, that is, collecting data for a research study. At the conclusion of this project, as the university researchers said the usual "thanks and farewell," the Gardner teachers and administrators interrupted the leave-taking with a request for assistance from the university in solving problems that were important to the school. They believed that issues related to students' health, safety, psychological well being, economic circumstances, immigration status, and family problems were interfering with the academic success of their students and expressed a hope that university professionals would provide them with "answers" and "solutions."

While daunting, the school's request seemed like a match for the interests of the university faculty group which had been meeting informally to address a common set of concerns about the condition of America's children and families, particularly those living in poverty (Brabeck, et al., 1998). This group consisted of self-selected faculty from across various professional programs (Law, Social Work, Nursing, Education, Psychology, Management) as well as from departments in Arts and Sciences. A continuing series of conversations among these faculty highlighted the isolated character of each profession's approach to working with what they variously referred to as "clients," "patients," or "students." Consistent with what many policy experts had been pointing out, these faculty discussions made clear that an individual seeking assistance from one or more of these professions would most likely experience fragmented and uncoordinated care (Lerner & Simon, 1998; Peterson, 1995; Schorr, 1997). Each profession acknowledged that it was singularly ignorant of the issues and approaches of other professions and of how these differences might impact the client.

To address the need to collaborate across professions, university faculty and administrators committed themselves to the development of a formal structure—the Center for Child, Family, and Community Partnerships—to promote interprofessional collaboration in the university as well as outreach scholarship in the community. However, despite this intensified activity at the university, faculty quickly realized that their efforts would remain abstract and ungrounded unless they were informed and shaped by professionals in the community who had experience "in the trenches." For this reason, they were seeking a community site serving children and families in which they could learn how to integrate the realities of practice with the theory of interprofessional collaboration. In this way, the Gardner school's plea for assistance in its efforts to respond adequately to the full range of its students' needs—social, psychological, health and educational—merged with the university's desire to work in a community site. This convergence of goals marked the beginning of the school-university partnership.

In the years that followed, university and school professionals engaged in a dialogue that would attempt to co-determine not only the answers and solutions, but more fundamentally, the very definition of the problem (Walsh, Buckley & Howard, 1998). In keeping with their professional practice focus on the individual person, the university faculty viewed "the problem" as located within the child, or at least, within the school. While they recognized that the barriers to learning experienced by each of these children were the product of numerous external forces, they were accustomed to employing a traditional clinical model that located the problem almost exclusively within the particular child. As a consequence, they understood the "problem" to be each child's level of academic achievement and suggested that the changes that would benefit the children and families of the Gardner School could be made within the context of the school building. In simplest terms, their defined objective was to "fix" the child.

The school principal, however, quickly challenged this definition. "The problem is not located in the child," she said, "but in the many worlds that the child must traverse." She clearly saw the child as embedded in many contexts and located the problem in the relationship between the child and those contexts. Similarly, she viewed the school's difficulties as part of the problems of the larger community and suggested that the school should play a vital role in helping to build stronger families and communities that, in turn, would better support the development of their children. She pointed to particular stressors which interfered with parents' ability to support their child's education (e.g., inadequate after-school care, limited English proficiency, lack of access to necessary health care, immigration-related legal difficulties). The principal argued that the school had a responsibility to alleviate some of these difficulties rather than to continue to view such problems as irrelevant to its objectives. For university professionals, these identified issues did not fit within the parameters of what they had always viewed clinically as "the problem" (Bibace et. al, in preparation). "Fixing the child" was a good distance from intervening in the systems which surrounded the child (Lerner, Walsh & Howard, in press).

What emerged from these discussions was a partnership that not only embraced the school and university, but, very importantly, the community. The community "brought to the table" the large number of community resources and agencies necessary to develop a concrete intervention strategy. The partnership, consisting of parents, community agencies, and university faculty, met weekly for two years to plan a response to the concerns of the school and community about their children.

Consistent with each partner's emphasis on the impact of context on development, and with funding from the DeWitt Wallace Reader's Digest Foundation, the intervention that seemed to the partners to flow logically from the needs of the children and families as well as the capabilities and resources of the partners was a transformation of the school into an Extended Services School. Adapted from the model of the Children's Aid Society Schools in New York City, this type of school would not only extend the school day into after-school, week-end, and summer hours, it would also focus specifically upon integrating academic instruction with opportunities for enrichment, career exploration, youth development, and family support services (Dryfoos, 1994). By forging a link between the school and larger community, it would not only respond to the needs of children, but also those of adults. To mobilize and coordinate the involvement of other agencies in the community and neighborhood, the partnership reached out to a local YMCA to serve as its lead agency.

GOAL-RELATED ACHIEVEMENTS

Since its inception, the Gardner Extended Services School has launched a number of programs of significance to the community. For example, it now not only offers an extensive after-school enrichment program for children and adolescents, but it also provides parents and community members with health-care, legal assistance, mental health services, job counseling, ESL courses, and computer training. In addition to the development of these programs, this partnership has also been successful in addressing policy issues that significantly impact the project. For example, it has been able to secure janitorial coverage for the late evening hours by working with the local unions and Boston public school system. Critically, for the project, partnership members are gaining a larger voice in city and state policy issues regarding comprehensive, coordinated care for children. Finally, while it is too early in the project to measure long-term outcomes, the partners expect eventually to see changes in academic achievement, social development, and other areas important to the participants. Evaluating these types of programs has been recognized as a difficult and complex task (Schorr, 1997). The project will be assisted in this effort by serving as one of the sites of a formal evaluation conducted by its primary funder, the DeWitt Wallace Foundation.

CRITICAL FACTORS ASSOCIATED WITH THE SUCCESS OF THIS PARTNERSHIP

Many factors have contributed to the short-term success of this fledgling project. For example, the ability to partner successfully has been aided in no small part by a shared set of beliefs among both university-based and community-based partners about the nature of human development. Their conceptual agreement that, (a) development occurs in relationship to various contexts, (b) development is reflected at multiple levels (e.g., biological, social, and psychological), and (c) development involves a pattern of both strength and deficits, greatly facilitated their ability to negotiate with one another (Lerner, 1996).

The potential success of the project was also significantly enhanced by a shift in the usual arrangements for funding. In contrast to the usual university-school collaborations in which either the university or the public school most frequently serves as the recipient of and fiscal agent for the funding, the partnership located the largest of its grants in the community partner, that is, the local YMCA. This represented a fundamental shift for the school which recognized that locating the grant in the community meant sharing control of the program with the community. It also required a fundamental change in the orientation of the university which typically received the "overhead" from faculty-authored grants. As a Jesuit university, whose mission statement explicitly calls for the generation of knowledge that can make a difference in human lives, Boston College recognized the central importance, for faculty and students, of engaging in outreach scholarship. For this reason, it was willing to relinquish both the control and the funds related to this partnership.

University students have also made a significant contribution to the positive outcomes which the project has enjoyed. The project has served as a practicum site for graduate and undergraduate students in a wide range of professions and disciplines. They have engaged in learning experiences that focus on inter-professional collaboration in a setting that requires their working together. In addition, students seeking service-learning projects have enhanced the ability of the project to reach a larger number of children and parents (Brabeck, Walsh, Kenny & Comilang, 1997).

KEY LEARNINGS FROM THIS PARTNERSHIP

By partnering with the school and community in the identification of the problem and the design and implementation of interventions, university faculty have come to view "co-learning" as an essential component for a partnership. The members of the partnership realize that no one partner is *the* expert, but that the work will require different expertise at different times. Sharing the role of the "expert" as a function of the task allowed for the dissolution of a permanent hierarchy and the creation of flexible hierarchies which could respond to the needs of the moment (Bibace, et. al, in preparation). What had begun as a vertical relationship became a horizontal one in which each partner brought a different type of knowledge and expertise.

Through the process of co-learning, the partnership has become clearer about identifying the strengths of each partner. For example, it relies on university faculty to coordinate and implement the program evaluation but, in the design of that evaluation, it relies on parents and children to define the project outcomes which are important to the community (Walsh & Madaus, 1997). There is a recognition that the work necessitates such an interplay of distinct professional capabilities. While the university partners were able to draw upon knowledge of research to inform the development and implementation of an effective program for children and families, they required the involvement of the community in order to design a program that spoke to the particular needs of this locale. Similarly, while the school partners had immediate experience in "what worked" in daily practice, they benefited from the university's expertise in what have been identified as "best practices" for youth and family programs on a more national level.

PROSPECTS FOR LONG-TERM SUSTAINABILITY

The relationship between the Gardner School, the community, and Boston College has now existed for several years. All participants recognize the challenge of sustainability and have taken steps to insure the survival of the project. A Steering Committee, including an equal number of representatives from each member of the partnership (school, community, and university), provides a process for making decisions, for problem-solving, and for proposing new areas for growth. In addition, institutional commitments have been secured by this Steering Committee. That is, the leadership of the partners' larger organizations—in particular, the university president, the director of the area YMCA, and the superintendent of schools—have each publicly supported this collaborative effort. The public support of the university was demonstrated when the Gardner School principal was awarded an honorary degree by the university for her efforts to address the barriers to learning experienced by so many of these children. Perhaps of greatest importance in sustaining the project is each partner's repeated efforts to place the common goals of the project ahead of their individual, institutional goals. This is a particularly difficult stance for small, underfunded agencies that are struggling to survive financially.

The partners recognize both the necessity and the perils of "going to scale." At the same time, they do not want to confine the learnings of this project to an isolated pilot program. They have begun a process of dialogue in the community with other public schools, agencies and universities, as well as with potential funders about which aspects of this project would be essential in any community-wide replication. While the project has received funding from the DeWitt Wallace Reader's Digest Foundation and has other sources of support, the leaders of this partnership appreciate that in order to sustain and replicate this program, it will be essential to develop financial strategies that go beyond grant support or "soft money." They realize that they will need to determine how to drive existing funding streams (both national and local) into the project, and recently have begun to work with the current state legislature to enact legislation that may eventually assist these projects.

The project has not been without challenges. While the institutions involved may share a common conceptual framework, they have different histories, cultures and immediate purposes (Eccles, 1996). Involving parents who speak such a variety of languages and whose undocumented status makes them afraid to approach any public institution has been a slow and difficult process. Court-ordered school busing to achieve racial integration has resulted in a school population that comes from not one, but multiple communities that are spread over the entire City of Boston. "Linking school and community" in this complicated context remains a continual challenge to the partners.

The university faculty have also confronted their own set of challenges in their efforts to participate in this work. That is, the current reward system of universities promotes independent scholarly contributions and provides little incentive, particularly for untenured faculty, to invest time in the collaborative efforts required for outreach scholarship. Efforts to modify these and other university structures in order to promote an increase in outreach scholarship occur in slow, small steps. Despite these challenges, project participants have come to realize that in a partnership, however imperfect, they can negotiate the problem and proposed solutions, learn from and teach one another, and in a struggle that parallels that of the larger human community, provide some positive responses to the issues faced by children and families.

REFERENCES

Bibace, R., Dillon, J., & Dowds, B. (Eds.). (in press). Partnerships in research, clinical, and educational settings. In I. Sigel (Series Ed.), *Advances in Applied Development Monograph Series*. Hillsdale, NJ: Erlbaum.

Brabeck, M., Cawthorne, J., Cochran-Smith, M., Gaspard, N., Hurd-Green, C., Kenny, M., Krawczyk, R., Lowery, C., Lykes, M. B., Minuskin, A. D., Mooney, J., Ross, C. J., Savage, J., Soifer, A., Smyer, A., Sparks, E., Tourse, R., Turillo, R. M., Waddock, S., Walsh, M., & Zollers, N. (1998). Changing the culture of the university to engage in outreach scholarship. In R. M. Lerner & L. A. K. Simon (Eds.), *Building university-community collaborations for the twenty-first century: Outreach scholarship for youth and families* (pp. 335-364). New York: Garland Press.

Brabeck, M., Walsh, M., Kenny, M., & Comilang, K. (1997). Interprofessional collaboration for children and families: Opportunities for counseling psychology in the 21st century. *The Counseling Psychologist, 25*(4), 615-636.

Bronfrenbrenner, U., & Crouter, A. C. (1983). The evolution of environmental models in developmental research. In P.H. Mussen (Ed.), *Handbook of child psychology: History, theory, and methods: Vol. 1* (pp. 357-414). New York: Wiley.

Dryfoos, J. G. (1994). *Full service schools: A revolution in health and social services of children, youth, and families.* San Francisco: Jossey-Bass.

Eccles, J. (1996). The power and difficulty of university-community collaboration. *Journal of Research on Adolescence, 6*(1), 81-86.

Lerner, R. M. (1996). Relative plasticity, integration, temporality, and diversity in human development: A developmental contextual perspective about theory, process, and method. *Developmental Psychology, 32*(4), 781-786.

Lerner, R. M., & Simon, L. A. K. (1998). *University-community collaboration for the 21st Century: Outreach scholarship for youth and families.* New York: Garland Press.

Lerner, R. M., Walsh, M. E., & Howard, K. A. (1998). Developmental-contextual considerations: Person-context relations as the bases for risk and resiliency in child and adolescent development. In A.S. Bellack & M. Hersen (Eds.), *Comprehensive clinical psychiatry: Vol. 5. Children and adolescents: Clinical formulations and treatment* (pp. 1-24). New York: Elsevier Science.

Peterson, G. (1995). The need for common principles in prevention programs for children, adolescents, and families. *Journal of Adolescent Research, 10*(4), 427-448.

Schorr, L. (1997). *Common purpose: Strengthening families and neighborhoods to rebuild America.* New York: Anchor Books.

Walsh, M. E., Buckley, M., & Howard, K. A. (1998). Critical collaborations: School, family, and community. In R. Haney & J. O'Keefe (Eds.), *Conversations in excellence: Providing for the diverse needs of youth and their families* (pp. 63-84). Washington, DC: NCEA.

Walsh, M. E., & Madaus, G. (1997). Evaluation of an extended services school in Boston. *The Evaluation Exchange, 3*(2), 10-11.

Wang, M., & Kovach, J. (1996). Bridging the achievement gap in urban schools: Reducing educational segregation and advancing resilience-promoting strategies. In Williams, B. (Ed.), *Closing the achievement gap: A vision for changing beliefs and practices* (pp. 10-36). Alexandria, VA: Association for Supervision and Curriculum Development.

26 FAMILY T.I.E.S. FAMILY SUPPORT PROGRAM FOR ADOLESCENT MOTHERS AND THEIR CHILDREN: A COLLABORATION BETWEEN MOTT CHILDREN'S HEALTH CENTER AND MICHIGAN STATE UNIVERSITY

Laura Bates
Tom Luster
Michigan State University

Donna Massie
Judith Peck Key
Mott Children's Health Center

BACKGROUND OF THE PARTNERSHIP

Like many successful relationships, the partnership between Michigan State University (MSU) and Mott Children's Health Center (MCHC) began as a short-term, informal collaboration that expanded and evolved over time into an ongoing relationship that is now in its seventh year. From simple beginnings the partnership grew to include several university departments and a variety of health center programs; however, this chapter will discuss the original collaboration formed to address the problem of adolescent parenthood.

In 1990 Flint, Michigan and the surrounding area were struggling with a deteriorating economic situation brought on by many years of downsizing in the auto industry, the area's major employer. Between 1980 and 1990 the proportion of children in Genesee County who lived in poverty had grown from 14.3% to 24.9%. Moreover, in 1990 about 30% of the children lived in single parent families, and 69% of children under 6 who lived in female-headed households were living below the poverty level (Kids Count in Michigan, 1995). During the same period, the Genesee County rate of births to teens 15-17 years old was over 30% higher than the state average (Priority 90's, 1991).

MCHC, a privately endowed health center with a long history of service to low income children and youth in Genesee County, decided to respond to concerns about the rising rate of adolescent parenthood and resulting child poverty by launching a major, community-wide initiative to assist low-income teen mothers and their children to overcome the negative consequences of early childbearing. Adolescent mothers are less likely than their peers who delay childbearing to complete high school or receive postsecondary education, and thus, are at risk for living in poverty. The children of adolescent mothers tend to lag behind their peers on cognitive assessments in the preschool years, and many of these children arrive at school with academic skills that are not on par with those of their classmates. Although teenage mothers and their children, on average, do less well than their peers, there are marked individual differences within samples of teenage mothers and their children. Some do well while others struggle. MCHC hoped to increase the number of teenage mothers and their children who fared well despite the challenges of early childbearing.

GOALS OF THE PARTNERSHIP

Seeking to design an intervention program that would reflect "best practice" in the field, MCHC convened a community advisory committee made up of professionals from their own staff and the Flint community, as well as the second author, a professor in the MSU Department of Family and Child Ecology who had done previous research on teen parenting and early intervention. His initial role was to offer the committee insights gleaned from research regarding adolescent parents and their children and about what "works" in early intervention programs.

The program resulting from this initiative was Family T.I.E.S. (Trust, Information, Encouragement, Support), a five-year family support program based on the principles developed from the experience of professionals and recent research (Olds & Kitzman, 1990; Schorr, 1988). Both sources of information suggested that Family T.I.E.S. was most likely to be successful if: a) the primary person providing the intervention establishes a close relationship with the young mother; b) the program is long term; c) case loads are small; d) the person working with the families is able to cross traditional service delivery boundaries; and e) the program is ecologically oriented, that is, it focuses on the infant, the mother, the mother's support system, and the larger context rather than on any one of these components. Services were provided by Family Advocates, paraprofessional workers who lived in the Flint community.

At the outset it was decided that evaluation of the program's success in achieving the stated goals would be an integral part of the design and MSU was asked to design and oversee a five-year program evaluation. The outcomes of interest for the mothers included completing high school and eventually finding adequate employment, avoiding additional unintended pregnancies, and providing high quality care for their children. The psychological well-being of the young mothers was also emphasized in this program, because teens' ability to nurture their children and to take advantage of services that are available are likely to depend on their psychological adjustment (Schorr, 1988). The primary goal for the children was to help them deal successfully with developmental tasks during the first five years of life so that they arrived at school prepared to succeed in that setting.

The goals of the partnership were not formally stated at the outset but gradually expanded from initial sharing of information in an advisory capacity to full cooperation in an extensive program evaluation. Over time, other goals were added, such as coordination of community services and identification of service gaps, and the development of an assessment tool that would help programs to identify individual teens referred for service according to their level of risk. At the same time, the longitudinal nature of the study allowed the university to conduct basic research on the factors contributing to successful outcomes for teen mothers and their children.

At a time of increasing need and diminishing resources, program evaluation was seen by MCHC as a means by which they could assess the impact of their investment and allocate resources in the most effective manner. Finally, the partnership could be used to bring all aspects of the community together to define a common strategy for supporting young families.

BENEFITS OF THE PARTNERSHIP FOR MSU

What was gained by MSU as a result of the collaboration? As noted in our Mission Statement, MSU is committed to "developing new knowledge and conveying that knowledge to its students and to the public...and to contributing to the understanding and solution of significant social problems." Family T.I.E.S. provided us with an opportunity to gain new insights into adolescent parenthood. It also provided us with opportunities to do a number of things that are valued at the University: a) publish in peer-reviewed journals; b) obtain external funding for research; and c) train students to do research. The findings from Family T.I.E.S. also raised new questions that led to further research. In this section, we will provide some examples of how the collaboration between MSU and MCHC contributed to the Land Grant Mission of MSU.

Family T.I.E.S. offered to us an unusual opportunity to conduct longitudinal research about young mothers and their children because the program and its evaluation lasted for five years. Without the assistance and persistence of the Family Advocates, who were all local residents with a network of sources within community, we would never have been able to keep track of this transient group of teens, many of whom had lived in unstable or even chaotic circumstances.

The longitudinal nature of the study allowed us to address questions that could not be addressed with cross-sectional data. For example, we were able to determine if the adolescents' childrearing beliefs, which were assessed before the children were born, were predictive of the adolescents' parenting practices in subsequent years (Luster, Perlsadt, McKinney, Sims, & Juang, 1996; Luster, 1998).

Because data were collected at nine points in time, the data set is an unusually rich source of information about adolescent parents. We learned a great deal about the adolescents, their developmental history, and their current circumstances. The Family Advocates who worked with the young mothers on a weekly basis proved to be a particularly valuable source of information. Working with the families for five years, the Family Advocates had insights into the young mothers and their families that we could not hope to obtain from our interviews with the young mothers or our brief observations of their parenting practices during assessments in the home. In fact, the advocates' assessments of the teens and their circumstances six months after the children were born were far more useful for predicting later outcomes for both the young mothers and their children than was the information we collected from the adolescents at the same time (Luster, 1998; Luster, Fitzgerald, Bates, Key, & Walton-Ramsey, 1998). This rich data set was an important factor in obtaining funding from the Spencer Foundation to conduct a follow up study of the children in early elementary school.

Another valuable outcome of this collaboration was that the information we gained from working with adolescent mothers in Family T.I.E.S. led to further research questions that we explored with other data sets. Our early conversations with the Family Advocates led us to think more about who becomes a teenage mother (i.e., selection factors). Clearly, many of their clients lived in challenging circumstances and had known challenging circumstances in the years before their children were born. It is important to understand more about the characteristics and circumstances of teens who become parents if we want to understand how they parent and other outcomes such as educational attainment. This led to research on the antecedents of adolescent pregnancy (Luster & Small, 1994; Small & Luster, 1994; Perkins, Luster, Villarruel, & Small, 1998). The Family T.I.E.S. research also piqued our interest in the role of sexual abuse in teenage parenthood (Luster & Small, 1997).

Part of our mission is to train the next generation of researchers. Family T.I.E.S. provided opportunities for graduate and undergraduate students to be involved in data collection, data analysis, conference presentations, and publications. In addition, interaction with program workers helped students to understand more fully the difficulties of translating research results into effective programs and in applying theoretical knowledge to actual people. We hope that it also made them more sensitive to the fact that research is an intrusion into the lives of its subjects and should always be conducted with respect for the individuals involved.

BENEFITS OF THE PARTNERSHIP FOR MCHC

Important benefits were gained from this partnership for MCHC and the Flint community. A major benefit from the health center's point of view was tapping into the expertise of the university to develop program outcomes based on current knowledge and in evaluating the efficacy of service programs. In an era of diminishing resources, evaluation of program outcomes is essential for more efficient use of existing resources and for securing new resources. In 1991, systematic evaluation of program outcomes was a new endeavor for the health center, and through the partnership MCHC learned a great deal about developing measurable outcomes and program objectives. The skills developed by staff in defining and evaluating program outcomes have been invaluable in writing program proposals to attract new monies in support of innovative programs. For example, MCHC won the contract from the state welfare agency to provide services to pregnant and parenting teens who are welfare recipients in Genesee County.

Information from the Family T.I.E.S. data set has been used by program supervisors to more accurately assess the service needs of adolescents entering this new program. With assistance from MSU staff they have developed an assessment tool that identifies factors we found to be associated with poor outcomes for the teens or their children. These teens are then given greater support from staff, while those with fewer risks can be served less intensively. In addition, both research and practice have indicated that the mental health status of the teen does predict her parenting practices and her own success; this has led to a greater understanding of the need for mental health services for teens in the Flint Community.

The young mothers in Family T.I.E.S. had been randomly assigned to one of two treatment groups when they enrolled. Although there was clear evidence that many young mothers in each group benefited from the services they received, the program evaluation did not demonstrate significant advantages of an intensive social support model for teens in producing successful outcomes. Young mothers who received less intensive service were as successful as those who received more intensive services in this study.

MCHC is now modifying its program for teen mothers, in part based on the Family T.I.E.S. evaluation, and has put resources into new programs of family support. A major new initiative has been launched to provide education and employment assistance, support in relationship-building, responsibility training, and parenting education to young fathers. Girls who enter the teen mothers' program may refer their child's father for services as well.

The partnership also proved to be a valuable resource for staff development. It exposed Family Advocates and other health center staff to recent research on adolescent parenting, and to knowledge about program interventions for teen parents and young children. In addition, MCHC staff were frequently included in training for data collectors on the use of various assessment tools they could use in their own work. For example, Robert Bradley, one of the developers of the Home Observation for Measurement of the Environment (HOME) inventory, came to Flint to train staff on his widely-used instrument.

Equally important were the opportunities the university contact provided for staff to interact informally with university personnel, forming mutually beneficial relationships. The Family Advocates were all paraprofessional staff who brought considerable life experiences to their work but who had varying degrees of experience with university-level education. Not only did they learn about the university as a resource for their own professional development, but they also contributed to the university programs by making presentations to classes and to researchers about the realities of work with teen parents. While this exposure is only one of many factors that may have contributed to their personal career decisions, it is worth noting that six of the original seven Family Advocates are still working in a human service field, and a majority have pursued additional university training. Several have already achieved distinction in academic pursuits. For example, one former Family Advocate recently won a Dr. Charles Drew International Research Fellowship to conduct field research in Africa.

The partnership also helped the health center and the university to increase their communication with the shapers of social policy in the state. Through periodic MSU/Mott research policy rounds, both institutions had the opportunity to meet with members of local and state governmental entities and to share research-based information about the needs of adolescent parents and the impact of social policy decisions on real people. These meetings provoked a lively interchange of ideas and helped to bring the families to life for policy makers.

BUILDING A SUCCESSFUL COLLABORATION

Although both institutions have been pleased with the benefits of this partnership and continue to work together, there were important issues that had to be dealt with along the road in order to make the collaboration work. Some of the issues that had to be resolved were related to the differing missions of the two institutions (provision of health services vs. knowledge generation). The early decision to compare two levels of services in Family T.I.E.S. provides a good example of the need to find solutions that are workable for both parties in a collaboration. The health center traditionally provides the most intensive services to clients who are identified as having the greatest needs. Some members of the Community Advisory Committee (CAC) favored assigning the adolescents who were at highest risk to an intensive treatment group and the adolescents who were at lowest risk to a less intensive treatment group. If this strategy had been followed, it would have been very difficult to evaluate the program because the two treatment groups would have been so different at the start of the study. The ideal design for researchers is to randomly assign the adolescents to either a treatment group or a no-treatment control group. However, the use of a no-treatment control group was unacceptable to the CAC. They believed strongly it was unethical to study adolescent mothers and their children without providing services if problems were detected. The compromise solution that was acceptable to everyone involved was to randomly assign the young mothers to one of two treatment groups (more intensive vs. less intensive services). In this way the two groups would be comparable and no family would go without needed services if needs were identified. This research design is not ideal for evaluation purposes since the risk of concluding that the program was not effective (when, in fact, it was effective) is greater when two treatment groups are compared rather than when a treatment group is compared with a no-treatment control group. However, researchers must conduct their studies in ways that are acceptable to the community.

Other key components of a successful collaboration include mutual respect and trust. Because universities tend to be concerned with long term outcomes while service agencies are charged with helping people right now, often on a crisis intervention basis, there was some concern that the university had more to gain than did the community from the evaluation of Family T.I.E.S. Some members of the Flint community believed that poor people are "studied to death" to obtain information for publication, without apparent benefit for the people studied.

This is a legitimate concern and, therefore, it is imperative that evaluators provide feedback to service providers in a timely manner so that information can be used to make course corrections in the program, and so that the special needs of individual families (e.g., a child who is having problems in the area of language development) can be addressed as expeditiously as possible. We recognized and acknowledged that research was an intrusion into the lives of the participants and into the work of the health center; therefore, we worked to minimize the impact of the research on program operations and regularly sought feedback from the MCHC staff about how the research was being perceived.

Research-policy rounds were another avenue for bringing research results to the community in a more timely manner. At the same time, community leaders could respond to the findings before publication and sensitive issues could be addressed. We found that to be successful, university personnel who work in the community must possess sensitivity, willingness to listen, and respect for the study participants in addition to good research skills.

Developing trust among individual staff persons was also important, because, as any good administrator knows, the success of a new project is largely dependent on the support and cooperation of the persons who carry out daily activities. Initially the program staff did not see the research as benefiting the teens currently in the program; therefore they had reservations about the time they were asked to spend scheduling research assessments. In addition, they were concerned that the data collectors might be judgmental about their clients or insensitive to cultural differences.

The evaluation team began to give Family Advocates feedback from the child assessments as soon as they were done, so that they could celebrate successes and address concerns with family members. The information helped advocates direct families to appropriate resources for early intervention. In addition, the researchers sought input from the Family Advocates in planning each wave of data collection. They reviewed research instruments that the evaluators developed and questions that they thought were confusing for the teens or culturally biased were revised or eliminated. Interviews with the Family Advocates about their perceptions of the impact they were having on the young mothers also led the research teams to measure additional outcomes, such as the adolescents' sense of trust in others. Assessments were shortened after they reported negative feedback from the teens, and questionnaires and consent forms were reviewed by the MCHC reading specialist to ensure they were at an appropriate reading level for our group.

Over time we learned that housing the research staff in the same location as the program staff, and having them participate in some of the staff functions helped greatly to overcome initial mistrust. Giving each staff a thorough orientation to the purpose and activities of the other organization helped to build a sense of being members of one team, as did training local residents or students from the Flint community to do the data collection. These changes not only alleviated some staff concerns but also improved the quality of the data collected.

CONCLUSION

Although the two organizations have different missions, we shared a common goal in this enterprise. The health center and the university were both committed to improving the life chances of adolescent mothers and their children. Even though we were particularly concerned about the well-being of the 142 families who enrolled in the program, all parties involved hoped that the insights we gained from this project would be valuable to adolescent mothers and their children generally and to those who provide services to this population. Because of this common goal, there were few issues that could have undermined our working relationship, and it was relatively easy to arrive at consensual decisions. However, even when a collaboration works well, addressing a complex social issue, such as early childbearing, is a challenging task.

Urie Bronfenbrenner (1979) is fond of quoting one of his mentors, Walter Fenno Dearborn, who said, "If you want to understand something, try to change it" (p. 37). The wisdom of those words became apparent to us during Family T.I.E.S. We learned a great deal about early childbearing by trying to improve the outcomes of adolescent mothers and their children. We also gained a new appreciation for the complex lives of teenage mothers. Family T.I.E.S. did not achieve all of the (probably unrealistic) goals that we set when the program was created. However, the successes that we experienced in the program depended upon the expertise and resources of both institutions, and in particular, the tireless efforts of the Family Advocates.

REFERENCES

Bronfenbrenner, U. (1979). *The ecology of human development.* Cambridge, MA: Harvard University Press.

Kids Count in Michigan. (1995). Produced by Michigan's Children, Michigan League for Human Services, and Michigan State University. Retrieved March 22, 1998 from gopher://genesee. freenet.org:70/00/comserv/prio/fa/Genk/kc95.

Luster, T. (1998). Individual differences in the caregiving behavior of teenage mothers: An ecological perspective. *Clinical child psychology and psychiatry, 3,* 341-360.

Luster, T., Fitzgerald, H., Bates, L., Key, J. P., & Walton-Ramsey, T. (1998). *Findings from a five-year family support program for adolescent mothers.* Paper presented at the Society for Research on Adolescence, San Diego, CA.

Luster, T., Perlstadt, H., McKinney, M., Sims, K., & Juang, L. (1996). The effects of a family support program and other factors on the home environment provided by adolescent mothers. *Family Relations, 45,* 255-264.

Luster, T. & Small, S. A. (1994). Factors associated with sexual risk-taking behaviors among adolescents. *Journal of Marriage and the Family, 56,* 622-632.

Luster, T. & Small, S. A. (1997). Sexual abuse history and number of sex partners among female adolescents. *Family Planning Perspectives, 29,* 204-211.

Olds, D. L. & Kitzman, H. (1990). Can home visitation improve the health of women and children at environmental risk? *Pediatrics, 86,* 108-116.

Perkins, D. F., Luster, T., Villarruel, F., & Small, S. A. (1998). An ecological, risk-factor examination of adolescents' sexual activity in three ethnic groups. *Journal of Marriage and the Family, 60,* 660-673.

Priority 90's. (1991). *The quality of life for children and their families in Genesee County*. Flint, MI: The Mott Children's Health Center.

Schorr, L. (1988). *Within our reach: Breaking the cycle of disadvantage.* Garden City, NJ: Anchor Press/Doubleday.

Small, S. A. & Luster, T. (1994). Adolescent sexual activity: An ecological, risk-factor approach. *Journal of Marriage and the Family, 56,* 181-192.

27 CHECKPOINTS: BUILDING CAPACITY TO ENHANCE PROGRAM IMPACT THROUGH EVALUATION

Hiram E. Fitzgerald
L. Annette Abrams
Mary Andrews
Francisco Villarruel
Michigan State University

Robert Brown
United Way of Michigan and University Outreach Partnerships

Celeste Sturdevant Reed
Institute for Children, Youth, and Families

American society is faced with pervasive problems confronting individuals, families, and communities. Issues of child and youth development, of economic competitiveness, of environmental quality, of violence and crime, and of health and health care, require creative solutions and the design, deployment, and evaluation of innovative public policies and intervention programs. There is increasing pressure for universities to take an active role in the development of innovative solutions to these societal problems. Michigan State University has responded to such pressures to design and deliver knowledge applications, in part, through its Applied Developmental Science Program (Fitzgerald, Abrams, Church, Votruba, & Imig, 1996; Lerner, Lerner, Nguyen, Pease, Reiling, Firlan, White, & Freel, 1994). The overarching goal of the ADS Program is to establish university-community partnerships that focus on resolution of community-defined problems.

NATURE OF PARTNERSHIP

Consistent with the strategic plan of United Way of America, United Way of Michigan (UWM) and Local United Ways (LUW) in Michigan were attempting to implement outcome-based evaluation as part of their funding strategy. The idea was simple; outcome-based evaluation could provide a data base to document program performance and, over time, lead to greater accountability of United Way allocations. Implementation of the idea, however, proved to be far more difficult. Few individuals within the United Way system had received training in outcome-based evaluation. UWM, therefore, defined a need for continuing education based on the desire to build capacity for evaluation at the volunteer and professional levels of local human service agencies, with the expectation that such knowledge would lead to improvements in service delivery, program quality and resource allocation, the construction and utilization of developmentally and contextually appropriate assessment instruments, the design and evaluation of developmental interventions and enhancement programs, and the dissemination of knowledge at the level of the individual, family, and community (Abrams, McCrohan & Hembroff, 1995).

In December 1994, a multidisciplinary team of evaluation specialists met to discuss ways to build capacity within human service agencies for evaluation, including various aspects of program evaluation. Michigan State University's representative to the UWM Board (Annette Abrams) reported that UWM had strong interest in outcome-based evaluation. In January 1995, the team met with the UWM Chief Professional Officer (Robert Ivory) and Director of Agency Services (Robert Brown) and forged an agreement to work collaboratively to develop curriculum components and instructional models for an outcome-based evaluation training program. The partnership was based on ADS' model for university-community partnerships which emphasizes shared responsibility for all facets of partnership activities, including funding (Fitzgerald et al., 1996).

ANALYSIS OF THE PROCESS

The planning process began with the creation of a team composed of local United Way representatives and self-selected faculty and staff across disciplines. The team met bi-weekly to discuss recommended content and sequencing. The group agreed that training sessions should be grouped into five areas: Understanding evaluation, designing evaluation, implementing evaluation, using evaluation, and culturally-competent evaluation. Four content areas were suggested for each category, for a total of twelve training days. Faculty and staff, based on their interest and expertise, volunteered to outline essential learning goals for particular training days. What emerged was the curriculum outlined in Table 1. This curriculum outline became the vehicle for eliciting "customer" reactions through focus groups in five Local United Ways. Focus groups brought together United Way directors, staff volunteers, and funded-agencies to share their preferences regarding teaching methods, locations, and fees. The focus group reports (Abrams, 1995, Reed, 1995) provided clear guidance for the creation of a year-long training program to be offered one day each month by faculty and United Way staff. Program recommendations emerging from the focus groups included: 1) New training cohorts should begin every six months in order to accommodate demand, including the high staff turnover in human service agencies; 2) Allow participants to choose a content-only curriculum or an extended curriculum that could lead to certification as a trainer; 3) Avoid homework! Because of time constraints and inadequate agency staffing, homework should not be used. All exercises should be completed in the training sessions.

4) Cultural competence should be integrated throughout the curriculum. It should also, like other essential content areas, be presented in its own in-depth session. 5) A university program should not abandon participants at the end of training. Rather, technical assistance should be offered both during and after training. Technical support and consultation should occur by telephone, electronic mail, and/or facsimile transmission. 6) The training approach should appeal to adult learners, be user friendly, and frequently use case studies and in-basket exercises. Table group interactions should be a predominant form of teaching and learning. 7) The program should certify the competency of program graduates to become local trainers and advisors. This training-of-trainers allows the development of local teams whose members can benefit from exposure to similar information and techniques. All of these recommendations were incorporated in the curriculum design.

Table 1. *CHECKPOINTS: Model Curriculum for Teaching about Evaluation*

A. UNDERSTANDING EVALUATION			
Defining evaluation	Purpose of evaluation	Types of evaluation	Standards for evaluation
B. DESIGNING EVALUATION			
Understanding evaluation methods	Defining outcome objectives	Identifying indicators	Instrument development
C. CULTURAL COMPETENCE			
Definitions	Cultural diversity	Impact on design	Impact on evaluation
D. IMPLEMENTING EVALUATION		**E. USING EVALUATION**	
Collecting data	Analyzing and interpreting data	Communicating evaluation results	Linking evaluation results to program development or improvement

Failed attempts to garner foundation grants for program development led to a request that University Outreach provide start-up funds. The business plan used to justify this investment included projected annual revenues and a schedule for repayment of the University's investment. Upon receipt of University Outreach funding, a small design team began meeting weekly to write training manuals and to hash out details. One design team member was retained (Celeste Reed) to design and implement an assessment of the program's long-term impact on the behavior and decision making within participants' organizations. A series of competency questionnaires were developed to evaluate aspects of the learner, the curriculum, and the trainer (Seabrook, Reed, & Abrams, 1997). In other words, evaluation of the effectiveness of the training program was an integral part of the planning process from the beginning.

ACHIEVEMENTS RELATED TO GOALS

The CHECKPOINTS curriculum is composed of a six-session series of workshops focusing on the basics of outcome oriented program evaluation, and another six-session series of workshops emphasizing the skills and professional context of evaluation that would allow participants to serve as "trainers." The two series are linked together for those individuals who wish to share their skills with others as "train-the-trainer" preparation.

Part I

The basic CHECKPOINTS series of training workshops focuses on the application of evaluation processes and techniques to the realities of today's accountability arena. Hands-on exercises assist participants in recognizing the evaluation and accountability needs and opportunities available within their agencies. A goal of the training experience is to incorporate a proactive strategy within agencies so that the capacity and potential of programs can be documented and predicted for agency-wide and community-wide planning. This entails a careful articulation of the programming activities of the agency along with the theory or logic underlying programs that provide the rationale for various expected outcomes and impacts. A characteristic of CHECKPOINTS is emphasis on the development of cultural sensitivities. Programs are viewed within their cultural context and program evaluations are designed to be consistent with cultural norms and experiences.

A critical portion of the CHECKPOINTS curriculum focuses on the articulation of outcome and impact indicators and potential strategies of measurement. Participants are involved in discussions and case studies of evaluations using various types of indicators and various strategies for measurement or documentation. Both research-oriented and "home-made" indicators are discussed along with the issues of reliability, validity, and efficacy that pertain to quality measurement. Evaluations are viewed as opportunities to document contextual and programmatic features at various stages of programming and for various purposes. A practical approach is reinforced so that agency staff can foresee designing, managing, and institutionalizing evaluation processes using their own expertise. The need for outside expertise and contracting with evaluators is discussed briefly, but reserved for the second six-session series (PART 2). It is anticipated that participants will begin to develop a set of reference materials and sources of assistance to call upon in the future. CHECKPOINTS and other inter-agency collaborations can provide on-going reinforcement and access to evaluation networks to assist participants in building a sense of community around evaluation materials.

Methods of data collection and analysis are divided into two sessions. In the first session, various methods are reviewed and tips on predicting management and budgeting requirements are included. Interviewing, focus-group techniques, questionnaire construction, logs and documents, and observational techniques are discussed with examples provided from various local agency experiences. The second session provides a hands-on experience of coding and manipulating data, techniques of data reduction and summary, and a basic review of analysis strategies and computer programs. This session also reviews various design issues and the presentation of data for various reporting styles and purposes.

In total, the CHECKPOINTS series highlights the basics of designing, implementing, and reporting in-house program evaluations, building upon an awareness of the accountability issues facing agencies, and the need for culturally sensitive and practical approaches so that evaluation processes can become an on-going aspect of agency management. At the end of the series, participants are expected to not only have a good understanding of the issues and approaches that can be taken in creating outcome-oriented program evaluations, they will also have the skills and sensitivities to evaluate their work and link it with the wealth of literature on evaluation.

Part II

The second six-session series focuses on the professional needs of those anticipating serving as evaluation consultants, trainers, or organizational managers of evaluation services. The six-sessions of this series include discussion of: 1) Professional evaluation roles—the skills and sensitivities needed to serve as consultant, mentor, teacher, peer expert, or manager. Participants undertake a self-analysis of their own experiences and competencies, try to get-in-touch with their own and their agency's expectations for their involvement in evaluation, and begin to plan as well for their own professional development needs. This session highlights the experiences of other peers and agency staff to illustrate the breadth of roles and needs that exist, as well as the diversity of ways to approach working in teams and networks. 2) Cultural relativity—a review of principles and experiences to ground evaluations within cultural contexts. A set of case studies and discussions help participants learn from others' experiences and begin to assess their own and their agency's cultural competence. The session attempts to enhance multi-cultural skills and to develop awareness of the cultural issues affecting program evaluations. 3) Evaluation standards—ethical and professional standards of practice in program evaluation. A series of issues are reviewed to highlight professional standards of practice, privacy and informed consent issues, the proper use and management of data, and other proprietary and ethical issues. The discussion of professional practice also includes issues of developing agency policies and stakeholder oversight processes. 4) The development and presentation of evaluation training activities. Each participant is required to design an evaluation training activity and implement that activity in the presence of one of the evaluation training staff to complete certification procedures. The peer and professional feedback provided through this process assists participants in recognizing their strengths and weaknesses, helps to focus on ways to work with audiences, and structures a natural bridge to serving in training roles and being recognized as trainers!

In total, the six-session professional trainer series offers a forum for participants to network with peers and other evaluation professionals, to begin to define roles for their future involvement in evaluation, and to recognize some of the responsibilities of professionals in the field of evaluation.

PROSPECTS FOR LONG-TERM SUSTAINABILITY

CHECKPOINTS was inaugurated in April 1997 with new groups of participants entering the program every six months. In 1997, registrants represented United Ways, United-Way funded agencies, private foundations, MSU-Extension, school personnel, nonprofit human service agencies, private consultants, faculty, graduate students, and health staff. The majority of participants remained in the program for 12 months, thus receiving essential content, as well as professional development experiences and preparation for becoming a certified trainer. By the end of 1998, over 300 individuals will have received CHECKPOINT training, either in the extended original version, or in various tailor-made short courses or summer institutes. Moreover, ADS will sponsor annual reunions of its trainers as part of its effort to build a state-wide network of outcome-based evaluation consultants with a special focus on human service agencies that serve children, youth, and families.

In mid-1997, an unexpected demand to customize training for specific audiences became apparent as state government and AmeriCorps sought out the CHECKPOINTS program. Six-month, non-certificate sequences were jointly designed and offered to local and regional public health officers, community-based recipients of minority health grants, and Michigan's AmeriCorps grantees. Customization, we soon learned, requires intensive knowledge of participants job functions, operating philosophy, and organizational culture. Quality customization requires the commitment of funders' time to inform CHECKPOINT trainers about funder policies and desired outcomes. For example, before training AmeriCorps personnel, CHECKPOINT trainers first had to become sufficiently familiar with AmeriCorps operations to inform curriculum developers about the degree of match between CHECKPOINT's content and trainee needs.

In addition to ongoing and customized training, CHECKPOINTS offers training to faculty and students at other institutions of higher education, week-long institutes for those unable to travel monthly, and "retainer" relationships to grant making organizations wishing to enhance grantee capacity by linking them with CHECKPOINTS' campus-wide infrastructure.

WHY WAS THIS A SUCCESSFUL PARTNERSHIP?

CHECKPOINTS emerged from collaboration, both within the university and the community. Key to the emergence were the roles that the internal and external champions of the project played. Externally, United Way of Michigan's Director of Agency Services generated exposure, interest, and support from the United Way system. During initial development phases, local United Way staff from key communities were identified and asked to participate on advisory committees and to host focus group discussions. Additionally, UWM created a special newsletter to keep the development of the project in front of all the United Ways in Michigan. The Director of Agency Services also ensured that CHECKPOINTS became a regular topic of discussion among United Way fund distribution staff at their regular peer meetings. Last, the Director of Agency Services devoted significant time to maintaining individual dialogues concerning CHECK POINTS with the staff of larger United Ways in the states. All of these actions culminated in 7 out of the top

12 United Ways in Michigan participating in CHECKPOINTS during the first year of actual training.

In addition to the development of an evaluation curriculum and a delivery system of evaluation trainers, the assessment of the impact of the training program is an essential part of CHECKPOINTS success. Throughout the process of curriculum development and delivery, assessment of the training program itself has been a shared responsibility of trainers and trainees. Evaluation of the training program was designed to provide both quantitative and qualitative indicators of organizational change, effectiveness of human service delivery, and best practices with respect to application of evaluation strategies in human services programs.

Finally, as reported by Robert Brown, "From the perspective of UWM, CHECKPOINTS is a prime example of successful collaboration that strengthens the United Way system. In 1997 UWM developed a strategic plan for transition to the next century. As part of that planning process, focus group evaluations were conducted with United Way staff and volunteers throughout the state. CHECKPOINTS consistently was identified as a value added to local United Ways. In the eyes of UWM, ADS has successfully crafted a partnership that delivered a needed product to a hungry audience in a timely fashion."

REFERENCES

Abrams, L. A., Fitzgerald, H. E., & Sandmann, L. (1996, July). *Enhancing the impact of service programs: An evaluation training program for practitioners.* Paper presented at the quadrennial meeting of the World Association for Infant Mental Health, Tampere, Finland.

Abrams, L. A., McCrohan, N., & Hembroff, L. (1995, Oct.). *United Way investments in the children of Michigan.* Institute for Public Policy and Social Research, East Lansing, MI: Michigan State University.

Fitzgerald, H. E., & Abrams, L. A. (1998, Feb.). *Applied developmental science: A scholarship based approach to university-community collaborations.* Presented as part of symposium (C. R. Cooper, Chair), "The role of research in promoting positive change in youth: Challenges and new strategies for university-community partnerships," at the biennial meeting of the Society for Research in Adolescence, San Diego, CA.

Fitzgerald, H. E., Abrams, L. A., Church, R. L., Votruba, J. C., & Imig, G. L. (1996). Applied developmental science at Michigan State University: Connecting university and community via programs for children, youth, and families. *Journal of Research on Adolescence*, 6, 55-66.

Lerner, R. M., Lerner, J. V., Nguyen, H., Pease, M. L., Reiling, D. M., Firlan, U.S., White, M.D., & Freel, M. A. (1994). *Using community-collaborative evaluation research to build the capacities of youth, families, and communities to promote positive youth development: a community-university model of outreach scholarship* (Progress Rep. 1). East Lansing, MI: Michigan State University, Institute for Children, Youth, and Families.

Reed, C. S. (1995). *Enhancing impact through developmental evaluation: An empowerment agenda for human services agencies. Feedback from community partners' review session.* Applied Developmental Science, East Lansing, MI: Michigan State University.

Seabrook, L., Reed, C. S., & Abrams, L. A. (1997). *CHECKPOINTS Competency Questionnaires.* Applied Developmental Science, East Lansing, MI: Michigan State University.

Villarruel, F. A. (1997). *Outline for culturally relevant dimensions of program evaluation: Applied developmental science at Michigan State University.* Applied Developmental Science, East Lansing, MI: Michigan State University.

Ziazi, Z. (1998). *CHECKPOINT quarterly report: Feedback for the design team.* Applied Developmental Science, East Lansing, MI: Michigan State University.

28 THE YOUNG SPARTAN PROGRAM: PARTNERS WITH STUDENTS

Joanne G. Keith
Karen McKnight Casey
Charles A. Blackman
Michigan State University

Two third-grade children living less than five miles from each other—different schools, different communities—were asked about their career aspirations. One selected fast food work, the other chose pediatric cardiology. Either choice could be a worthy occupation, but both children illustrate that they are developing their sense of future by what they could experience and see around them.

Mark entered the Young Spartan project office as a freshman, unclear of his college major and career goals. He wanted opportunities to work with kids, to work in community. Four years later he is a competent and confident young leader ready to graduate—with both classroom and community-based knowledge and learning. He is a dual major in education and pre-law.

PURPOSES AND GOALS

Educational aspirations. Learning in community. Expansion of boundaries. Creating a sense of future possibilities. Career exploration. Understanding diversity. Seeing academic work in action. These activities are vital to educational goals for school age children, and for university students. How are they learned? How are they enhanced? Can students do this task alone or is community-based learning necessary? Are they learned best by default—or can they be designed?

If universities are to develop young adults with such skills and abilities, they need to provide not only academic support units but also authentic field opportunities. In these settings real success and failure can occur (Jacoby, 1996; Kolb, 1984; Lerner & Simon, 1998; Wingspread, 1993). If public schools are to expand the opportunities for children who experience limited opportunities to see beyond their neighborhoods, who have few role models and foresee restricted career options, the public schools need to work with the community to enhance student learning. One way to enhance the learning of both college students and elementary students is through partnerships between universities and local elementary schools (Greiner, 1994; Hackney, 1994; Harkavy, 1998). The Young Spartan Program is designed to be one such opportunity for this urban community.

NATURE OF THE PARTNERSHIP

The Young Spartan Program grew out of two visions for how a university could better serve the community: 1) The vision of a university president and provost who wanted to recapture the land grant mission and looked for innovative ways to invest in the surrounding community, and 2) the vision of elementary principals who saw ways in which the university could enhance learning in local urban public schools. Combining these visions, a proposal was written by area elementary principals and an outreach representative from state government outlining a program to be implemented in the schools. The proposal formed the impetus for formalizing the development of the Young Spartan partnership (Keith, Knox, Perkins, & Blackman, 1995).

The Young Spartan Program is a broad-based collaborative effort designed to enhance educational outcome with the vision of increased academic achievement and career awareness for elementary and higher education students. The principal partners in this effort are from a metropolitan area of Lansing (the capital city of Michigan, a large industrial state) with a population of approximately 150,000. Partners include: (a) Eight elementary schools in Lansing, a public school district with approximately 19,000 students in kindergarten through 12th grade; (b) Michigan State University, a land grant, research-intensive university with more than 40,000 students enrolled in 14 degree granting colleges; (c) state government; (d) the Lansing Regional Chamber of Commerce; and (e) the City of Lansing. The shared vision of this collaborative body is increased academic achievement and career awareness for elementary and higher education students.

ANALYSIS OF THE PROCESS

To reach the above-noted objectives, the Young Spartan Program creates a spectrum of opportunities for elementary school students to experience the community and its members as educators in a reciprocal exchange. For example, elementary students often come to the university for planned learning experiences. Likewise, university faculty, staff, students, retirees and other community members go to the school sites and share their expertise in a variety of ways. While the main focus of this project is academic and social development for elementary students with leadership and service opportunities for university students, the benefits extend to other participants including community volunteers and businesses, teachers and principals, and university staff and faculty (Young Spartan Program, 1995). This article focuses primarily on the benefits for the university and elementary students.

ACHIEVEMENTS RELATED TO GOALS

The Young Spartan Program is an educational and socially powerful intervention that holds great potential for enhancing the learning and development of college students. The Young Spartan Program offers a wide spectrum of learning experiences designed for students at different levels of education and at various stages of development. These opportunities extend across a variety of academic majors and career paths; placements are not contingent on a major in education, but instead relate to a specific area of interest or career exploration. Each year more than 400 university students from more than 50 academic and non-academic units within the university participate in the Young Spartan Program. The learning experiences fall into several categories: Involvement in single events, educational series, specialized content clubs and extra-curricular activities, course-related assignment, coordination of educational experiences, and partnership administration. The benefits for university students vary depending on the level of student investment, structured reflection and learning, and time involvement. On one end of the involvement continuum is the one–time event which may lead to further exploration and a search for additional opportunities. On the other end of the continuum is the intensive involvement of project coordinators and assistant administrators, which has contributed to adjustment of career goals and greatly enhanced career placements (Keith, Casey, Adams & Simpson, in press; Keith, Perkins, Greer, Casey, & Ferrari, 1998).

All levels of student involvement use experiential education as a core strategy in enhancing student learning. From our data collection over the past three years, both formal and informal through surveys, focus groups, student portfolios, reflection papers, case studies, and telephone interviews, we found some basic recurring themes. These themes illustrate the benefits to university students: Expanding horizons and boundaries, clarifying one's purpose, building individual skills, creating relationships and community connections, and enhancing understanding of communities as systems (Keith et al., in press).

Certainly, the impact upon the elementary students is paramount. The Young Spartan Program has been particularly successful in expanding career awareness and exploration opportunities through experiences such as job shadowing and speech contests on the topic of career goals. Academic performance has been emphasized through educational experiences such as reading tutors; school clubs for math, video, media, language, computer and writing; science experiments and curricular-based lessons; and career exploration activities. A total of over 4000 elementary students participate annually in one or more of the educational activities. Standardized tests demonstrate improving achievement scores and the Young Spartan Program has been one of the players (Haas, 1996).

LEARNINGS FROM THIS PARTNERSHIP

The Young Spartan Partnership has existed formally for over five years; during this time we have observed, discussed, thought, evaluated, and reformulated our progress. Through interviews, discussions, and reflection we have observed several significant factors that we think are essential in understanding the nature of such a university/school partnership.

Observation 1: Partnership phases reflect basic development or growth characteristic of organizations including entrepreneurial, growth, decline or renewal stages (Oakley & Krug, 1992). The learnings for the students, for the project administrators, and for the partnership as a whole have been intentional and serendipitous, positive and negative, idealistic and realistic. The phases of the partnership have not necessarily occurred sequentially or separately. The prospects for future growth and development remain positive in that support from central administration of both institutions remains strong. Staff from both the university and school system remains committed to the partnership. There are signs of growth and renewal occurring.

Observation 2: Embracing ambiguity and course corrections are imperative. The "best laid proposals" for programming through university/school partnerships are bound to go awry. All systems involved in the partnership are dynamic and in constant change—personnel turnover, funding priorities, dependability of staff and students, political climate within and surrounding the institutions, and generation of new ideas are but a few of the changing variables impacting the partnership. With ambiguity and the unexpected nature of events in plentiful supply, developing tolerance for and even embracing ambiguity as an opportunity for innovation is necessary (Keith et al., 1995).

Observation 3: The work will expand beyond the capacity to deliver. As well, there is the corollary: Time available to devote to the partnership will be far less than the time needed. The needs and wants of students in this urban public school district are great—academically, socially, and financially. Fifty to 70 percent of the students receive free and reduced-price lunches. Most schools have means on standardized tests that are well below the state average. Setting limits to programming and to numbers of schools involved is an ongoing challenge. There is a constant tension between the struggle to maintain the quality of educational experiences while responding to community needs and requests.

Observation 4: Logistics, logistics, logistics—they require constant attention. Dependability of people—students, teachers, and university professionals—cannot be assumed. Transportation, placement, and scheduling challenges occur daily. Building in redundancy (i.e., back-up systems), and meeting expectations in spite of people not carrying out responsibilities becomes a major challenge for the partnership. This is the nature of an organization with members whose primary responsibilities are not necessarily central to their required work, be they university student or professional. To keep the partnership system running smoothly, the treatment and care of its "volunteer" participants requires considerable nurturance and support.

Observation 5: Faculty at the university and in the public school classrooms need to see the pay-off to their students and to themselves. One primary advantage to the partnership is that it paves the way for connections between busy and sometimes overloaded teachers and professors. It provides a service and skill which many professors and teachers find daunting—both for lack of time and ability. If this connection works well, professionals on both sides of the partnership are pleased and become increasingly involved in working with the project.

Observation 6: Stressful relationships are inevitable—within and between institutions. Trust between the university and school systems takes time but results in strong social capital development. These relationships help weather the inevitable points of disagreement between and within institutions. Our experience suggests that the most difficult battles are not always those between the two different institutions, but within the university or school system. Partnership personnel often perceive their internal differences as more difficult than those between institutions. With a strong trusting relationship between the partnership members, we have been able to meet these challenges with some degree of success.

Observation 7: A base level of commitment of human and financial resources is necessary for sustainability. The time spent finding funding can become an overarching and time consuming responsibility and task; if possible, a base level of commitment is needed. Program personnel can then focus on programmatic issues. In this partnership, because of the high impact on students' education, the university provides financial resources for a full-time academic outreach specialist, part-time support for a faculty member's time, some student support, and operating dollars. The level of support has evolved with increasing roles for the outreach specialist and decreasing and more narrowly defined roles for the faculty liaison.

Observation 8: A community champion or community wizard (McLaughlin, Irby, & Langman, 1994) is the best project director. Interested faculty are invaluable for increasing credibility within the university, just as teacher involvement is essential for increasing credibility within the school district, but the role of project leader requires a different set of skills. This person's strength needs to lie in knowing the community, especially the resources and operating procedures of the university and school district. This person needs to know how to engage, work with, and motivate volunteers from a wide range of abilities and backgrounds. Careful attention to details and budgeting skills are required. An imagination to see the application of higher education academics to the lives of school age children is necessary. Chemistry for kindergartners, physics for fifth graders, mathematics everywhere, and athletes with life skills as well as athletic abilities are but a few examples of seeing the applications relevant for children. Furthermore, adults need assistance to gain and share these understandings.

CONCLUSION

These key observations are a sampling of the learnings from the Young Spartan Program—one partnership at work. It has been an iterative process—sometimes a roller coaster and sometimes a merry-go-round, sometimes an uphill battle and at other times a celebration of wonderful successes. Our experience with the Young Spartan Program leads us to conclude that students in the university and elementary schools can and should be taught by design, not only by default, through community-based learning. We would argue that for students this learning would be best advanced in a community of learners such as a university/school partnership where the responsibility is shared by faculty members and specialists who have the academic and community knowledge to lead and work within such an educational experience. Students, both children and young adults, want to advance their leadership skills and career opportunities. What is needed are universities and public school systems willing to commit to developing, maintaining, and sustaining long-term partnerships.

ENDNOTE

1. The name "Young Spartan" was selected because the Spartan of Greek mythology is the mascot of Michigan State University and its students and alumni are known as Spartans. The elementary students participating in the program were viewed as "young" Spartans to emphasize the role of education in their lives.

REFERENCES

Greiner, W. (1994). In the total of all these acts: How can American universities address the urban agenda? *Universities and Community Schools, 4*(1-2), 12-15.

Haas, B. (1996). *Young Spartan Program Evaluation, 1994-1997.* Lansing, MI: Human Service Research, Inc.

Hackney, S. (1994). The roles and responsibilities of urban universities in their communities: Five university presidents call for action. *University and Community Schools, 4*(1-2), 9-11.

Harkavy, L. (1998). Organizational innovation and the creation of the new American university. In R. M. Lerner & L. A. K. Simon (Eds.), *University-community collaborations for the 21st century: Outreach scholarship for youth and families* (pp. 275-287). New York: Garland.

Jacoby, B. & Associates. (1996). *Service-learning in higher education.* San Francisco: Jossey-Bass.

Keith, J. G., Perkins, D. F., Greer, J. C., Casey, K. M. & Ferrari, T. M. (1998). The Young Spartan Program: A bridge between the ivory tower and the community. In R. M. Lerner & L. A. K. Simon (Eds.), *University-community collaborations for the 21st century: Outreach scholarship for youth and families* (pp. 289-313). New York: Garland.

Keith, J. G., Casey, K. M., Adams, S. S., & Simpson, K. (in press). *The Young Spartan Program: A parallel vision for community enhancement and student learning.* Kappa Omicron Nu Forum.

Keith, J. G., Knox, A. A., Perkins, D. F., & Blackman, C. A. (October, 1995). *Building an educational collaboration on behalf of children, youth and families: A case study* (Research Report 539). East Lansing: Michigan State University Agricultural Experiment Station.

Kolb, D. A. (1984). *Experiential learning: Experience as the source of learning and development.* Englewood Cliffs, NJ: Prentice Hall.

Lerner, R. M., & Simon, L. A. K. (Eds.). (1998). *University-community collaborations for the 21st century: Outreach scholarship for youth and families.* New York: Garland.

McLaughlin, M., Irby, M. & Langman, J. (1994). *Urban sanctuaries: Neighborhood organizations in the lives and futures of inner-city youth.* San Francisco: Jossey Bass.

Oakley, E., & Krug, D. (1992). *Enlightened leadership.* Denver, CO: Stone Tree Publishing.

Wingspread Group on Higher Education. (1993). *An American imperative: Higher expectations for higher education.* Racine, WI: Johnson Foundation.

Young Spartan Program. (1995). *Annual Report.* East Lansing: Michigan State University.

29 FOSTERING COMMUNITY GUARDIANSHIP: SERVING CHILDREN AND FAMILIES THROUGH COMMUNITY-UNIVERSITY PARTNERSHIP

Lorilee R. Sandmann
Lou Anna Kimsey Simon
Michigan State University

NATURE OF PARTNERSHIP

> *The Dexter Elmhurst Family and Community Services Center is devoted to the economic, educational, social and cultural advancement of area residents with a focus on families. This center will be a beacon to serve, embrace and empower the greater central west community of Detroit.*

So proclaims the Dexter Elmhurst Community Council as they define the vision they hold for a multigenerational, community-operated, human service facility in their Detroit community of nearly 100,000. The Dexter Elmhurst residential area, developed in the 1950s, is the birthplace of many of Motown's superstars and continues to serve as a cultural center for the African-American community in the city of Detroit. Currently, female-headed households comprise 40 per cent of all households and 40 percent of all persons in the neighborhood live below the poverty status. Residents of this area are struggling to shape their community identity and face the challenges of contemporary urban existence. The emerging community-based and managed facility is designed to become a focal point for community restoration by strengthening families, serving seniors and supporting neighborhood youth.

To move from a neighborhood building abandoned by the state to the community's vision of a lively family and community services center, Wayne County Family Independence Agency (FIA) redirected its agency's priorities and resources. They created a partnership with Michigan State University (MSU), the Wayne County Human Service Coordinating Board, and a loose confederation of neighborhood residents. The primary purpose of the partnership is to establish the center as a self-sustaining operating facilitating that meets community health, human service, and recreation needs under the "guardianship" of community residents. A secondary goal is to establish a model for more effective public-private partnership organized for the purposes of community capacity building and transformation.

The Dexter Elmhurst case offers three primary areas where university scholars' work appears most pertinent: guiding planning for new initiatives; building capacity of individuals, groups and institutions to promote positive changes in their communities; and evaluating outcomes of intervention efforts to guide future activities in directions more likely to succeed. Specifically, the partners asked MSU to provide technical assistance, training, planning and evaluation services to support the Dexter Elmhurst Community Council during the council's transition period of preparation to assume full ownership of the center from Wayne County FIA. The university's programs in social work, criminal justice, anthropology, urban affairs, business, and Extension as well as its museum provide scholarly services through a cooperative effort. University Outreach provides administrative leadership. During this multi-year effort, Michigan State University has taken the lead in:

- Providing technical and organizational development assistance to the interim board of directors to help them establish a new community-based, non-profit organization to own and manage the Dexter Elmhurst facility and serve area families and children.
- Collaborating with the Dexter Elmhurst Community Council to develop a strategic plan that includes a community visioning process and a resource inventory that includes a cultural assessment of the target area.
- Developing a business plan for the Dexter Elmhurst Community Center to identify the center's operating and capital investment budget for the center, provide cash flow projections for the next ten years, and assess the resource development requirements of financing a ten-year operating capital investment budget.
- Designing a participatory evaluation strategy that will establish, monitor and assess community-based and human service delivery objectives.
- Creating training plans and technical assistance to integrate technology with community strengths to assist council operations and establish center educational programs.

ANALYSIS OF THE PROCESS: LESSONS LEARNED

There are two features of this partnership that are distinct, significant, and potentially useful to others involved in similar work. One is the movement from a traditional leadership-development, capacity-building training program to a collaboratively developed and enacted guardianship curriculum. The other is movement from parallel program development toward an interdisciplinary university team engaged in integrated thinking and acting.

From Leadership to Guardianship

Building on theoretical frameworks from community self determination, economic development, adult learning, cultural and urban differences, and successful university-community rebuilding initiatives (Crane, 1998; Fetterman, Kaftarian, & Wandersman, 1996; Johnson & Bell, 1995; Kretzmann & McKnight, 1993; Sandmann, 1997; Schorr, 1997; Walshok, 1995), university scholars and community-based staff proposed an 18-month leadership development, capacity building training program. As the monthly sessions were held and assessed, however, it became clear that the emphasis was incorrect.

The community council did not need classic "leadership" training for many were already highly experienced community and business leaders. Discussions with community leaders revealed that their anticipated role in the community center was that of "guardians." They were the elders, the keepers of the community's rich history, the knowers of families' resources and needs. This "naming" and recognition of a more plausible theory of change had broad implications for the relationship between the partners and for subsequent educational efforts. To develop a deeper understanding of this role, MSU anthropology faculty provided team members with information on how various cultural groups across the world interpret the guardian role.

This reconceptualization changed the focus and approach to monthly training sessions. Simulations became a more prominent pedagogy giving council members an opportunity to practice new interpretations of the community guardian role in a safe, culturally appropriate context and within the expectations of the community center's guiding policies, programming, personnel and procedures. This reframed set of training materials is compiled into a curriculum to be reviewed by the project team for the purpose of understanding what has been learned from the process, to be incorporated into future university-community collaborations, and to serve as a model for other communities.

From Parallel to Integrated Program Development

Universities, non-profit organizations and government entities have experimented for more than three decades with collaborative interventions designed to improve the quality of community life. Large-scale social welfare and economic redevelopment projects have been conducted in all of the nation's major cities, based on varying concepts of structure, process and leadership for community collaborations. However, despite an impressive accumulation of experience and case study, it is still unclear which variables are likely to produce success in community-collaborations involving a university, non-profit organization or government partner.

Therefore, evaluation research was conducted that focused on three dimensions of collaboration: 1) the interactions between conflicting paradigms for interventions and changes represented by project partners and academic disciplines; 2) perception of partnership and change by community residents in the project; and 3) the leadership role played by the university project coordinator. These dimensions are significant because they reflect some of the major challenges to interdisciplinary, collaborative outreach by universities in projects involving community transformation.

In the highly sensitive area of urban redevelopment, success demands effective knitting together of public, university, community non-profit and grassroots activity in the context of blended academic skills and knowledge. The initial faculty team meeting, similar to most collaborative processes, was characterized by differing academic disciplines insisting on the dominance of a single change paradigm, mixed perceptions of improvement or goal attainment, and poorly resolved group tension. When these differences become apparent to the non-academic project partners and impeded fulfilling the university's responsibilities, it was evident that mere coordination of faculty involvement was insufficient.

Evaluation research on the project showed that intense and persistent leadership—by MSU and cooperating partners—was key in moving the program development efforts of faculty involved in complementary, but parallel intervention processes to a more integrated pattern of thinking and acting. (An example is the unlikely linkage of MSU Museum's neighborhood cultural assessment and the criminal justice faculty member's evaluation of the community-policing program.) Over time, the process has integrated competing perspectives, developed a shared sense of power and change among participants, and demonstrated a leadership role that was well defined and replicable. The end result was to merge the perspectives of seemingly unrelated academic disciplines into a new whole and to generate and apply scholarship to a community setting.

ACHIEVEMENT RELATED TO GOALS

Community council members have begun to wear the mantle of guardians both symbolically and operationally. They have achieved non-profit organizational status and draw from the community resource inventory to make programmatic decisions. The center is open, programs are offered, and an on-going monitoring and evaluation system is in place. Further, community members are taking on guardianship roles beyond those based in the center. For example, they are guiding a major "Paint the Town" initiative, involving thousands of volunteers and businesses collaborating in a housing renovation effort of over 500 neighborhood homes. The center has attracted additional resources as well. The City of Detroit Police Department was awarded a substantial grant to create a presence and programming at the center.

In addition to impact in the community, collaborating partners have attained their own goals. While espousing citizen empowerment, sponsoring government agencies, such as the Family Independent Agency, are struggling with their changing role. They are learning how to turn over authority and responsibility to local citizens. From a higher education perspective, this partnership's long-term nature is providing an ideal setting for documenting impact of scholars' engagement in communities both internally on scholarship and externally on public issues. Products, such as the curricula, training programs and manuals, planning and evaluation designs and methodologies, and policy round tables have resulted from this scholarship that can be generalized and disseminated to other communities to implement and guide public policy. Faculty and community partner co-presentations at professional meetings, peer reviewed journal articles, and student dissertations are being accomplished.

REASONS FOR SUCCESS

This collaboration of community participants, government, and higher education stands as a model of community renewal and self-determination that enhances the capacity and quality of community life and serves as a model of outreach scholarship. Several defining characteristics of this partnership distinguish it from individual community-based projects. The passionate backing of an intermediary organization, Wayne County FIA, inspired development of an imaginative, context-sensitive approach to welfare reform that builds on the existing community social infrastructure. Stakeholders agreed on values and outcomes and to continuous negotiation and development of the means to achieve them. Community members put aside differences to take an active role in creating a new model and in accepting the mantle of responsibility implied in the guardianship paradigm. The University was prepared to engage in a new model of interdisciplinary outreach scholarship and to act with the same passion as those who live in the neighborhood. A critical mass of resources—human and financial—labored for an intense period of time to build capacity for long term sustainability. Partners provided mutually reinforcing interactions that enriched their own organizations and the environment. This blending of expertise has insured that all partners learn as well as teach. By aggregating researchers, disciplines, projects and organizations within a single community, this partnership fostered synergy and change to achieve a deep and complex understanding of how this community works—understanding that is the key to insuring positive impacts on the lives of Dexter Elmhurst families.

REFERENCES

Crane. J. (Ed.). (1998). *Social programs that work.* New York: Russell Sage Foundation.

Fetterman, D. M., Kaftarian, S. J., & Wandersman, A. (Eds.). (1996). *Empowerment evaluation: Knowledge and tools for self-assessment and accountability.* Thousand Oaks, CA: Sage.

Johnson, D. M., & Bell, D. A. (Ed.). (1995). *Metropolitan universities: An emerging model in American higher education.* Denton, TX: University of North Texas Press.

Kretzmann, J. P., & McKnight, J. L. (1993). *Building communities from the inside out: A path toward finding and moving a community's assets.* Evanston, IL: Northwestern University, Center for Urban Affairs and Policy Research.

Schorr, L. G. (1997). *Common purpose: Strengthening families and neighborhoods to rebuild America.* NY: Anchor Books/Doubleday.

Walshok, M. L. (1995). *Knowledge without boundaries: What America's research universities can do for the economy, the workplace, and the community.* San Francisco: Jossey Bass.

Sandmann, L. R. (Ed.). (1997). *Points of distinction: Planning and evaluating quality outreach.* East Lansing, MI: Office of the Vice Provost for University Outreach, Michigan State University.

30 BEYOND JUST SAY NO: THE MICHIGAN ABSTINENCE PARTNERSHIP

Shelly E. Schadewald[1]
Jackson Non-Profit Support Center

NATURE OF PARTNERSHIP

The Michigan Abstinence Partnership (MAP) began in 1993 and is led by the Michigan Department of Community Health. The Partnership is a broad-based group with members from across the state, including health professionals, parents, teens, educators, and representatives from business, government, volunteer organizations, and advocacy groups. It targets 9-14 year-old children with the concept of staying healthy by avoiding risky behaviors, such as sexual activity and the use of alcohol, tobacco, and other drugs. MAP also focuses on parents in order to reinforce the importance of the family in making healthy choices.

MAP utilizes a media campaign, educational and promotional materials. Community training, technical assistance, and funding are also used to establish supportive environments and educational systems for helping children remain abstinent. The Partnership provides funding, technical assistance and evaluation support to twenty Michigan communities. MAP celebrated its fifth anniversary in May 1998, citing successes including contributing significantly to the 19% reduction in teen pregnancy rates in Michigan (MDCH, Division of Vital Records and Health Statistics, 1996). This made Michigan one of the top five states for teen pregnancy reduction in the country.

PURPOSES AND GOALS

The goal of the Partnership is to reduce adolescent risky behaviors, particularly sexual activity, and promote positive, healthy choices for Michigan's adolescents and their families.

The Partnership is committed to several key guiding principles:

- The Partnership supports abstinence-based programs, meaning that the focus is on the concept of staying healthy by avoiding risky behaviors such as sexual activity and the use of alcohol, tobacco, and other drugs.
- Programs target 9-14 year-old children and must be developed in a culturally-competent, age, and gender appropriate manner.

- Parents are an essential part of helping their children learn that abstinence is a healthy behavior. Youth need the support of communities in which they reside to reinforce this message.
- Programs must be skill-based, meaning that in addition to information, methods and skills for dealing with pressure must be taught and practiced.
- Each community is different. Community members, parents, schools, and children must determine their own needs in using abstinence-based programs to help children lead more healthy and productive lives (Michigan Abstinence Partnership: Promoting Healthy Behaviors for Michigan's Children, An Action Primer, 1996).

Furthermore, the MAP integrates sound health education principles which include the following:

- Programs must be broadly supported by the community. Consensus is essential to the success of the program.
- All segments of the community must be committed to working together to provide consistent messages.
- Programs must focus on increasing knowledge and skill building so that young people not only know the reasons for abstinence, but also know how to deal with pressure.
- Young people must be motivated to build self-confidence so that they can effectively choose to abstain despite pressure from peers and the media to engage in risky behaviors.
- Programs should be long term and multifaceted. Short term solutions such as one-time presentations with no community involvement and support are ineffective. Instead, successful programs require ongoing educational opportunities about abstinence, goal setting, and skill-building for young people and their parents are needed.
- Structured recreational opportunities and programs where supervision and "free-time" are provided.
- Programs must have an evaluation component to learn what does and does not work.
- Children themselves must be a part of the program development and evaluation.

The Partnership's principles are basically consistent (while maintaining a focus on abstinence) with the findings of Kirby (1997), who reviewed more than 80 teen pregnancy prevention programs. His research suggested that components such as parent-child communication, youth development programs, and programs with multiple interventions including education, media, and community involvement are essential for successful outcomes.

The Partnership provides funding, technical assistance and evaluation support to each of twenty funded communities. The communities are selected through a Request for Proposal process based on a community action plan unique to their own needs. Through this process and support, communities are enabled to develop exciting and unique initiatives to positively impact adolescent health in their community.

ANALYSIS OF THE PROCESS

The Partnership developed a model of excellence by creating and maintaining a diverse campaign committee structure with over 100 members. In April of 1993, careful planning was done to ensure membership diversity. This included invitations to Planned Parenthood, Right To Life, Michigan Family Forum, the educational community, Michigan State University's Institute for Children, Youth and Families, and representatives from substance abuse prevention, local prevention programs, mental health, the faith community, health care and the business community. At the initial meeting, the guiding principles were discussed and consensus was reached. Leadership for the Campaign Committee as well as the subsequent formation of three subcommittees were carefully selected. The Co-chairpersons were selected to represent diverse sectors, health and education, one male and one female, and different ethnic and political backgrounds. One was a Representative of the State Board of Education; the other, the President of Mott Children's Health Center. They agreed to lead the Partnership for at least a five-year period. Subcommittees, including Family/Community Relations, Program Content and Curriculum, and Media are also led by outstanding and diverse individuals.

The Family and Community Relations Subcommittee is led by the former Director of Family Services Administration, Michigan Family Independence Agency and the Director of the Michigan Association for Local Public Health. The purpose of the subcommittee is to provide a forum for community support of abstinence initiatives. This subcommittee developed the Community Training Workbook (1998) and the Partnership Catalog (1997-98), and provided input into media messages. This subcommittee also provides representatives for the Request for Proposal review process.

The Program Content and Curriculum Subcommittee was co-chaired by the Director for Middle Level Education of Detroit Public Schools and the former Director of the Institute for Children, Youth, and Families at Michigan State University. The latter person has now been replaced by a Comprehensive School Health Education Coordinator. The Program Content and Curriculum Committee develops and revises the Partnership's educational products, including the Action Primer, Program Review Checklist, and Resource Bibliography. It also provides feedback on media and other content-related messages.

The Media Subcommittee is currently co-chaired by a producer for WXYZ-TV (ABC Detroit) and the President of Seyferth and Associates, a public relations firm. Their task is to develop a media plan, evaluate/update the media campaign, and supervise the purchase of air time for the commercials.

The Campaign Committee and the subcommittees utilize a consensus model to reach decisions about the Partnership's direction through several strategies including:

- following the guiding and health education principles
- maintaining focus
- maintaining balanced leadership
- nurturing ownership of the Partnership by members
- discussing issues and striving for compromise
- reaching agreement through consensus without voting

- maintaining a forward focus, meaning that MAP as a whole seeks to look for growth and future direction.

The Partnership Campaign Committee oversees the direction of the Partnership, including support for community funding and activity, development of education and promotional materials, and the development and maintenance of the media campaign. Michigan State University's Institute for Children, Youth and Families played a pivotal role in the development of the Partnership's educational materials and media messages, which are now used statewide, nationally, and even internationally, with more than 750,000 in current distribution. Those products are referenced in this chapter.

ACHIEVEMENTS RELATED TO GOALS

MAP has achieved many successes beginning with the membership diversity, which has remained consistent over the last five years. To support that diversity and continually maintain "ownership" in MAP and its future direction, a consensus building model is utilized.

The development of educational products such as the Action Primer and the Resource Bibliography are used world wide and are serving as a model of excellence for abstinence programs throughout the country. More than 750,000 are in distribution throughout the world.

The promotional items, which contain messages such as "I Don't Have to Do It to Prove It," use positive, youth developed messages. These items reinforce educational programs and signify for youth a choice which can be stated to their peer group when wearing MAP t-shirts or shoelaces, for example.

The media campaign is an award-winning media campaign which was evaluated in 1995 (Moore and Associates, 1995). The report demonstrated that 75% of adolescents polled felt this advertising was helpful in encouraging youth their age not to have sex.

MAP provides competitive funding to 20 communities implementing community action plans which are unique to their community. Funded community activities include parent education programs, youth curricula, structured recreational programs with positive reinforcement of the abstinence message, peer education programs, mini-grant funding, youth rallies, family fun days, and local media campaigns. These communities receive considerable support from a team of technical assistants, which is a unique feature in abstinence programming. MAP provides evaluation support.

The Partnership has a unique success in cultivating an evaluation plan and implementing it through the Michigan Public Health Institute (MPHI). MPHI is a nonprofit corporation created under Public Act 264 of 1989. The MPHI is a cooperative venture of the Michigan Department of Community Health, the University of Michigan, Michigan State University and Wayne State University. Representatives of these four partner institutions serve on MPHI's 12-member Board of Directors. The purpose of MPHI is to provide an organization for collaborative research and programs with the goal of preventing disease, prolonging healthy life, and promoting sound public health practices. The evaluation model developed for MAP combines evaluation technical support for local communities, providing extensive evaluation training and tools to community initiatives, and tracking key health indicators related to the target population. MPHI released a Midterm Report (1996) that detailed the lessons learned thus far in the creation and implementation of the Michigan Abstinence Partnership.

In order to maintain long term sustainability, MAP has comprehensive funding combining federal, state, and local sources. Because of the successes enumerated in this section, the Partnership is serving as a model for excellence throughout the country in abstinence education programming.

Of course, the most important success is demonstrated in the health indicators. According to 1996 Pregnancy data, released by the Michigan Department of Community Health Vital Statistics, teen pregnancy rates are down 19% in Michigan from 1989 to 1996. Live birth rates and abortions have also fallen significantly. The Partnership's prevention efforts significantly contributed to this decline.

PROSPECTS FOR LONG TERM SUSTAINABILITY

MAP is sustainable in the long term due to three primary facets: Campaign Committee consensus, diverse funding sources, and community development and training.

The consensus building model has been very successful in creating ownership and commitment to the issue of promoting positive and healthy behaviors among Michigan's youth. MAP continues to maintain its focus and principles since its inception.

The funding sources now include federal, state, and local dollars. MAP originally was funded by state dollars, donations from major corporations, and from local citizens. Each community must apply and submit a community action plan. Funds are awarded competitively. As communities were funded, a local match of 20% was required. The local match is generally comprised of a combination of local funding and in-kind donations such as rent, office supplies, copying, volunteer time, and donations from businesses. In 1996 federal funding was sought under Title V legislation, bringing an additional $1.89 million dollars to the Partnership. The federal funding is available non-competitively to each state for five years beginning in Fiscal Year 1998.

The Partnership is perhaps most importantly sustained by the nurturing and support of local community, grass-roots efforts. Through community funding, technical assistance and evaluation support, communities develop their own community action plans. In addition, the Partnership developed a Community Training Workbook (1998) to provide non-funded communities with a workbook to establish community initiatives, utilizing a "Train the Trainer" approach. These communities benefit from Partnership strategies, educational products, lessons learned (MPHI Midterm Report, 1997), and promotional items.

LEARNINGS FROM THIS PARTNERSHIP

The lessons learned thus far in the implementation of the Michigan Abstinence Partnership are detailed in the MPHI Midterm Report (1997).

Critical to the success of a partnership such as MAP is establishing and maintaining an active committee with diverse philosophies and representation. The members must be dedicated to the purpose and principles of the partnership and committed to a focused campaign. Leadership for the committee and subcommittees must be carefully selected to be diverse and balanced. To bear the workload to balance the committee or subcommittees, and maintain consensus building, having co-chairs is essential. Because of the importance of leadership, each co-chairperson must be committed to serve long term and to be actively involved.

The consensus model for direction and decisions at the campaign committee level and subcommittee levels allows for discussion and ownership. Voting may distract and divide the members when considering issues. Minutes and meeting summaries document the discussion and what conclusion was reached.

The involvement of children in planning activities is essential. Positive messages without scare tactics are most effective for youth. The media campaign is useful and effective in influencing peers to consider and make healthy decisions (Moore, 1995).

Local coalitions with detailed action plans specific to their communities can be successful in impacting parents and children. Such coalitions must also maintain membership diversity in their representation and use of a consensus building model. A clear, concise community action plan provides proper guidance and necessary steps for implementation of successful community activities. In addition, staff support, technical assistance, clear expectations and evaluation technical assistance are critical to a successful community initiative.

Funded community coalitions have learned that providing information and skill-building opportunities to parents are essential to help them develop good parent-child communication on the issue of abstaining from risky behaviors. In addition, children need skill-building activities and multiple interventions which will ultimately result in influencing behavior, such as choosing abstinence as a lifestyle during adolescence. Multiple intervention activity is critical. Providing curricula, after-school programs, and parent education to the same target population will more effectively help youth build and maintain the necessary skills to avoid sexual pressure.

WHY WAS THIS A SUCCESSFUL PARTNERSHIP?

The Michigan Abstinence Partnership is successful because the Campaign Committee and subcommittee structure utilizes a consensus model for decision making. The committees also maintain diverse representation in its membership who all agree to the primary focus and principles of MAP. Careful planning and well-balanced leadership are also essential to the ongoing success of this initiative.

It is also successful because of nurturing grass-roots level activity through competitive funding of community action plans, the team of technical assistants and evaluation support on a long term basis. The communities have each learned lessons and honed their own skills in the implementation of abstinence programs. Lessons learned include the need for adequate staff time devoted to the program, carefully focusing evaluation components, and the importance of multiple intervention activities to really impact youth. Regarding the latter, the various intervention strategies include media, educational products, promotional items, training, community funding, and technical assistance. To maintain those activities, quarterly Campaign Committee meetings and involvement of the diverse membership representing all sectors in the direction of the Partnership has kept the momentum of the campaign strong. Diverse funding sources from federal, state, and local sources financially supports all efforts.

Ultimately, the Partnership is committed to the concept that our children *can* lead healthy lives by avoiding risky behaviors, such as sexual activity and the use of alcohol, tobacco and other drugs. Working together, we can do great things.

CONCLUSION

Community collaboration on many levels is the cornerstone of the Partnership and its continued success. Collaboration can be challenging, but also can produce excellent rewards (Keith, 1993, Keith et al., 1995). The Michigan Abstinence Partnership has proven the importance of collaboration and the strength it can provide in achieving impact on youth. MAP displays many important characteristics for success, including utilizing consensus, maintaining diverse membership with balanced leadership, investing in and nurturing grass roots activities, involving youth in developing messages, and evaluating all aspects of MAP efforts.

ENDNOTE

1. The author was project consultant to MAP when this chapter was written.

REFERENCES

Michigan Department of Community Health. (1997). 1989-1996 Michigan Resident Birth File, Division for Vital Records and Health Statistics.

Michigan Abstinence Partnership. (1996). *Promoting healthy behaviors for Michigan's children: An action primer for families, schools, and communities.* Lansing, MI: Author.

Kirby, D. (1997). *No easy answers: Research findings on programs to reduce teen pregnancy.* Washington, DC: The National Campaign to Prevent Teen Pregnancy.

Michigan Abstinence Partnership. (1998). *A community training workbook.* Lansing, MI: Author.

Michigan Abstinence Partnership. (1996). *Michigan Abstinence Partnership catalog, 1997-98.* Lansing, MI: Author.

Michigan Abstinence Partnership. (1994). *Promoting healthy behaviors for Michigan's children, program review checklist.* Lansing, MI: Author.

Michigan Abstinence Partnership. (1998). *Promoting healthy behaviors for Michigan's children, resource bibliography for families, schools, and communities.* Lansing, MI: Author.

Moore and Associates. (1995). *Michigan Abstinence Partnership media campaign evaluation.* Lansing, MI: Author.

Davidson, W., Naegeli, M., Schadewald, S., Aponte, G. (1997). *Michigan Abstinence Partnership midterm evaluation report.* Lansing, MI: Michigan Public Health Institute.

Keith, J. G. (1993). *Building and maintaining community coalitions, on behalf of children, youth and families: Project report, community coalitions in action.* Lansing, MI: Michigan State University Institute for Children, Youth and Families.

Keith, J. G., Knox, A. A., Perkins, D. F., Blackman, C. A. (1995). *Building an educational collaboration on behalf of children, youth and families: Project report, community coalitions in action.* Lansing, MI: Michigan State University Institute for Children, Youth and Families.

31 SKIPPED GENERATION PARENTS: BUILDING COLLABORATIVE PARTNERSHIPS TO SUPPORT CUSTODIAL GRANDPARENTS

Andrea B. Smith
Linda L. Dannison
Western Michigan University

NATURE OF THE PARTNERSHIP

Social service caseworkers observed a significant number of custodial grandparents who appeared isolated from typical community support networks. These grandparents, for one reason or another, were actively involved in parenting their children's children. Many issues of re-parenting were of significant concern. Some grandparents presented poor parenting skills and others were frustrated with their circumstances. Resources typically available to support foster care families were not available to these families. These observations were numerous enough to bring the matter to the attention of others, including supervisors and other caseworkers.

Discussion during a *Strong Families/Safe Children* County Community Coordinating Council meeting focused on this issue. Coordinating Councils are county-wide representative bodies, formed under gubernatorial mandate, that bring diverse agencies together with consumers to focus on local issues. The County Extension Director, a member of the Council, volunteered to conduct focus groups with available custodial grandparents. Following initial data collection, a partnership was formed with faculty members from a local university who were approached to facilitate support group sessions for this population. A review of the literature was conducted by faculty, and information obtained from focus groups was analyzed.

BACKGROUND

Grandparents comprise a unique group of skipped generation parents. Recent statistics indicate that well over three million children currently live with their grandparents in a home where no biological parent is present. This represents a two-thirds increase in numbers during the past decade (Children's Defense Fund,

1997). A very high rate of teenage pregnancy, incarceration, parental alcohol and other substance abuse, the death of one or both parents, divorce, child abuse and neglect, and other conditions are contemporary problems of national concern. (Becklund, 1993; deToledo & Brown, 1995; Jendrek, 1994; Yorkey, 1993). Elder individuals have always played an important part in extended family support roles, but grandparents are called upon in increasing numbers to provide support and assistance to families in need of outside help (Burton, 1992; Creighton, 1991; Minkler, Driver, Roe & Bedeian, 1993; Minkler & Roe, 1993). This support and assistance often involves full-time parenting of grandchildren.

Many grandparent caregivers find their personal resources stretched to the limit. Issues of health, financial stability, and parenting are salient to these individuals (Smith, Dannison, & Vacha-Haase, 1998). Almost one-half of those caring for grandchildren are grandmothers without partners (Creighton, 1991), and serving as primary caregiver for more than one dependent is not unusual (Minkler & Roe, 1993). Employment may not be feasible with the added caretaking responsibilities, and financial resources planned for retirement years can quickly be depleted as the children's needs are addressed. Often grandparents are encouraged by social service agencies or courts involved with the parent(s) of these children to become custodial caregivers for one or several young siblings. Limited public funding often pressures agencies to place at-risk children with relatives to avoid more costly out-of-family placement.

PILOT SUPPORT GROUP

An eight week pilot program for custodial grandparents was conducted during the summer of 1995. Funds to support this initiative were provided through the Department of Social Services (DSS). Focus group sessions provided information about topics considered important for inclusion into this type of educational support group. Sessions were facilitated by a Family Life Education graduate student and a social worker whose agency volunteered his time. Each class session was evaluated for grandparents' satisfaction with content, delivery style, and extent of grandparents' learning. Grandparents' input about additional information they would like to receive was also solicited.

CREATING A TEAM TO DESIGN A CURRICULUM

Analysis of evaluation information led the facilitators and supporting faculty to conclude that the service provided was effective and important, but also revealed a lack of any formalized curriculum for custodial grandparents. The second phase of this project, development of a curriculum resource for custodial grandparent support groups, was funded by the Michigan Family Independence Agency (formerly the State Department of Social Services) through the Strong Families/Safe Children program. The project directors, chairperson of a University Family and Consumer Sciences Department, and the local Director of County Extension, developed an interdisciplinary Curriculum Design Team who authored the original curriculum and subsequent revisions. This six-person team represented the professional areas of law, early childhood, psychology, adult education, parenting and family economics.

The Curriculum Design Team worked under the direction of a 22-person Project Advisory Committee which included content experts, representatives of agencies serving grandparents, and grandparents. This Advisory Committee identified topic areas for inclusion in the curriculum, defined pertinent terminology, made suggestions about session format, and provided ongoing feedback to curriculum authors. This group took their responsibilities very seriously and worked diligently to insure project quality and success. They chose to meet monthly throughout the duration of the project and provided invaluable suggestions and advice.

The final version of the curriculum was called *Second Time Around—Grandparents Raising Grandchildren: A Curriculum for Grandparent Support Groups.* The curriculum is organized into eight chapters and includes a facilitator's guide, instructional activities and materials, resource materials for grandparents, participant feedback forms, and suggestions for facilitator assessment of grandparents' learning. The eight chapters are: 1) Understanding Your "Not-So-New" Role; 2) Promoting Personal Well Being; 3) Refining Parenting Skills; 4) Building Relationships; 5) Working With School and Community; 6) Managing Finances; 7) Exploring Legal Issues; and 8) Looking to the Future. An editor was hired to insure that the authors' writing styles were consistent and that all utilized a similar editorial format. A graphic artist worked with the editor to develop a creative and attractive final product.

ANALYSIS OF THE PROCESS

An independent evaluation team was hired and provided ongoing evaluation throughout this project. Evaluation activities began prior to project start-up (e.g., with a focus group with grandparents and a preliminary pilot conducted with a grandparent support group) and were ongoing throughout the curriculum development process. Approximately 30 reviewers from the local community, including Advisory Committee Members, representatives of organizations serving re-parenting grandparents, and custodial grandparents examined individual chapters or the entire curriculum. Using semi-structured questionnaires, they provided critical feedback to the Curriculum Design team regarding structure, content, and language. Expected outcomes or learning objectives were re-stated to improve clarity and measurability. Various evaluation tools were incorporated to assess service delivery and participants' progress in the grandparent support program.

ACHIEVEMENTS RELATED TO GOALS

The grandparent curriculum was pilot tested with two grandparent support groups, one meeting in a rural area sponsored by Senior Services and one meeting in an urban area sponsored by a local, inner city church. A total of 17 grandparents attended these sessions and represented diverse socioeconomic and ethnic groups. Grandparents who participated in the pilot programs were informed that this was the introductory utilization of the curriculum and that a key expectation was their provision of critical feedback about the content and materials, enabling revisions prior to dissemination. Grandparent participants felt strongly motivated to carry out this role and eagerly provided feedback and suggestions for improvement. The entire evaluation process continuously sought and obtained feedback from a large number of people representing a great variety of perspectives. This formative evaluative approach enhanced the success and effectiveness of the final curriculum. (Vacha-Haase, Ness, Dannison and Smith, manuscript submitted for publication).

WHY WAS THIS A SUCCESSFUL PARTNERSHIP?

Lack of effective services for custodial grandparents defined the key issues of this project. Three main components contributed to the overall success of this project. The high level of involvement from custodial grandparent group participants, use of an interdisciplinary Curriculum Design Team, and the high degree of commitment and involvement from a diverse Advisory Committee were unique and positive features of this endeavor.

Custodial grandparents were included during every step of the process and were encouraged and empowered to guide the overall direction of the curriculum. These caregivers had unique and multiple needs and were often isolated from other families sharing similar concerns. They discussed their strengths and challenges in the focus groups, attended pilot support group meetings, and offered direct advice to the Curriculum Design Team. Their participation and input continued throughout the field testing of the curriculum. Local custodial grandparents were heavily invested in this project because they readily identified that their opinions mattered and that the information they offered had the potential to benefit many other grandparent-headed families.

It was readily apparent at the onset of the curriculum project that the content of the needed curriculum was very diverse and would require a number of authors with broad background expertise to address all the critical content areas. The interdisciplinary Curriculum Design Team held routine group meetings and also attended meetings of the Advisory Committee. Authors also met individually with project directors and the editor. The content of the curriculum was re-written several times before it satisfied the Advisory Committee, pilot groups, the evaluator and the editor. The authors became very flexible and willing to share their proprietary pride during the process. This collaborative exchange enabled the Curriculum Design Team to view the completed project as a group product, as opposed to an individual accomplishment.

The Advisory Committee formed the central core of this project. This group, comprising academicians, professional practitioners, and custodial grandparents, willingly contributed ideas and suggestions during the entire project. The committee felt a strong level of responsibility to assist in developing a high quality curriculum that would be appropriate for diverse custodial grandparent audiences. They continually encouraged the Curriculum Design Team to provide extensive curricular options which would enable group facilitators to select activities to meet specific group needs. Advisory Committee Members' enthusiasm, dedication, and candor were outstanding and provided a continuing source of motivation to the project directors and the Curriculum Design Team.

What began as a grassroots community need driven by a cooperative venture of professionals and lay persons emerged as highly developed curricular resource for custodial grandparents. *Second Time Around—Grandparents Raising Grandchildren* is currently in its third printing and is being used by grandparent support groups nationwide. The success of this endeavor will continue to be measured by the numbers grandparent-headed families whose life circumstances are positively impacted by the results of this project. The simple observations made by professionals, when communicated to others within the profession, sparked this solution-oriented cooperative project.

REFERENCES

Becklund, L. (1993, March 14). I wanted somebody to love. *Los Angeles Times.*

Burton, L. M. (1992). Black grandparents rearing children of drug addicted parents: Stressors, outcomes and the social service needs. *The Gerontologist, 32,* 744-751.

Children's Defense Fund. (1997). *State of America's children yearbook.* Washington DC: Children's Defense Fund.

Creighton, L. L. (1991, December 16). Silent saviors. *U. S. News and World Report,* pp. 80-89.

Dannison, L., & Nieuwenhuis, A. (Eds.). (1996). *Second time around: Grandparents raising grandchildren.* Kalamazoo, MI: Western Michigan University Press.

deToledo, S., & Brown, D. (1995). *Grandparents as parents: A survival guide for raising a second family.* New York: The Guilford Press.

Jendrek, M. P. (1993). Grandparents who parent their grandchildren. *Journal of Marriage and the Family, 55,* 609-621.

Minkler, M., Driver, D., Roe, K. M., & Bedeian, K. (1993). Community interventions to support grandparent caregivers. *The Gerontologist, 33*(6), 807-811.

Minkler, M., & Roe, K. (1993). *Grandparents as caregivers: Raising children of the crack cocaine epidemic.* Newbury Park, CA: Sage.

Smith, A., Dannison, L., & Vacha-Haase, T. (1998). When "Grandma" is "Mom": Strategies for teachers. *Childhood Education, 15*(1), 12-16.

Vacha-Haase, T., Ness, C., Dannison, L., & Smith, A. (Manuscript submitted for publication). Grandparents raising grandchildren: A psycho-educational approach.

Yorkey, M. (1993, September). Picking up the pieces. *Focus on the Family,* p. 13.

32 A BROAD AND DYNAMIC PARTNERSHIP: MINNESOTA'S CHILDREN, YOUTH AND FAMILY CONSORTIUM

Martha Farrell Erickson
Richard A. Weinberg
University of Minnesota

In Minnesota, university researchers, community leaders, concerned citizens and local media are working together to sow "seeds of promise" in the lives of children and families. Building on the University of Minnesota's groundbreaking research on risk and resilience, the Children, Youth & Family Consortium (CYFC) joined forces with a major Twin Cities newspaper and a local network television affiliate to deepen public understanding of the factors that enable children to thrive and succeed, even in the face of high risk circumstances. *The Star Tribune* contributed nearly a full page in each of four Sunday editions of their paper for op-ed pieces written to educate and motivate readers as to how they can make a difference for children in their communities. On the Monday evening following each of the newspaper pieces, the local CBS affiliate telecast a related summary of key research findings and an engaging family story that brought the research to life. Readers and viewers then were invited to study a more detailed photo-journalistic report and to use it as a starting point for considering how they could become activists for the well-being of children and families in their own communities. Seeds of Promise reports continue to be used by individuals and community groups around the state—and around the country—as they seek direction for building strong, supportive networks for their children.

Taking the Seeds of Promise concept to the next level of action, CYFC now is coordinating a university-wide initiative to engage faculty, students, staff, and alumni in working to improve learning outcomes for young children in two urban schools. Each school site has established a leadership team that includes the principal, a lead faculty member from the U of M, a family liaison hired from within the community, and the U's Seeds of Promise coordinator. Addressing needs identified by families and teachers, the Seeds initiative so far has included an immunization campaign for young children in the school community; personal outreach to families of entering kindergartners; home visits aimed at improving school attendance and family involvement; after school activities for school-aged children; a family literacy program using university students as tutors; and a variety of parent education and support programs.

Seeds of Promise is just one example of the exciting work that can evolve when a university opens its doors to the surrounding community. And it is just one of many examples of the partnership activities that have defined the University of Minnesota's Children, Youth & Family Consortium since its inception in 1991. Here we briefly describe how and why the Consortium was established, present highlights of the Consortium's recent achievements, and discuss the challenges that we have faced—and continue to face—as we strive to build on the Consortium's early successes.

SIMPLE BEGINNINGS

The University of Minnesota has a long history of distinguished research and teaching on a wide range of child and family issues. And, as a land-grant university with a strong Extension Service, the university has a tradition of outreach and applied science. Nonetheless, in 1991, there was a growing recognition that university departments and disciplines too often worked in isolation, missing critical opportunities for collaboration and synergy as they studied the pressing issues facing today's children, youth and families. Similarly, many faculty, as well as colleagues outside the university, were concerned that the university's resources were not sufficiently focused on the harsh realities of life in the 1990s. There was a need for new partnerships to link research, practice and policy to strengthen communities and improve the well-being of children and families.

It was in that context that the CYF Consortium was established. Early in 1991, with leadership from dedicated faculty in education and human development, human ecology, and health sciences, the university hosted a planning retreat for 50 faculty and community leaders. Strongly affirming the need for an "all-university community consortium," this group drafted a mission statement, identified guiding principles, and developed a preliminary plan to translate ideas into action (Erickson & Weinberg, 1998; Weinberg & Erickson, 1996). Then, with seed money from the university's central administration—and with a commitment to find creative ways to leverage the resources of participating departments and community organizations—the Consortium opened its doors, staffed by one part-time director and a secretary. With the guidance of an eager advisory council made up of diverse faculty and community representatives, and with oversight from a council of deans, we turned on our lights, plugged in the phone, and announced to the world, "Here we go!"

UP AND RUNNING

Our phones started ringing immediately, with countless requests for information and offers to join with us as we began to operationalize the vision set forth in the planning retreat. As first steps in establishing an identity and creating mechanisms for sharing information, we did three things: 1) published a quarterly newsletter with a distribution of about 9,000; 2) organized periodic conferences or seminars to bring university and community people together around topics of mutual concern; and 3) building on new internet technology, began to create an "electronic rolodex" to help users locate experts or resources on topics of interest. (Note that the "rolodex" soon mushroomed into what is now known as CEC, described in a later section of this paper.)

Initially we also invited university and community folks to come together monthly in work groups around the three parts of the university's land-grant mission (research, teaching, and outreach/service). These groups generated many ideas—and implemented some—as we figured out new ways to work together through interdisciplinary seminars, collaborative research projects, and special events. But above all, these groups were about building new relationships, often across a chasm that separates the cultures of town and gown. As these face-to-face relationships developed, and mutual trust and respect deepened, the initial working groups gradually dissolved or were transformed into a wide range of vibrant, working partnerships built around common concerns, such as adoption issues, father involvement, school-family partnerships, and adolescent health needs. Through each of these partnerships, more and more people began to see themselves as a part of the Consortium.

With strong momentum, we experienced extraordinary growth in the scope of work, number of participants, opportunities for new partnerships—and, not surprisingly, number of staff employed in the Consortium office (now 8-14 people in any given quarter). Through a combination of proactive outreach (both in and out of the university) and diligent responsiveness to community-identified needs, the Consortium within its first two years became well-known as a place for CYF professionals, public officials, journalists, and concerned parents to turn for information. And by our third year of operation we had been invited into a partnership with the Vice President of the United States, putting us on the national and international map as a connecting place for those who want to create family programs and policies that are grounded in good research.

The Consortium's activities are broad, varied and constantly evolving, but highlights from our first six years include:

- **Consortium Electronic Clearinghouse (CEC)**, an on-line resource and networking center that has become the nexus of many university-community partnership activities. CEC is home to such collaborative websites as KidsCount, FatherNet, AdoptInfo, and Minnesota's Early Childhood Training Network.
- **Adolescent Health Partnership**, which designs and implements creative, interdisciplinary evaluations of community interventions and proposed youth policies at the local, state and national level (see Weinberg & Erickson, 1996, for a more complete description).
- **DHHS Project on Father Responsibility**, through which we convened a national panel of scientists and family support professionals to help us synthesize research on fathering and develop a theoretical framework to guide federal agencies in their efforts to encourage father involvement and responsibility (Doherty, Kouneski & Erickson, in press).
- **Family Re-Union**, an ongoing series of annual family policy conferences moderated by Vice President Al Gore and co-sponsored by the Children, Youth & Family Consortium. Topics have included work and family, family and the media, families and learning, families and health, and the role of men in children's lives. Each year, the conference becomes a springboard for other

exciting local, national and international activities, many of them coordinated by the Consortium.

CHALLENGES

Despite the overall success of the Consortium, our journey is not without challenges. As discussed elsewhere, we are ever mindful of these barriers that sometimes impede our progress (Erickson & Weinberg, 1998):

- **Cultural differences** between academia (with a focus on generating knowledge and seeking long-term solutions for long-term problems) and the community (with a need to provide prompt, direct service with short-term results).
- **Community distrust of the university**, sometimes grounded in experience with academic researchers who seemed arrogant, over-directive, and insensitive to the needs and strengths of community participants.
- **A university reward system** that fails to create adequate incentives for faculty members to work across disciplines and/or in community partnerships.
- **Turfdom between academic departments**, often exacerbated by management and accounting systems that effectively pit one unit against another.

Beyond those common barriers to university-community partnerships, the Consortium also faces a somewhat unique challenge in demonstrating its own value. Because it is our intent to work as a *catalyst* for partnership, rather than always *managing* the work within our own office, we are never quite sure how—or if—to claim credit for activities. On the one hand, at its best, the Consortium may be nearly invisible in a project, with funding and recognition going to other academic units and/or community organizations. But on the other hand, if we are too invisible, we may jeopardize our own existence. Struggling with how to even describe what the Consortium is, some of our founding fathers and mothers refer to the Consortium as an "attitude" or even a "fragrance." That is hard to measure, but you would miss it if it were gone!

LOOKING TO THE FUTURE

From the beginning, the Consortium was fueled more by passion than dollars. That continues to be the case today. The faculty who participate do so more because they believe it is the "right" thing to do than because of any obvious, short-term rewards in the work. (However, some faculty definitely have reaped material benefits, including opportunities for external funding for research, through their work in the Consortium.)

To continue to nurture and extend the partnerships we have built thus far, we need the commitment of the university to sustain funding for basic operations—understanding that the Consortium is accountable for "value added" that will justify the university's investment. And we need to continue to seek deeper system change that will create more obvious incentives for faculty participation in university-community partnerships.

We have accomplished much in our first six years; and there is much still to accomplish. Our hope is that the Consortium attitude will continue to be contagious, infecting faculty, students and administrators across campus with the desire to focus knowledge and energy on improving the well-being of children and families.

REFERENCES

Doherty, W., Kouneski, E., & Erickson, M. F. (1996). *Responsible fathering: An overview and conceptual framework.* A report prepared for the Administration for Children and Families and the Office of the Assistant Secretary for Planning and Evaluation of the U. S. Department of Health and Human Services.

Erickson, M. F. & Weinberg, R. A. (1998). The Children, Youth and Family Consortium: A University of Minnesota/Community Partnership. In R. M. Lerner & L. A. K. Simon (Eds.), *University-community collaborations for the twenty-first century: Outreach scholarship for youth and families* (pp. 185-201). New York: Garland Publishing.

Weinberg, R. A. & Erickson, M. F. (1996). Minnesota's Children, Youth, and Family Consortium: A University-Community Collaboration. *Journal of Research on Adolescence, 6*(1), 37-53.

33 BUILDING PARTNERSHIPS: THE UNIVERSITY AND COMMUNITY UNITE

Ann P. Blackwell
Anne M. Stanberry
The University of Southern Mississippi

NATURE OF PARTNERSHIP

The efficacy of joining forces with others sharing similar goals and purposes to more effectively create change is an established phenomenon. It is particularly important to remain alert and receptive to opportunities for collaboration with persons and groups beyond one's typical horizon. In many cases, the foundation for such partnerships is established over a considerable length of time, allowing for credibility and trust between persons and groups to develop. This chapter provides one example of collaboration between faculty members in a School of Family and Consumer Sciences in a public university and personnel in a public school system. The partnership was formed to secure grant money for enhancing the education of young children and their parents.

BACKGROUND

The Mississippi Coalition for Change: Quality of Life Issues was formed in 1993 and comprises eight professional organizations whose goals and purposes include improving quality of life for individuals and families in our state. Coalition members include organizations in family and consumer sciences, early childhood, marriage and family therapy, nutrition and dietetics, and professional education. Each year, the present authors integrate activities of the Coalition into the family and consumer sciences curriculum to stress the professional's role in public policy. Experience with the Coalition undergirds the philosophy that achieving a higher quality of life for individuals and families requires a collaborative effort.

Each year, representatives of the Coalition are invited to participate in a focus group sponsored and planned by a graduate level class taught by one of the authors at our public university. Undergraduate students observe the focus group and participate in open discussion following the formal discussion. The endeavor introduces students to the focus group process and promotes dialogue among university students, faculty, and Coalition members. Perspectives from a variety of persons representing organizations that are diverse, yet connected in their commitment to families, promote students' thinking beyond their normal boundaries. In turn, Coalition members witness faculty and students in action; perceptions of student and program credibility are positively affected; trust relationships between professionals involved in the process develop; and links between formerly distant groups emerge. This effort is coupled with other activities involving students and the Coalition to promote public policy engagement and enhance students' skills and confidence in the public policy arena.

Benefits resulting from conscious and persistent communication and involvement on the part of university faculty with the Coalition include additional opportunities for partnership initiated by individual members of the Coalition. In 1997, the authors were approached by a Coalition member who directs a parenting center in a contiguous community. The director of the parenting center was aware of a grant opportunity and had ideas for pursuing it; she sought university faculty perceived to have vision and grant-writing skills. The concept of successfully working together on additional projects, which required four years to germinate, was embraced by the individual. The boundary between public school educators, who often stay behind their "privacy fences," and university faculty, who often are accused of being "locked in the ivory tower," was altered to allow this collaborative effort to proceed.

PURPOSES AND GOALS

The guidelines of the grant invited rich integration of the public school program and the university curriculum. The grant also afforded the opportunity to meet one of the major requirements for successful partnerships, i.e., all parties involved could make significant contributions and reap significant benefits. After several meetings between the parenting center director and the authors, the following purposes for the collaboration were identified:

1) Better utilize resources available through the public school district and the university to serve parents and children in our community.
2) Strengthen the relationship between the representatives of the public school district and the university program.
3) Enhance and expand community involvement with the public school parenting center.
4) Provide preservice university students with field-based opportunities early in their university program.

ANALYSIS OF THE PROCESS

The Mississippi State Department of Education grant, which came through the United States Department of Education, provided $70,000 per school year for a Reaching New Heights in Local Innovations proposal. The parenting center director, with the help of the authors, based the grant on the national educational goals of school readiness and parent/community involvement. A major component was the expansion of the home/school/community partnership program, Parents as Teachers (PAT). Specific objectives of the partnership and the grant were to recruit more participants in the Parents as Teachers program, assist families in gaining the necessary parenting skills to improve children's school readiness, and identify children's developmental delays and handicaps. The authors wrote a separate sub-grant that established a paid graduate assistantship for a family and consumer sciences student to work with the parenting center and that provided other opportunities for student involvement in the Parents as Teachers program.

ACHIEVEMENTS RELATED TO GOALS

Results of the partnership have been extremely favorable. In addition to the focus on the purposes of the collaboration and specific objectives of the grant, additional benefits have been derived. The partnership revealed opportunities for practicum and volunteer placement for undergraduate and graduate students in family and consumer sciences. Students have been afforded opportunities to connect theory to practice and witness the impact of their education on others in the community. Specifically, students have benefited from working with educators, community personnel, parents, and children in different environments. They have experienced personal and professional growth and gained confidence by applying knowledge and skill gained through university coursework in authentic situations. In turn, the public school district and families in the community have benefited from the students' involvement. With the additional human resources available through students, more lives can be touched and more progress achieved.

For faculty members, several benefits have resulted from the collaborative effort. The curriculum has been enhanced and strengthened by additional opportunities for students to engage in active learning. In addition, students can observe training for Parents as Teachers personnel on the Denver Developmental Screening and Learning Accomplishment Profile-Developmental (LAP-D) conducted by university faculty as a component of the partnership. In addition, the opportunity to conduct longitudinal research on the effects of the PAT program on children's school readiness and achievement has been identified through the partnership. Last, the partnership serves as a wonderful addition to illustrations in classroom discussions regarding the need for students to be involved as professionals in public policy and open to partnerships with diverse groups.

In conclusion, the present partnership meets the challenge issued by the National Association of State Universities and Land Grant Colleges (NASULGC) (1997) for universities to revitalize their partnerships with school systems, strengthen the link between students' education and careers, and provide active learning. Through volunteer and paid service at the parenting center, students learn to value that small ways of helping others can make a big difference. Students grasp the important contributions they can make to improve the quality of life for individuals and families in our community. These are vital concepts for students to embrace and for university faculty to reinforce on a consistent basis. Partnerships that allow students to share their caring and expertise with others in real-world situations provide an ideal tool for this reinforcement. The authors are committed to sustaining and improving the aforementioned partnership, complete with benefits for several groups, and to actively pursue others in order to more effectively create change and improve quality of life for individuals and families in our state.

PROSPECTS FOR LONG-TERM SUSTAINABILITY

Due to the benefits derived from this partnership for all persons involved, the prospects for long-term sustainability are excellent. The positive evaluations regarding implementation of the established goals provide excellent endorsement for continuation of the grant money. In addition, proposed longitudinal research that will compare the achievement scores of children participating in the Parents as Teachers program with nonparticipating children will invite local school district funding and the possibility of research funding.

Sustainability is also foreseen in the growth and development of university students seeking to impact the lives of young children. The experiences afforded through this partnership have impressed upon the students the realities of life for children and families in our communities, the critical need for effective parent education, and the contributions that students can make to the actual outcome of another's life. They are better equipped to share their expertise and better educated regarding the need for this expertise in society today.

The sustainability of collaboration among the professionals involved in this partnership is also clearly anticipated. As a result of the initial partnership, relationships are further cemented, strengths are clearly identified, and synergistic efforts are strongly encouraged. The successful collaboration prompts investigation of additional opportunities to join forces and share resources to improve the quality of life for individuals and families in our sphere of influence.

LEARNINGS FROM THIS PARTNERSHIP

Persons involved in the partnership effort experienced considerable affirmation concerning the value of diversity. Participation by persons from a variety of economic, educational, and ethnic backgrounds underscored the verity that opportunities multiply when collaboration is embraced. University students, in particular, developed broadened perspectives when exposed to the benefits of diversity and when encouraged to reflect on its impact. This perspective was nurtured through experiential learning that revealed the richness of resources available through a variety of individuals and groups.

Additional insight was afforded to separate entities involved in the collaborative effort. For example, university students learned that academic theory has real-world application; parents involved in the Parents as Teachers program learned that there is significant potential for improved cognition in their children; and Parents as Teachers personnel realized that working together creates a greater impact because more people can be served and more needs can be met. Also, as a result of the partnership, the university students and the university program gained credibility as interaction occurred in the community.

WHY WAS THIS A SUCCESSFUL PARTNERSHIP?

The partnership proved successful because everyone involved made important contributions. The university faculty possessed expertise needed by the Parents as Teachers program and also possessed resources available through their students.

The director of the parenting center had information regarding grant opportunities and also placement opportunities for the university students. The university students contributed expertise as well as human capital for the Parents as Teachers program.

Success of the partnership also resulted from tangible benefits received by each of the participating parties. As described in the section, "Achievements Related to Goals," each member of the partnership realized gains as a result of the effort. The ultimate success of the partnership, however, was derived from the knowledge that many young lives were positively touched and improved by the collaboration. Opportunities for these children to experience success in school and success in life were enhanced. Because everyone involved in the partnership shares a passion for children, this understanding denotes true success.

REFERENCES

The National Association of State Universities and Land-Grant Colleges. (April, 1997). *Returning to our roots: The student experience*. Available: http:/www.nasulgc.nche.edu.

34 PREPARING STUDENTS FOR COLLABORATION: THE MU INTERPROFESSIONAL INITIATIVE

Tracy K. Dranginis
Kathy Thornburg
University of Missouri

During the 1990s in Missouri, as in much of the rest of the country, trends in social policy have continued to reflect the desire to devolve decision-making, responsibility, and resources to local communities. The process of devolution not only necessitates that different individuals, professions, organizations and institutions will be developing, testing, and implementing social policy, it also necessitates that these same individuals and groups will be required to collaborate in decision-making and be accountable for resource allocation and use in more immediate and complete ways than ever before. It is through the recognition of this trend that the administrators, faculty, students, and their community partners perceived the need to train pre-service professionals for collaborative practice.

NATURE OF PARTNERSHIP

The nature of the MU Interprofessional Initiative (MUII) partnership may best be described through the MUII's vision statement:

> To create an approach to interprofessional education at the University of Missouri that graduates students in the development and human services professions with the intellectual capacity and professional skills needed to work effectively within a collaborative community environment. To systematically change the way colleges, departments, faculty, and students work together to prepare for service to Missouri's children, families, and communities.

The MUII vision statement was created by its membership that includes faculty, administrators, undergraduate and graduate students, and community-based service providers representing eight colleges, 18 departments and programs, 11 state, community, and agency providers, more than 60 faculty members, and approximately 25 students.

PURPOSES AND GOALS

The purpose of the MUII is to create efficiencies and encourage cooperation and shared resources among faculty, departments, colleges and community-based professionals that train teachers, social service providers, health care providers, and human development professionals so that MU's graduates will be able to work collaboratively in the field. The concept for the MUII can be traced to the Missouri Caring Communities model, a collaboration among seven Missouri state agencies: the Department of Social Services, the Department of Elementary and Secondary Education, the Department of Health, the Department of Mental Health, the Department of Labor and Industrial Relations, the Department of Economic Development, and the Department of Corrections.

The Caring Communities model was designed as a mechanism to address the anticipated impact of federal welfare reform policy on Missouri's communities. The core goal of Caring Communities is to coordinate the efforts and resources of these agencies so that they may deliver improved, comprehensive services to Missouri's children and families even in an era of a reduction in resources.

However, the model, like similar collaborations in other states, was impeded by a lack of experience in collaborative activities among agency professionals as well as by local service providers and community-based organizations. Historically in Missouri, as elsewhere, services to children and families have been delivered by a smorgasbord of health, educational, and social service providers, both public and private, with little or no coordination among them. Services often overlap, efforts are duplicated, gaps in needed assistance occur, and comprehensive solutions to complex problems are impossible for reasons of both logistics and culture of professions barriers. The leadership of the Caring Communities model recognized these potential barriers to coordinated service delivery and asked the University of Missouri to address one aspect of this issue by consciously and systematically developing, piloting, and institutionalizing collaborative practice learning through an interprofessional initiative.

Through support from Missouri Caring Communities and the Ewing Marion Kauffman Foundation, MUII has set and implemented or is in the process of implementing the following goals:

- Identifying the potential barriers and opportunities for interprofessional/interdisciplinary campus-based courses as well as field placements and developing a mechanism for coordination that addresses discipline-specific issues such as credentialing and licensure requirements.
- Developing a better understanding by faculty and students of the needs, strengths, and limitations of community-based professionals to provide collaborative learning experiences.
- Developing in the MU administration an understanding of the necessity of interprofessional education and creating mechanisms for institutionalization.
- Identifying a set of core competencies for interprofessional and collaborative practice. These core competencies will be used to inform the multiple efforts of MUII participants.

- Identifying and providing opportunities for MU faculty to learn of and implement emerging pedagogical techniques that encourage collaboration.
- Designing and implementing a multi-level evaluative process that addresses: 1) the needs of community-based providers for entering professionals trained in collaborative practice skills; 2) the logistical and intellectual development needs of students with these skills; 3) the opportunities for and barriers to participation in an interprofessional curriculum by faculty, programs, and colleges; and 4) the development of the organizational structure of the MUII.

ANALYSIS OF THE PROCESS

To achieve its goals the MUII has implemented a purposefully loose and flat network of opportunity for participation that is open and inclusive to faculty, students, community-based providers, and administrators. The MUII can best be described as having three basic units of participants: A board of deans and directors, a management team, and ad hoc teams to address specific planning or programmatic goals.

The board of deans and directors, representing the colleges and programs that train human service and development professionals, provides direction to the initiative in regard to policy development and institutionalization through the professional recognition of faculty involvement, and by securing and committing internal resources to the initiative. The management team includes faculty representation from varied disciplines including human development and family studies, educational and counseling psychology, community sociology, nursing, family and community medicine, and education. It also includes a "student" and a professional staff position. This group provides logistical support to the work teams including the distribution of funds for planning and implementing interprofessional activities, serves as liaison to external funders, advises the board of deans and directors on policy issues and resource needs, and communicates and hosts opportunities for increasing participation in the initiative through campus-wide meetings.

The community-advisory team meets with MUII faculty several times a year to provide new and reality-based ideas on issues related to developing an interprofessional curriculum. The membership of this team comprises education, social service (both private and public sectors), and health care practitioners, representing multiple levels of managerial and clinical responsibility. The community-advisory team helps MUII faculty understand and bridge the gaps between pre-service and in-service education. Additionally, they provide critique of and support for interprofessional field placements and field research.

The ad hoc teams come together on a temporary basis to address specific planning or programmatic goals. To date the teams have met as necessary to complete their work and then disbanded, joined with other teams working on variations of the same set of issues, or reconfigured around a follow-up or implementation issue. All of these teams are multi-disciplinary and all include community-based professionals and students. Membership in these teams remains open and newly interested parties are encouraged to join at any point in the process. The MUII professional member provides support to these teams in regard to communications, logistical arrangements, accessing funds, and reporting to the larger MU community. Examples of the ad hoc teams include the team that determined the core competencies of interprofessional and collaborative practice, the team that developed and is conducting the MUII evaluation process, and the team developing an interprofessional curriculum to be used in conjunction with coordinated, multi-disciplinary field placements.

Finally, interdisciplinary teams of faculty and community-based professionals, or individual faculty working with students on interprofessional/collaborative practice issues, may apply for MUII funds to support their specific projects. These funds may be used to 'buy' a small amount of their salary, to hire staff (typically student assistants) to perform some of their duties, to pay for materials and supplies, and to support travel directly related to interprofessional education and collaboration. Some examples of the work of these teams/individuals include: An interdisciplinary graduate seminar developed a comprehensive, multidisciplinary literature review in the area of interprofessional education and collaborative practice for the Internet; an interdisciplinary team of faculty traveled to another state university to benchmark the use of problem-based learning techniques in a collaborative practice setting; and support was given to a faculty member to administer a community-based, mentoring literacy program that places MU students and community volunteers in the local schools to work with at-risk children on reading skills.

ACHIEVEMENT RELATED TO GOALS

The MUII has been successful in implementing a number of interprofessional and collaborative activities in the arenas of teaching and research to date. The following examples, although not comprehensive, give a good indication of the nature of the MUII activities:

1) The cataloguing and profiling of existing interprofessional and collaborative practice initiatives on campus. This was done to avoid duplication of effort and to share the resources of the MUII.
2) The cataloguing of the existing community service activities and requirements by MU degree programs and departments. This catalogue is used to identify opportunities for collaboration in field placements.
3) The piloting of an undergraduate, interdisciplinary service learning course delivered through the MU Office of Service Learning.
4) The development of virtual case studies to be used by interdisciplinary student teams during their field placements.
5) The development of an interprofessional health core that includes credit and non-credit activities to prepare professional educators and health care practitioners.
6) The development of a comprehensive literature review in the area of interprofessional education and collaborative practice through an interdisciplinary graduate seminar.
7) The implementation of a literacy mentoring program that places MU students as well as community volunteers with at-risk pupils.

8) The planning of a partnership with Kansas City, Missouri elementary schools to place interdisciplinary teams of MU students for extended, collaborative field placements.
9) The development and implementation of a multi-level MUII evaluation process.
10) The development of an MUII web site to inform the MU community of the Initiative's actions and to encourage participation.

PROSPECTS FOR LONG-TERM SUSTAINABILITY

The potential for the long-term sustainability of the MU Interprofessional Initiative is quite high due to the commitment of administrators and faculty across the colleges that train human service professionals as well as from community-based agencies and organizations that hire these MU graduates. This commitment is based in the realization of the necessity to adapt to the trends in social welfare policy regarding both the devolution of services and the reduction in resources at the federal, state, and local levels.

There are, however, several issues that have yet to be fully addressed in regard to the long-term sustainability of the MUII. One of these issues is the need for the internal commitment of real and permanent funding to interprofessional training at both the main administrative level as well as within colleges and departments. Second, there is the need to address the issue of credit for participation in interprofessional activities (both teaching and research) by faculty while on tenure track. The existence of these barriers to participation potentially means a generation of faculty who need to know how to train students in collaboration although they currently cannot be part of the process of developing the MUII and may not be successful in developing their careers at the same time. The third issue is the need to address the reality of the increasing number of and contribution made by non-tenure track faculty across the university system who require real dollars for participation in the MUII.

LEARNING FROM THIS PARTNERSHIP

If it were possible to begin the MUII process over again, there are two primary issues that were not foreseen that could be addressed differently. The first is described above regarding the barriers to participation faced by untenured, tenure-track faculty, and non-tenure track faculty. Second, is the need to be consciously aware of and sensitive to the organization and professional culture of the various schools and programs involved. Not only are there ongoing internal debates over the value of interprofessional education, but there are ongoing territorial issues regarding service provision. Thus, the concept of collaboration, sharing information, clients, and tasks, can be threatening to those professions that have had to work very hard to achieve their credibility with the public and other professions.

CONCLUSIONS: WHY IS THIS A SUCCESSFUL PARTNERSHIP?

The MUII is an example of a successful university-community partnership for many reasons, not the least of which is the time, energy, and creativity put forth by numerous faculty, administrators, community-based professionals, and students. From this experience, the MUII can offer the following suggestions as helpful in creating an effective approach to training students to work collaboratively across professional boundaries for the good of children, families, and communities:

- Let the process evolve. The most effective MUII teams have been those that were self-selected and that followed their own path.
- Be flexible regarding the methods of participation by faculty, students, and community-based professionals at both the individual and organizational (departments/programs, agencies, etc.) level.
- Build strong relationships and have commitment from key decision-makers at the beginning of the process and throughout its evolution. This enhances the likelihood of successful institutionalization.
- Include community-based professionals and students in the development of an interprofessional and collaborative practice curriculum. Ultimately, these are the individuals who put learning into practice.
- Be open and inclusive to participation from all that are interested. Healthy children, strong families, and sustainable communities are the result of caring and commitment from the whole community not just those who provide direct services.

REFERENCES

Blank, M. J., & Lombardi, J. (1991, June). *Towards improved services for children and families: Forging new relationships through collaboration.* Washington, DC: The Institute for Educational Leadership.

Casto, R. M. (1987). Preservice courses for interprofessional practice. *Theory into Practice: Interprofessional Education, 26*(2), 103-109.

Casto, R. M. (1993). Defining, supporting and maintaining interprofessional education. *Journal of Education Policy, 8*(5-6), 153-155. (ERIC Document Reproduction Service No. EJ 475 840)

Chaskin, R. J., & Richman, H. A. (1992, Spring). Concerns about school-linked services: Institution-based versus community-based models. *Future of Children, 2*(1), 107-117.

Cyphert, F., & Cunningham, L. L. (1987). Interprofessional education and practice: A future agenda. *Theory into Practice: Interprofessional Education, 26*(2), 153-156.

Houle, C. O., Cyphert, F., & Boggs, D. (1987). Education for the professions. *Theory into Practice: Interprofessional Education, 26*(2), 87-93.

Knapp, M. S., Barnard, K., Brandon, R. N., Gehrke, N. J., Smith, A. J., & Teather, E. C. (1993). University-based preparation for collaborative interprofessional practice. *Journal of Education Policy, 8*(5-6), 137-151. (ERIC Document Reproduction Service No. EJ 475 849)

Lawson, H., & Hooper-Briar, K. (1994). *Expanding partnerships: Involving colleges and universities in interprofessional collaboration and service integration.* Oxford, OH: The Danforth Foundation and the Institute for Educational Renewal at Miami University.

Winton, P. J. (1992). *Working with families in early intervention: An interdisciplinary preservice curriculum* (2nd ed.). Chapel Hill: University of North Carolina Frank PorterGraham Child Development Center.

35 RESEARCH-BASED PARENTING EDUCATION FOR DIVORCING PARENTS: A UNIVERSITY-COMMUNITY COLLABORATION

Mark A. Fine[1]
Marilyn Coleman
Sara Gable
Lawrence H. Ganong
Jean Ispa
Johnetta Morrison
Kathy R. Thornburg
University of Missouri - Columbia

Focus on Kids (FOK) is a mandated parenting education program for divorcing parents in central Missouri. Although the program is facilitated by faculty in the Department of Human Development and Family Studies (HDFS) at the University of Missouri, its ultimate success relies on an extensive collaboration with many community partners.

NATURE OF PARTNERSHIP

The FOK partnership includes the University, University Outreach and Extension, the 13th Judicial Circuit Court in central Missouri, and community members who are mandated to participate in the parenting education program. The Family Court, with the approval of the commissioners and judges, established a rule in 1995 that requires all parents with minor children who are currently divorcing or filing a motion to modify their original divorce decree to attend a 2.5 hour parenting education session.

The Department of Human Development and Family Studies was given the responsibility of developing the program and for providing the parenting education sessions. At present, we have three teams of two faculty members who facilitate the sessions. One other faculty member and three graduate students have been trained as facilitators. The FOK faculty regularly review the curriculum and make changes as needed. Because of the close working relationship with the Court, curricular issues and possible changes are discussed with the Court representatives.

University Outreach and Extension is involved in several ways. First, one of the faculty facilitators is a state Extension specialist. Second, University Extension is currently extending the program to other parts of the state. Towards this end, a number of regional Human Development Extension specialists have finished a training regimen that exceeds 20 hours of preparation, observation, and co-facilitation and are working within their own communities (e.g., by contacting judges and other court personnel) to determine if they can provide FOK to divorcing parents.

PURPOSES AND GOALS

The primary purpose of the program is to help parents facilitate their children's adjustment to the divorce process. Of course, we also hope to improve parents' well-being, but this objective is secondary to our central goal of helping the children. Specifically, five research-based objectives have informed curriculum development and presentation: 1) To encourage ex-spouses to resolve conflicts pertaining to their children directly with each other and without putting children in the middle of their disputes; 2) to encourage both parents to remain actively involved in the lives of their children following divorce (within limits discussed below); 3) to provide concrete suggestions of helpful parental behaviors (e.g., talking directly with one's ex-spouse about child-related issues) and potentially unhealthy parental behaviors (e.g., criticizing one's ex-spouse in the presence of the child); 4) to provide information on how divorce affects children's socioemotional adjustment, with some attention to differing effects on children of various ages; and 5) to provide information on self-help organizations, self-help groups, human service agencies, and other organizations that may be helpful to children and parents as they attempt to adjust to the process of divorce.

The session itself consists of the following components. First, we introduce ourselves, review the purpose and objectives of the program, distribute readings for later use, share assumptions that underlie the program, and describe the course of the session. Second, we play a portion of a videotape that shows a number of children describing what the divorce experience has been like for them and engage the group in a discussion of the children's comments. Third, we show a series of four vignettes on the videotape. In each vignette, family members are engaged in a divorce-related dilemma (e.g., involving visitation, child support, transitions from one home to another for children, and one parent becoming romantically involved with a new partner). In the first part of each vignette, the situation is not handled well and, in some way, the children are placed in the middle of the parents' conflicts. After the first part of the vignette is played, the tape is stopped and the participants are engaged in a discussion of what did not go well, what the issues are that led to the conflictual interaction, and what might be done to resolve the situation. After the discussion, the second part of the videotaped vignette is played, which shows the family members attempting to resolve the conflict. After the vignette is completed, another discussion ensues with group participants. After the four videotapes, and with time permitting, we show a final segment of the videotape that shares some more impressions from children and parents regarding the process of divorce, present information on parenting plans, and/or answer any specific questions that participants came to the session with. Finally, the participants are asked to complete a written evaluation of the session.

ANALYSIS OF THE PROCESS

Working with the Court

After meeting at a national conference on family mediation, several HDFS faculty and representatives from the Family Court met to discuss the idea of developing a parenting education program for divorcing parents. Our mutual interest in developing a program for divorcing parents was furthered by preliminary findings that such programs can lead to positive child outcomes (Kramer & Washo, 1993). As a faculty, our strategy was to work on curriculum and program details and to present proposals to the Court representatives. Through this process, we came to agreement on what topics would be covered, who would teach, how registration would operate, and funding procedures. Court representatives were actively involved at every stage of the planning process. In addition, since the inception of the program, the Court has taken responsibility for fee collection and participant registration.

Program Planning and Development

Eight HDFS faculty volunteered to develop and implement the program. After initial planning meetings, several subcommittees were formed: 1) curriculum, 2) logistics/budget, and 3) evaluation. The curriculum committee was particularly active, as it reviewed a large number of commercially produced videotapes, selected topics that would be covered, and planned how the session would be structured. All three committees made recommendations to the FOK faculty group as a whole.

Curriculum Development for a Diverse Audience

We felt that it was important that our curriculum be acceptable and accessible to program participants, who vary considerably in educational and socioeconomic background. In particular, we wanted the vignettes in our videotape to represent different races, ages of children, parental educational levels, and socioeconomic statuses. Where existing materials (e.g., a videotape) were deficient, we determined how we could compensate by presentation or discussion during the session.

Program Funding

The budget was designed to create an incentive for faculty to provide the instruction, to buy teaching and resource materials, to provide refreshments for participants, and to establish a fund that could be used for program development (e.g., making our own videotapes). We based the budget on estimates of the number of parents in the two counties who would be required to participate. Faculty do not receive additional compensation, but rather receive access to funds that can be used for professional purposes, such as travel, books, and equipment. We charge the Court a set fee per participant who attends a session. Those developing similar programs should take into account that there are likely to be substantial costs up front, before income is received (e.g., purchasing videotapes for review).

Session Scheduling

Sessions are scheduled a year in advance, and are held at the university. There are benefits to having the sessions on campus (e.g., availability of rooms free of charge, proximity for faculty) and challenges (e.g., parking can be difficult, some participants are not familiar with the university campus). We schedule four sessions per month based on an estimate of approximately 20 participants per session.

It is important to make sure that the room is appropriately set up for the session. For us, this means having tables in a U-shape, having a VCR and television set, and having an overhead projector and screen. We serendipitously fell upon the benefits of having participants sit around a table after the room had been incorrectly set up for one session (we had previously placed chairs in a semi-circle with no table). We think the group dynamics improved substantially after making the table a standard part of our room set up.

Gaining the Acceptance of Important Constituencies

The success of collaborative programs depends on acceptance from affected constituencies. In our case, we worked extensively with the court representatives, but, in hindsight, we could have worked more closely with lawyers in the two participating counties. We gave presentations on the program to representatives from the local bar associations, but it might have been better had we involved lawyers in the early planning. This might have resulted not only in an improved educational product, but also more support from lawyers after the program started.

In the early phases of the program, court representatives observed a number of sessions and they have an open, standing invitation to observe any session at their discretion. We also allow selected others to observe (e.g., graduate students, lawyers, Extension specialists) with permission of both the Court and the faculty team teaching that particular session.

ACHIEVEMENTS RELATED TO GOALS

Since the program began in 1995, we have served over 2,000 divorcing parents. At the end of each session, participants evaluate the usefulness and value of different aspects of the program. The evaluations have been consistently positive (mean ratings on almost all items above 4.0 on a 1-5 scale), particularly given that participants are mandated to attend and have to pay a fee. Thus, we feel that we have been successful in meeting our educational goals.

Nevertheless, we recognize that our goals are primarily attitudinal and educational in nature rather than behavioral. We do not know if we have been successful in effecting behavioral changes in parenting practices following divorce. To address this issue, guided in part by calls in the literature for sounder evaluations of divorced parenting programs (Braver, Smith, & DeLuse, 1997), we have recently conducted focus groups of past participants to determine not only what their impressions were of the program itself, but also if they believe that they have behaved differently as a result of attending the session (Morgan, 1998). Qualitatively, FOK participants reported feeling overwhelmingly positive about the program, most felt that a more extensive program would be appropriate, and most supported an optional program for children. They identified the three most valuable components of the program as the focus on keeping children out of the middle of parental disputes, provision of practical information that would help them during the process, and the opportunity to interact with others in similar situations.

Focus groups were also conducted with a comparison group of demographically-similar divorcing parents who did not participate in Focus on Kids. With respect to qualitative comparisons between the groups of parents who participated in FOK and those who did not, most FOK parents felt that they were able to keep their children out of the middle, while comparison group participants were more likely to report putting children in the middle. Further, FOK parents were more likely to report that both parents were staying active in the children's lives. However, both sets of parents were equally likely to report difficulty communicating with former spouses and reported that their children's outcomes were better after time had passed. In terms of quantitative comparisons between parents in the two groups, relative to those in the comparison group, FOK parents reported less conflict and reported providing and receiving more support from former spouses.

We also have plans to conduct pre- and post-evaluations with psychometrically sound instruments to assess whether there are positive behavioral changes after participating in the session. Ideally, included in these assessments will be behavioral observations (before and after the FOK) of parent-child interaction while processing divorce-related issues to allow us to determine if parents are responding to their children in a more sensitive and responsive manner.

PROSPECTS FOR LONG-TERM SUSTAINABILITY

Focus on Kids will continue as long as the Court system, the legal community, and the citizens in the area support the notion of mandating parenting education for divorcing individuals with minor children living in the home. Given that parents are required to pay a fee, financial viability is not a major concern. Thus, sustainability will depend on public sentiment about the usefulness of the program and our ability to demonstrate that it is effective in meeting the Court's charge to us.

LEARNINGS FROM THIS PARTNERSHIP

Gender Composition of Teaching Teams

Whenever possible, we have mixed gender faculty teams. Our sense is that having both female and male presenters has been helpful because it allows all participants to have someone of the same gender with whom they can relate.

Sensitive Issues

In virtually every session, at least one participant raises an issue or shares an experience that is not addressed in the curriculum (or in others around the country, based on our review of other programs). For example, our curriculum emphasizes that it is beneficial to children if both parents remain actively involved in their children's lives after the divorce *and* that both parents want to remain actively involved. We know that there are situations when children may suffer from contact with a parent (e.g., an abusive parent) and that a large number of parents are not actively involved in their children's lives. We tell participants that, although our program encourages active parental involvement, we recognize that such involvement may not be desirable or possible for some children. In such cases, we encourage parents to talk about their experiences to the extent that they are comfortable in doing so.

Facilitating a Balance Between Didactic Presentation and Group Discussion

As with any group-based educational program, we struggle with finding a balance between presenting didactic information and encouraging group discussion. Because learning takes place most effectively when participants apply newly learned information to their own personal situations, limited didactic information is presented. For those seeking additional information, we also provide participants with written materials on the effects of divorce on children and adults and community resources.

Addressing Individual Needs

A dilemma arises when an individual in the group asks for extensive feedback on a particular concern. Because this is an educational group, we provide individual attention only as long as we think that other participants will benefit from the discussion. At the point where our judgment is that the exchange is no longer benefitting the group as a whole, we ask the individual if we can discuss the issue privately during the break or after the group session.

Being Sensitive to Participants' Diverse Experiences

Participants span a wide range of educational (46% have 12 or fewer years of education; 31% have either a bachelor's or graduate degree) and income levels (67% have annual family incomes below $35,000; 15% have incomes exceeding $50,000), presenting a number of pedagogical challenges, including: 1) Being careful not to present research-based information as if were applicable to all participants; 2) trying to be sensitive to those whose needs may not be optimally addressed by the curriculum (e.g., those who believe that child abuse is taking place; those whose ex-spouse may not be involved in the child's life); 3) respecting reasonable differences in parenting values held by the participants; and 4) presenting material in a way that is beneficial to individuals with a range of learning abilities and styles.

Meeting the Needs of Participants Filing Motions to Modify the Divorce Decree

Approximately 20% of our participants participate because a motion to modify the original divorce decree has been filed by either the participant or his or her ex-spouse. Most of these motions request changes in child custody, visitation, or support. This subgroup of participants has different needs (because they may have divorced as many as 10-12 years ago) than those who are presently divorcing *and* because our program (as do all others that we are aware of) focuses on those who are currently in the process of divorcing. We have attempted to address the needs of those involved in a motion to modify by: 1) Addressing more directly issues that may be relevant to them (e.g., discussing situations that may lead to a motion to change the amount of child support or when one parent wishes to move to another state); 2) showing respect for and an appreciation of the value of their experience; and 3) asking them to share experiences and insights as a way of helping those who are currently divorcing. A number of these individuals have responded quite positively to the program and have told us that they wished that it had been available when they had originally divorced. Nevertheless, we are considering forming separate groups for those who are currently divorcing and those who are involved in a motion to modify.

REASONS WHY FOK REPRESENTS A SUCCESSFUL PARTNERSHIP

Several factors are responsible for our successful partnership. First, we have an excellent working relationship with our primary partner—the local family Court. We maintain regular contact with Court representatives and involve them in all issues pertaining to the program, even those involving curriculum. Second, having faculty serve as facilitators is a tremendous strength. The faculty are not only well-versed in the literature on divorce, but have also conducted a number of studies that have contributed to our knowledge base on divorce. Not only are the program materials academically sound, but our status as university faculty gives us credibility that we might not otherwise be granted.

Third, FOK provides faculty with the opportunity to provide an important community service and to provide research-based information directly to a targeted audience, as opposed to more traditional college student audiences. In addition, the faculty benefit from the knowledge that they are providing an important community service, learn from participants in the program, and have their other research and teaching activities enriched by participating in the program.

Fourth, we have been buoyed by recent involvement with graduate students. Several graduate students who are in our master's program in family mediation have been trained to facilitate FOK sessions. Their training consists of observing several sessions, co-teaching with a faculty team, and participating in biweekly seminars. The seminars are especially helpful to us as faculty because they provide us with an opportunity to learn from each other, to share experiences from the program, and to gain more detailed knowledge about certain topics (e.g., parenting plans, new laws regarding child custody and visitation, child support guidelines).

Finally, the partnership has benefitted from the cultural milieu that is increasingly supportive of children's needs and parenting education courses for divorcing parents. This program is part of a nationwide trend of mandating attendance at similar courses for divorcing parents (Blaisure & Geasler, 1996). Were this a mandated educational experience that did not exist elsewhere, we might have more difficulty retaining the public support that we need to sustain the program.

ENDNOTE

1. The authors express their appreciation to the 13th Judicial Circuit Court, Columbia, Missouri, particularly Mary Mueller, for its financial, administrative, and pedagogical support for this program.

REFERENCES

Blaisure, K. R., & Geasler, M. J. (1996). Results of a survey of court-connected parent education programs in U.S. counties. *Family and Conciliation Courts Review, 34*, 23-40.

Braver, S. L., Smith, M. C., & DeLuse, S. R. (1997). Methodological considerations in evaluating family court programs: A primer using divorced parent education programs as a case example. *Family and Conciliation Courts Review, 35*, 9-36.

Kramer, L., & Washo, C. A. (1993). Evaluation of a court-mandated prevention program for divorcing parents: The Children First program. *Family Relations, 42*, 179-186.

Morgan, M. (1998). Unpublished master's thesis. University of Missouri-Columbia.

36 KIDS' TEAM: STATEWIDE AGENCIES MODEL FOR BUILDING COMMUNITY LEVEL COALITIONS

Georgia L. Stevens
Kathleen A. Lodl
University of Nebraska Cooperative Extension

NATURE OF PARTNERSHIP

As educators, we build coalitions to identify and address community problems. We aim to bring a sometimes diverse group of people together to study an issue and explore information on alternatives. While simple coalitions address a single issue, complex coalitions are multi-issue and are mobilized for a longer time. This paper describes building a complex coalition at the state level, in a project titled KIDS' TEAM, as a model for developing and guiding formation of community coalitions to address specific local needs.

Nebraska's Third Congressional District covers nearly 63,000 square miles and is sparsely populated; most of the 62 counties lack a single town with population above 5,000. The District lacks many of the concentrated family services that an urban or metropolitan area may provide. There were, however, five programs already organized around family or children's issues that had footholds in locales within the District (see Figure 1). These include the Family Preservation Team/Office of the Governor, the Nebraska Department of Education Federal Before and After-School Child Care Project, Family Community Leadership teams directed by Cooperative Extension, the Nebraska Department of Social Services and Cooperative Extension Child Care Provider Training Program, and Nebraska Cooperative Extension Educators.

PURPOSE AND GOALS

The project was initiated to help further develop the network and cooperation of these five organizations already involved in addressing youth-at-risk issues, build a statewide coalition, and utilize the coalition in serving as the model for nurturing the formation of local youth-at-risk coalitions.

Figure 1. *Organizational structure for implementing a coalition for KIDS' TEAM*

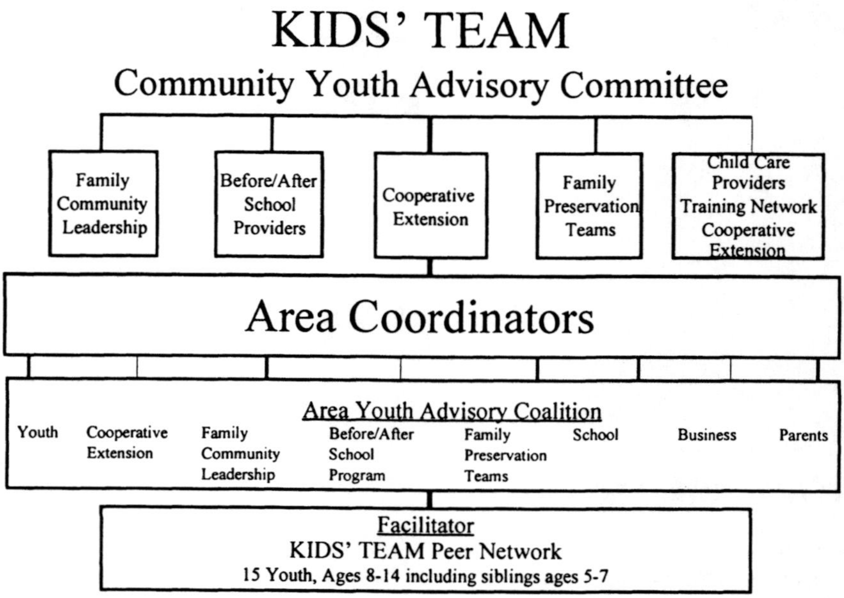

DEVELOPMENT OF A STATEWIDE MODEL COALITION

To initiate the project, the statewide coalition of 25 people from the five organizations met monthly in the first year of planning at a community in the center of the District. This meant asking statewide agency persons located in the capital city, Lincoln, to drive four hours to North Platte. This was a first step in equalizing distances and relaying commitment to the project because many of the representatives of the District drove at least four hours from the opposite end of the state to attend these meetings. These meetings brought the five partner groups together to identify other potential coalition members, review materials for local coalitions to use, develop job descriptions for the partners, and share the successes and stresses of project implementation.

ANALYSIS OF THE PROCESS

Using the statewide coalition as a model, Extension Educators served as Area Coordinators to facilitate the recruitment, implementation, training, and overall management of local community coalitions (see Figure 1). Each of the eight Area Coordinators were provided with the names of potential coalition partners within their area who belonged to these five member cooperator groups. These coalition partners served as a nucleus for the Area Youth Advisory Coalitions forming in local communities.

Area Youth Advisory Coalitions were encouraged to build local community coalitions with members from the five cooperator groups, school, business, parents and youth. These Area Youth Advisory Coalition members identified older youth and area adults who were willing to receive training and commit to facilitating one, or perhaps two, groups of 10 to 15 youth, ages 8 to 14 as KIDS' TEAM peer networks. The KIDS' TEAM peer network was the essence of the project as the children themselves were involved in planning, organizing, and experiencing activities on school release days.

ACHIEVEMENTS RELATED TO GOALS

Newsletters were mailed to 500 members of the five coalition partners during the first year to apprise them of the project and its goal. These newsletters provided a networking mechanism for community coalitions to share expertise.

Monthly conference calls linked the geographically distanced local coalitions and their projects. This allowed for personal dialogue on the trials and errors being experienced in local communities.

Four interactive satellite conferences provided content on various concepts of interest to coalitions. These topics included an ecological approach to addressing the needs of youth at risk, elevating school-age child care as a community concern, training of community members in coalition building, and family communication strategies for youth at risk coalitions.

As coalitions matured, they recognized their strengths and abilities to tackle community problems. Along with this growth came the need for coalitions to do strategic planning in order to be more effective. A two-day interactive satellite workshop on the strategic planning process was held with coalition members. The workshop provided opportunities for them to develop their goals along with the strategies to implement and sustain themselves. KIDS' TEAM coordinators reviewed the strategic plans developed by the local coalitions; in many instances the coordinators were able to link the coalition with state agency experts that could provide additional resources. This process encouraged community coalitions to sustain themselves through outside grant funding.

Many communities experimented with finding solutions for the school-age child care issue on a small scale, and then expanded the efforts of their coalition to tackle more difficult issues. Most now address a broad range of needs through programs such as parenting education, summer recreation, school-age child care, substance abuse and drunk driving prevention, farm safety, and cultural diversity.

EVALUATIVE RESULTS AND PROGRAM IMPACTS

While KIDS' TEAM was implemented in rural Nebraska, the model is adaptable to other settings. It brought together agencies at state and at local levels that have expanded efforts to assess local needs, built small scale programs that opened the doors to more difficult issues, and generated support from local, state, and national sources for these coalitions to sustain themselves.

More than 55 KIDS' TEAM local coalitions were put in place with over 500 adult and youth volunteers dedicating more than 39,000 hours and 430,262 volunteer contact hours. Almost $260,000 was generated in support from local, state, and national sources. It is anticipated that 85% will continue their efforts as community coalitions.

In measuring the impact of KIDS' TEAM on adolescent facilitators involved in the project, findings revealed that adolescent facilitators showed strengthened life skills, increased self-esteem, a heightened sense of career direction, and increased awareness of community citizenship (Lodl, Stevens, & Mesecher, 1995). Another study identified changes community coalition members perceived as a result of training and being a coalition member. Results of paired T-tests showed that participants had significantly greater skills in coalition building and in actions on public policy (Stevens & Lodl, 1998).

CURRICULUM AND RELATED INSTRUCTIONAL MATERIALS

KIDS' TEAM curriculum (Lodl, Stevens, & Steffens, 1995) has garnered a great deal of acclaim for the activity cards youth can use in planning and organizing their school-release days. In addition, videotapes, a facilitator's guide, and a trainer's manual are available for adult facilitators. Resources were also developed to assist in parenting education, facilitators training, coalition building, and coalition sustainability.

LEARNINGS FROM THIS PARTNERSHIP

This project has been a very successful partnership. University faculty on campus and throughout the state continue to dialogue and readily partner on projects with agency representatives. There is a broader recognition of the need to include local representatives on statewide task forces. Local coalitions have gained the confidence to go beyond simple issues to tackle more complex issues and to garner financial and community support that sustains their efforts.

REFERENCES

Lodl, K. A., Stevens, G. L., & Mesecher, C. (1997, Summer). Video-based interactive training: A model for reaching isolated audiences. *Journal of Family and Consumer Sciences, 89*(2), 2-5, 10.

Lodl, K. A., Stevens, G. L., & Mesecher, C. M. (1995, Winter). KIDS' TEAM: A case study of adolescent development through participation in a rural community program. *Journal of Family and Consumer Sciences, 87*(4), 53-56.

Lodl, K. A., Stevens, G. L., & Steffens, P. (1995). *KIDS' TEAM: Curriculum Cards, set 1-2.* National 4-H Curriculum Jury. National Recognition.

Stevens, G. L., Gerhard, G. W., & Sullivan, K. (1991). *KIDS' TEAM Facilitators' Guide, Trainer's Manual, Videotape.* University of Nebraska-Lincoln Cooperative Extension and USDA Youth at Risk Grant.

Stevens, G. L., & Lodl, K. A. (Submitted 1998). Community coalitions: Identifying changes in coalition members as a result of training. *Journal of Extension*.

Stevens, G. L., Lodl, K. A., Rockwell, S. K., & Burkhart-Kriesel, C. (1994, October). Do local realities clash with federal expectations? A case study of youth-at-risk funding. *Journal of Extension, 32*(3) [On-line]. Available http://joe.org/cgi-bin/mktoc/joe/1994october.

37 FIELD TRAINING IN APPLIED DEVELOPMENTAL PSYCHOLOGY: FORDHAM UNIVERSITY'S EXPANDING COMMUNITY PARTNERSHIPS

Ann Higgins-D'Alessandro
Celia Fisher
Fordham University[1]

Graduate study in Applied Developmental Psychology (ADP) at Fordham University was begun ten years ago to develop shared expertise and collaborative service and systems change efforts between the university and the multiple communities in which it lives. The ADP graduate program added courses to its advanced developmental psychology curriculum, specifically, a course in the approach and issues of Applied Developmental Psychology and revamped courses in research design, developmental psychopathology, and assessments to address applied work. The Fordham ADP doctoral program is uniquely defined, however, by its field experience courses—ADP Research Apprenticeship, ADP Practicum, and ADP Internship. The history and challenges of our ADP curriculum and field experiences are detailed in Higgins-D'Alessandro, Fisher, and Hamilton (1998) and Fisher, Rau, and Colapietro (1993).

The Fordham University ADP model of field training focuses on developing the following four competencies: Conceptualizing service delivery systems to include the goals and competencies of service providers and service recipients; recognizing the influence and dynamics of cultures and communities with the missions and regulations of agencies serving them; working successfully in multidisciplinary teams and in health care and social service settings; and becoming legitimate, integral members of the communities in which they work (Higgins-D'Alessandro, et al., 1998).

The field experiences in the Fordham ADP program include three formal components. The ADP Research Apprenticeship in the first year is mentored either by a Fordham ADP faculty person alone or jointly with a supervisor of one of our community partners. The doctoral student apprentice joins a project and team to learn first-hand about the challenges and rewards of real-world research. The ADP Practicum, in the third year, is a 12-hour a week field experience jointly supervised in which students refine their assessment and evaluation skills, learn skills related to the services and practices of the community partner, and utilize their research expertise to carry out a study addressing an issue of present concern to the site. The ADP Internship follows in the fourth year. The students come to these community partner field sites able to fully participate and contribute as emerging professionals.

THE NATURE OF FORDHAM'S PARTNERSHIPS WITH COMMUNITIES

Fordham is a Jesuit University with the explicit mission to educate students as "men and women for others." This goal of service is translated at the undergraduate level into extensive and successful outreach programs into Bronx and Manhattan schools, preschools, shelters, food kitchens, clinics, and even parks projects. At the graduate level, the Fordham mission is manifest by an administration that takes seriously the field placement and outreach work of graduate programs such as Applied Developmental Psychology. To support outreach research and training, Fordham provides tuition remission for graduate students working in field sites at least half-time. The University awards the ADP Research Apprenticeship, ADP Practicum, and ADP Internship full academic status as courses; this award recognizes the important didactic component involved in field experiences and gives both students and faculty credit for these efforts. Fordham has encouraged and supported the commitment to outreach scholarship of individual departments, faculty, and students, and has moved over the years toward the model that Chibucos and Lerner (Chapter 1, this volume) are recommending, demonstrating real commitment to systems change efforts. Fordham is positioned geographically but, more importantly, philosophically, to be a leader in demonstrating the power of community-university partnerships.

Current Types of Partnerships

Applied Developmental Psychology's partnerships with communities presently may be characterized into two types, those related to field experience courses, and those based in the ADP program, itself. The first type has been described; it comprises the three field experience courses, the ADP Research Apprenticeship, the ADP Practicum, and the ADP Internship. A wide range of community partners join us, such as acute and chronic care hospitals, preschools based in hositals and agencies serving developmentally delayed and disabled children, Headstart, nursing homes for elderly and individuals suffering from HIV/AIDS, the New York City-wide YMCA's Virtual Y After-School Program, middle and high school intervention programs, and residential care facilities for delinquent youth. The second type includes the efforts we make as the ADP faculty, both together and individually. As a program, we engage in multidisciplinary outreach efforts based at Fordham through our membership in the Consortium for Law, Social Service, and Psychology, the Third Age Center, and the Center for Schools, Families, and Communities in the School of Education. As individuals we do consultative and educative work in the community and within the university.

PURPOSES AND GOALS

The major purposes of our community partnerships are interrelated: 1) To train graduate students as ADP professionals; 2) to learn from communities and institutions about their own and collaborative goals and how they think ADP ideas and professionals can be useful to them; and 3) to demonstrate the power and effectiveness of applied developmental science research and education models to collaboratively create environments and systems in order to optimize human development and family well-being.

At this point, the relationships we have created with communities are individual and distinct, although we are beginning to plan how these partnerships may be interrelated into networks with shared missions. The social structures of New York City are complex and multi-layered as well as sometimes parochial and often political. These conditions seem to discourage the possibility that urban universities can be coordinators of change efforts; however, in this chapter we illustrate the role of university centers and suggest that they may be structures of university coordination, leadership, and advocacy for systems change efforts.

ANALYSIS OF THE PROCESS

The process of building community-university collaboration includes: 1) Identifying and creating honest communication and open processes between partners; 2) developing timelines and pace for projects; and 3) expanding the definition and usefulness of the ADS/ADP model in both outreach work with communities and in creating opportunities within the university.

One partnership component is honest communication, especially about issues of needs and requirements of each partner. For instance, our partnership with the Westchester Institute for Human Development (WIHD) necessitates clear, open discussion. We require that Practicum and Internship supervisors be Ph.D., licensed psychologists, whereas supervisors in paid work placements and multidisciplinary efforts need not be. WIHD, which provides assessments, foster care services, and other family services for children in need, offers beginning ADP students real-life applied research experiences as paid work, directly supervised by advanced students, social workers, or psychologists. WIHD also has a formal internship program and Fordham ADP students are highly competitive for the prized positions. As with our other community partners, WIHD has also agreed to accomodate our desire that students actively work on dissertations in their fourth year by freeing a block of time weekly for dissertation work by interns. Our partnership with WIHD is further strengthened and sustained when students choose to base their dissertation research at WIHD and Fordham mentors invite WIHD supervisors to be dissertation committee members. In the future, the ADP program will be seeking departmental and university support for enhancing this partnership by appointing qualified WIHD supervisors as clinical or field faculty.

The second partnership component is understanding that building each partnership takes time, and that the length of time and the pace will vary greatly. The partnership between Fordham University and the Lighthouse, the largest institute providing services and research for the visually impaired from preschool children to the elderly in NYC, developed in a relatively short period of time through fairly easy discussions. The initial placements of students in Research Apprentice positions were soon followed by ADP Practicum placements. This partnership was one of the earliest the ADP programs created. In contrast, a recent relationship among four partners (two universities, a private educational and housing authority in the Bronx, and a funding agency) has come into being only this past fall with the placement of students from both universities into an educational mentoring program serving the children in the housing projects. The partners began discussion two years ago and the collaboration is still developing; for instance, the funding agency recently increased its financial support based on its confidence in the developing partnership.

The third partnership component is extending the definition and practical meaningfulness of ADP. One example has been the development of Fordham's Consortium of Law, Social Services, and Psychology, an endeavor undertaken by the ADP program as a whole. It offers team-taught courses, multidisciplinary and discipline-based supervision, and work in Law Clinics for students from the three disciplines. Through the Law Clinics, student teams serve clients who seek legal help in obtaining educational services for their children, welfare services for their families, and for cases of domestic violence. In that capacity, the ADP student conducts necessary assessments and consults on their appropriate use, supervised by the Psychology faculty member. To help the Consortium develop, the current ADP student is using her knowledge of formative evaluation to assess this interdisciplinary effort. She is documenting and conducting an evaluation study of ways student teams work together as well as changes and growth in their professional identities and responsibilities. The development of the student teams is part of the Consortium's outreach effort to children service agencies and courts to offer new possibilities for treatment and adjudication. Soon, the Consortium will seek community placements for student teams rather than individual students.

Another example of this third partnering component, expanding the meaningfulness of ADP, is embodied in the ongoing work of defining ADP internships. Each ADP internship is negotiated between the student, the ADP program, and the site. Currently, we have had several ongoing relationships with approximately 75% of the sites, and 25% are new this year. Like our partnerships with Practicum sites, we feel these, too, are successful because the community partners have always invited us to send students in subsequent years. These invitations are usually accompanied with new ideas about the potential roles of ADP interns, whether in a hospital, clinic, or school for special children, showing that our interns have been excellent ambassadors, expanding the meaningfulness of ADP.

Consistent with her pre-doctoral and professional status, one intern is titled a "Developmentalist" at an agency in NYC in a Dominican neighborhood which provides more than 300 pregnant women and new mothers with resources and education so they can give their children the "best beginnings." This intern assesses infants and children, works with multidisciplinary teams, educates family support workers, and gives specialized workshops for staff. Client mothers are informed they will be placed randomly in either an intensive weekly or once-a-month track for visits, referrals, and other resources. Although blind to the assigned track of the families now, later on the intern will be able to use data from this program evaluation study as part of her dissertation research. The Ph.D. psychologist supervisor and administrators are pleased this intern is someone with sophisticated applied research skills who will be able to write a contextually detailed and sensitive article about the project and spell out the practical and policy implications of the findings.

An innovation by a school for autistic children last year was the creation of a Developmental Psychology Internship position, added to their existing Clinical Internships. The successful applicant was a Fordham ADP student, precisely because she was prepared and eager to use ADP knowledge and research techniques to help the school answer its own questions, one, about the cycles and changes in autism and two, about staff development, retention, and burn-out. This intern also conducts individual assessments, psychoeducational groups for the children, and extensive developmental education for the staff. This school is in rural New York State and serves all children to age 21 in its cachement area. All partners acknowledged that the applied research questions of this school cannot be adequately addressed in one year; however, they also understood the need to assess the successes of the first year of the new Developmental Internship. Thus, this final contract stipulated a one-year position with options for continuing for a second year.

In these examples, the community-university partnership is successful but still developing. All of us as stakeholders have begun to recognize that the "ideal ADP internship" will most often combine applied research with practice. This combination may, in fact, require a 2-year internship at some sites, instead of the usual 1-year internship required for clinical students. Secondly, both community partners and the ADP program have found that contracts are valuable means of ensuring reasonable protections and assurances which serve to strengthen the partnerships and foster long-term collaboration.

Individual Faculty Outreach

Our faculty-community collaborative efforts have been supported by large federal and private grants. Nancy Busch-Rossnagel and several students partnered with members of the community to develop assessment instruments for Latino infants and families based upon the community members' parental goals and values. Celia Fisher and her students have engaged adolescents and families in identifying best ethical practices in research and school-based interventions for high-risk adolescents. Ann Higgins-D'Alessandro and students collaborated with high school principals and teachers to design, implement, and evaluate programs for fostering student development and preventing risky behaviors in differing academic milieus.

ACHIEVEMENTS RELATED TO PURPOSES

The achievements of the first purpose, educating ADP students, are wedded to those of the second purpose, listening to and educating communities and stakeholders in order to utilize ADP ideas and talent to reach their own goals.

Two Practicum students placed at a large medical center were trained to conduct in-depth telephone interviews with grieving families as the initial part of an outreach and intervention program to prevent secondary malfunctioning in children who lost a parent to suicide. Although the program was clearly useful for participants, why some families and not others chose to utilize the program was unknown. In response, the ADP Practicum students' determined that conducting a utilization of services study using archival records of two years of telephone interviews with adult members would be most useful. That study identified barriers within families that prevented some from seeking assistance. It concluded that increased community outreach with facilitating access to the program as well as public education about suicide more generally were all warranted. Although initially they had thought they would conduct an intervention evaluation study, they listened to the needs of the site supervisor, were encouraged by her openness, and demonstrated their functional, working knowledge of what they had learned in their courses.

PROSPECTS FOR LONG-TERM SUSTAINABILITY

The third purpose, of expanding the definition and usefulness of the ADP model, is combined with the goal of sustaining long-term relationships with our partners. We have successful ones with three Fordham interdisciplinary centers, the Lighthouse, WIHD, Montefiore Hospital in the Bronx, and several schools. Long-term partnerships allow the community sites to learn what ADP can offer and allow us to learn about how our community partners conceptualize ADP. We both learn about the nature and issues involved at the level of systemic needs and changes.

For four years we have placed graduate students for Practicum and dissertation research with Fordham's Center for Schools, Families, and Communities. The Center conducts large-scale program evaluation projects and directs a national network of centers serving families through educational systems. The contributions and experiences of ADP students change as these projects move from design to completion. A successful partnership is sustained through discussions, matching interests, and defining the actual experiences and work at the Center for each ADP student each year. The yearly negotiations are greatly facilitated, as they are for all Practicum placements, by mutual mid-year and end-of-the-year evaluations of student performance and site opportunities as well as by faculty-supervisor discussions. In addition, a final luncheon is held in which students and supervisors talk about their challenges and achievements to the next year's class of Practicum students.

The partnership between a large nursing home and research institute in aging, Fordham's Third Age Center, and ADP has been very productive. The Center Director co-teaches the ADP Practicum course, and now three years into the partnership, one student is a full-time intern who has co-written a successful grant application at the nursing home. A second is a full-time intern at the Third Age Center, conducting research on healthy aging with Elderhostel. A third student is a half-time intern, and will be for two years, and a fourth is a Practicum student. They work with psychoeducational groups, carry out assessments, and conduct research. This level of coordination belies our usual skepticism and points out the clear potential for Fordham University to become a leader in research and service for the elderly.

Our relationship with Montifiore Hospital demonstrates how a student can begin as a paid work research assistant in her first year and continue working there throughout her graduate study, while still having very different training and experiences with other institutions for Practicum and Internship. In the last five years two students worked there, each for three years. Their responsibilities on a school-based asthma education project changed and expanded with their growing knowledge. Each has been the project liaison with the schools, coordinated and organized student groups, taught undergraduates to become educational health professionals, collected and analyzed data, written articles, and co-written grant applications.

LEARNING FROM PARTNERSHIPS

We have learned much from our community partnerships, and we hope some of this knowledge emerges from the examples in this chapter. Continuing the above example, we have specifically learned that Fordham University's Centers can link us with community partners and can be the forum through which the university coordinates services and research. This provides the opportunity for the university to serve and be seen as a community institution itself, becoming a visible and effective agent for social change on specific issues.

Another very important thing we have learned is to see ADP from the community partners' points of view. For instance, the Director of the Fordham Student Counseling Center thought that an ADP focus could address the problem of students awaiting therapy. Appreciating his belief but unable to imagine how this might be done, the Director, the Practicum professor, and a student embarked on a two-month long discussion. Using the ADP perspective and knowledge, the student designed a research study of the effectivenss of introducing journaling, a psychoeducational technique, into individual therapy. Positive results may indicate shorter-term therapy and with additional research have implications for offering journaling with support to students awaiting therapy.

CLOSING COMMENTS

We are continually learning because our community partners willingly engage with us in expanding the meaningfulness and usefulness of applied developmental psychology. Given reasonable, but not ideal, resources and a modicum of flexibility, current and new community-university partnerships will succeed to the extent that the process of building them utilizes the components illustrated here as well as important others. Coordinating partnerships so they may act together more effectively than singly to serve people and optimize human development is one important future challenge. An even bigger challenge will be to remain aware of the changing pictures of society as a shifting whole and use it to continually inform us of opportunities for universities to be coordinators, leaders, and advocates for social change.

ENDNOTE

1. Our faculty colleagues are Nancy Busch-Rossnagel, Aaron Hogue, Daniel Mrozcek, Kathleen Schiaffino, Reesa Vaughter, and Mary Ann Lewis, Director of the Third Age Center.

REFERENCES

Chibucos, T. R., & Lerner, R. M. (1999) Serving children and families through community-university partnerships: A view of the issues. In T. R. Chibucos & R. M. Lerner (Eds.), *Serving children and families through community-university partnerships: Success stories* (pp. 1-12). Norwood, MA: Kluwer Academic Publishers.

Fisher, C. B., Rau, J. M., & Colapietro, E. (1993). Models of graduate education in applied developmental sciences: The Fordham University doctoral specialization in applied developmental psychology. *Journal of Applied Developmental Psychology, 14*, 289-301.

Higgins-D'Alessandro, A., Fisher, C. B., & Hamilton, M. G. (1998). Educating the applied developmental psychologist for university-community partnerships: The Fordham model. In R. M. Lerner & L. A. K. Simon (Eds.), *University-community collaborations for the twenty-first century: Outreach scholarship for youth and families* (pp.157-183). New York: Garland.

38 POLICY SEMINARS FOR STATE AND COMMUNITY LEADERS

Charles McClintock
Cornell University

NATURE OF PARTNERSHIP

Spanning the campus-community boundary is one of the most challenging tasks for academia, and it is crucial over the long run to the evolving role of the professoriate in the scholarship of application, the financial health of academia, and the contribution of higher education to a broadly defined vision of societal well-being (Feller, 1986; Wolshok, 1995). One form of this campus-community connection is the policy seminar in which research findings are brought to bear on issues of immediate concern to legislative and agency audiences (Lewis & Ellefson, 1996). This chapter tells a story in progress about a policy seminar sponsored by Cornell University's College of Human Ecology that is building a sustained partnership among academia, government and community participants at state and local levels. The story has important successes to date as well as unmet challenges.

PURPOSES AND GOALS

The College of Human Ecology's Policy Perspectives Seminar offers opportunities for state and community leaders to interact with Cornell faculty around issues of concern to the well-being and future of New York State. Recent seminar events have centered around two broad themes—*welfare reform* and a wide range of factors critical to its success including financial support for children, child care, education and employment, and prevention of child abuse and neglect, as well as *community-based health planning.*

The policy seminars occur once each semester and published accounts of faculty presentations are posted on the College's website (www.cornell.human.edu) to facilitate wide access. There are two reasons for this structure. First, we want to build a network of relationships between faculty and policy makers via a set of regularly offered events. Second, our goal is to have specific seminar content emerge from these relationships, rather than unilaterally presenting a series of faculty experts on topics that might or might not be of current relevance to state or community needs. This collaborative model where expertise of practitioners and academicians is intermixed is more likely to produce results that are useful when applied to policy and program issues (McClintock, 1979). We also wanted to expand the seminar audience through Cornell's satellite conference downlinks at the community level across the state, and in that way serve as a catalyst to engage state and local audiences more directly with each other.

ANALYSIS OF THE PROCESS

Our general themes were selected for two strategic reasons. First, they both represent significant challenges to state and community leaders in the context of the "devolution revolution" in which greater financial and impact accountability is being shifted from federal to state and local levels of government (McClintock & Colosi, 1998). This shift has been underway for a decade or more and has been driven politically by federal deficit problems, state interests in experimenting with waivers from federal requirements in order to manage their own fiscal problems, broad changes in the financing and organization of health care, and a growing recognition of the need to involve local communities more effectively in a wide range of economic and social change efforts that will benefit children and families. The themes of welfare reform and health care are broad enough to include a variety of community concerns and campus expertise, and also create a focus that contributes to sustaining partnerships over time.

The second basis for selecting these policy seminar themes was to represent integrated areas of expertise at Cornell in relation to New York State concerns and priorities at both state and local levels. As the land-grant university for the state, Cornell's ability to use the county-based system of extension offices offered a related advantage. Our plan was to coordinate policy seminars in the state capital, Albany, with the Cornell Cooperative Extension (CCE) system located in each county and borough of New York City. The CCE system includes satellite downlink capabilities at local extension offices across the state that are regularly used for interactive conferences between campus and community-based participants. This educational delivery mechanism can be combined with internet and toll-free telephone connections to allow for exchange among local sites and with people located on the central campus.

The first seminar titled "Stemming the Tide of Children in Danger: Opportunities and Risks in New York State" was offered in October, 1995, and included cost/benefit perspectives on a set of related topics: 1) Training and research programs related to children and violence prevention in New York State; 2) needs of the foster care system in relation to protecting children in danger; 3) home visiting programs as long-term preventive interventions for a variety of poverty-related problems; 4) family violence prevention training; and 5) a demonstration of information technology aimed at linking human service professionals to administrative and archival data on their desktop computers that would permit better management of child welfare services. The program was intentionally broad in order to reach a variety of state agency staff, but it was also designed to portray a critical mass of expertise, both in research and training that might spark collaboration on emerging needs within the state.

In order to coordinate our state policy seminar with a local community downlink, and because a new academic department emphasizing family, health and consumer issues—Policy Analysis and Management—was being created at Cornell, our second seminar was delayed until October, 1996. This seminar, entitled "Supporting Children In An Era Of Welfare Reform" featured presentations on: 1) The correlates of varied sources of income for children including employment earnings, child support payments, and welfare payments; 2) how federal welfare reform legislation affects demand for child care in local communities, potential dangers of informal care arrangements, and child care as a job opportunity for adults receiving public assistance; and 3) family and employment demography of New York State since 1970, especially as it pertains to the role of education in labor market success for families on public assistance.

This second event was timed during the period when states were beginning to revise their legislation under federal welfare reform changes, and the degree of uncertainty among state and county groups was very high about which policy features could be shown to be effective in relation to employment, family strengths, and self-sufficiency goals. For this reason the seminar was focused on data and research-based knowledge specific to some of the key issues in welfare reform—education and employment, child care, and sources of financial child support.

The third seminar in May, 1997 continued under the welfare reform theme but with an emphasis on the need for data-based policy analysis and program management. In this case, New York State had already embarked on a social indicators project called Touchstones that was being developed by the New York State Council on Children and Families. The Council, working in close collaboration with its thirteen-member state agencies, was building a framework to link indicators in six broad areas—family, education, physical and emotional health, citizenship, economic insecurity, and community—to more specific state and community goals and objectives, and to related agency and inter-agency strategies and performance measures. Given the many changes underway in federal, state, and local welfare policies, the Touchstones Project was being designed to provide a means of monitoring the quality of life for children and families.

The approach taken for this seminar event was somewhat different from previous ones in that we agreed with the Council that our role would be to take a critical look at the Touchstones project and offer suggestions for its improvement. This stance, which we mutually referred to as the "group of ornery faculty," was based on a mutual desire to see improvements in how social indicators were conceptualized and used in comparison to similar efforts over the years.

The theme that united the faculty commentaries was the need to *contextualize* social indicators so that they will allow New York State and its communities to pose questions as well as report on performance. For example, our presenters discussed the need to:

- analyze an output indicator in relation to its inputs (e.g., children's graduation rate in the context of poverty rate or parents' education for a given locale) and make comparisons among communities with similar input profiles;
- group indicators in an array of problem types—from those that are well-structured and generally understood to those that are more complex, uncertain, and laden with value conflict—and develop processes by which local citizens can analyze and interpret data in relation to implications at the lowest meaningful level of community action (e.g., neighborhood, village, town);
- relate groups of health indicators to underlying causal models, identifying those that are sensitive to unanticipated environmental changes, and document the

economic and cultural/ethnic diversity that accounts for differences in outcomes;
- examine the inter-correlations among indicators as a means of seeing common underlying factors, while avoiding some of the statistical pitfalls of interpreting correlational data on individuals that is aggregated to the community level; and
- link agency-based indicators which typically identify problems and deficits with data from state and federal surveys that document positive behaviors and attitudes.

In November, 1997 and May, 1998 we presented the fourth and fifth seminars entitled respectively "Community-based Health Planning" and "Healthy Communities: Concepts and Collaboration Tools." These seminars were designed to follow up on a New York State Department of Health report emphasizing local community as the key locus for prevention programs and other efforts to improve the public's health. Faculty discussed "tools" that community groups could use to identify, prioritize and evaluate issues and efforts that were of greatest significance at the local community level. One of these planning and evaluation tools, the Concept Planning System, was already in use to help develop Rural Health Networks through the New York State Department of Health. The second tool, search conference methods, was being used with a group of very rural counties to help them conceptualize and plan efforts to deal with food insecurity for low income families. Other presentations focused on the benefits and costs of collaboration as shown through research-based and practitioner-based knowledge, and Cornell Cooperative Extension research and outreach projects on managed care enrollment for Medicaid populations, the economic impact on local communities of managed care and other broad changes in health care organization and financing, and the dynamics of family and community food decision making.

Plans for future seminars topics include an examination of how to improve linkages between the worlds of research-based and practitioner-based knowledge, and family and economic policy issues for elderly citizens.

ACHIEVEMENTS RELATED TO GOALS

There have been various successes from our three-year experiment with policy seminars and satellite conferences including legislative changes, the infusion of theoretical and empirical underpinnings into a wide set of discussions of social and health policy and program planning, and the prospects for continuing research and outreach partnerships on issues relevant to children and families. For these reasons we are likely to continue our college investment in support of this effort as part of our outreach mission.

The most important consequence of the first seminar on children in danger was to re-emphasize a contract with the college's Family Life Development Center to work directly with a state agency to draft legislation for the out-of-home placement of children at risk for catastrophic abuse. As mentioned earlier, the second event on welfare reform was timed to coincide with the major changes in federal legislation since there were many unknown implications for state policy and outcomes. One result of this seminar was subsequent opportunities for several faculty presenters to provide testimony before state legislative committees on program evaluation and child support issues in New York State. One of the positive outcomes from the third seminar on social indicators was the inclusion of a faculty member on the governor's "Task Force on Out-of-Wedlock Pregnancy and Poverty" evaluation committee. The charge of the committee is to recommend indicators that would be used by the state and local communities to monitor and improve the status of women and children most in need of support. The fourth policy seminar on community-based health planning has catalyzed the ongoing involvement of the Cornell Cooperative Extension network of county associations in an emerging state-wide alliance of groups called the New York State Community Health Partnership.

PROSPECTS FOR LONG-TERM SUSTAINABILITY

There are several factors that are working to sustain the Policy Perspectives Seminar program. First, the College of Human Ecology sees this kind of outreach activity as integral to its academic mission and therefore is able to justify the modest expenditure involved. Potential contracts that result from the relationships built through the seminars can bring direct support for the continuation of academic programs in seminar topic areas that also will be of direct relevance to state policy needs. This fact relates to a second reason for sustainability; state agency analysts, legislative staff and others are always in need of current research-based information as it applies to the pressing political and policy issues which they face.

Finally, there is a mutually beneficial outcome for faculty and policy-makers as they come to better understand the constraints under which the other group operates, as well as struggle with the complex interplay between scientific and political forms of rationality in the policy process. This realization motivates both the academic and the public policy participants to continue the relationship in order to sharpen their respective crafts and improve outcomes for the public at large.

LEARNINGS FROM THIS PARTNERSHIP

We have also learned several critical lessons that will improve the partnership in the future. First, the coordination of state-level seminars with community level satellite conferences is very demanding. We only were able to conduct a coordinated event for our seminar on supporting children in an era of welfare reform. Second, we had wanted to involve representatives from media and business in our events, both as planners and participants, but were unable to devote the resources necessary to nurturing these relationships. These two professional communities are critical given their power to focus public attention and marshal resources, and we are more convinced than ever of their value in future seminar events. At the same time, however, it is a challenge to include the media in a setting where open exchange is encouraged since both faculty and state officials might have reasons for wanting to avoid quotation or misattribution of findings in the give-and-take process of the seminar.

Finally, it is necessary to provide faculty support for this kind of scholarship of application, including helping them focus their expertise on problems and issues as defined by the community of policy and program practitioners, on preparation of visual and written materials, and on rehearsal of presentations with written feedback that is aimed at improving communications with the policy community.

WHY IS THIS A SUCCESSFUL PARTNERSHIP?

The Policy Perspectives Seminar partnership is successful mainly because it is educational across the campus-community boundary. As noted earlier, both faculty and policy makers come to respect each other's constraints and approaches to using knowledge in policy formulation. This awareness energizes faculty to communicate their findings in more accessible and more direct terminology, and also reminds state policy makers that research findings, while critical to sound decision making, rarely provide the specificity or certainty needed for particular public policy questions. Regular efforts such as this one that continue to educate and challenge the two communities of academia and policy represent the kind of collaboration that ultimately will improve outcomes for society at large.

REFERENCES

Feller, I. (1986). *Universities and state governments: A study in policy analysis.* New York: Praeger.

Lewis, B. J., & Ellefson, P. V. (1996). Evaluating information flows to policy committees in state legislatures. *Evaluation Review, 20,* 29-48.

McClintock, C., & Colosi, L. (1998). Evaluating welfare reform: A framework for including the urgent and the important. *Evaluation Review, 22,* 668-694.

McClintock, C. (1979). A program review and evaluation system: Framework for Congressional committees. In F. M. Zweig (Ed.), *Evaluation in legislation.* Beverly Hills, CA: Sage.

Walshok, M. L. (1995). *Knowledge without boundaries.* San Francisco: Jossey-Bass.

39 THE NORTH CAROLINA CHILD CARE CORPS: BUILDING A SUCCESSFUL UNIVERSITY AND COMMUNITY PARTNERSHIP THROUGH THE AMERICORPS NATIONAL SERVICE PROGRAM

Deborah J. Cassidy
Alice Henderson Hall
The University of North Carolina at Greensboro

Susan A. Hicks
Cornell University

In 1993 President Clinton signed into law the national service program, AmeriCorps. The AmeriCorps program, not unlike its predecessors, VISTA and the Civil Conservation Corps, was created to provide an opportunity for Americans of all ages and backgrounds to assist in solving problems that exist within American communities. AmeriCorps adopted a four part mission statement, consistent with the philosophy of encouraging and rewarding service in our country: 1) Getting things done in communities by working to meet their educational, public safety, and human and environmental needs; 2) encouraging responsibility in individuals for themselves, their families, and their communities; 3) strengthening communities by bringing individuals together to get things done; and 4) expanding opportunity by providing volunteers with specialized training, job experience, life skills, and an educational voucher. The AmeriCorps mission statement was at the forefront of formulating this university and community partnership designed to improve the quality of infant, toddler, and preschool child care in North Carolina.

NATURE OF PARTNERSHIP

The North Carolina Child Care Corps (NCCCC) was created in 1994 by faculty members from the Department of Human Development and Family Studies and the Vice Chancellor for Administration and Planning at the University of North

Carolina at Greensboro (UNCG). They envisioned a youth service program that would address two pressing needs for children and youth in North Carolina. The North Carolina Child Care Corps was designed to improve the quality of child care in North Carolina and provide an opportunity for young women and men to participate in full-time national service through a joint university and community partnership. Danzig and Szanton (1986) suggest that child care is a critical social need in our country that could potentially benefit from National Service Volunteers, specifically by reducing staff/child ratios. Indeed, staff/child ratios, as well as teacher education and training, and group size, are the factors most often cited as affecting the overall quality of child care programs (Feeny & Churn, 1985; Helburn, 1995; Phillips & Howes, 1987). Although the university faculty created and implemented the demonstration project, it was made possible by blending funding from a federal initiative, AmeriCorps, and a state initiative, Smart Start (North Carolina Partnership for Children).

The NC Child Care Corps collaborated with Smart Start, a North Carolina initiative established to blend state and local resources to ensure that young children have access to high quality early childhood education and developmental services. Smart Start provided the financial match required by AmeriCorps, with the remainder of the funding provided by the Corporation for National Service, which is the national nonprofit entity that operates AmeriCorps. In addition to supplying matching monies, Smart Start staff in local communities also assisted project staff recruit Corps members, determine appropriate placement sites for Corps members, and process the required paperwork. They also were invited to four half-day workshops with Corps members on the UNCG campus and informed Corps members of upcoming Smart Start board meetings and additional community service opportunities. The NCCCC administrative office was housed on campus at UNCG and all financial and budgetary services were provided by UNCG. Therefore, all Smart Start and Corporation for National Service (AmeriCorps) monies flowed through the university financial services department.

PROGRAM IMPLEMENTATION/TRAINING

During each year of the three-year project a new cohort of participants was recruited to the North Carolina Child Care Corps. Initially Corps members were provided an intensive four-week training program while housed in the campus dormitories at the University of North Carolina at Greensboro. While living on campus, Corps members ate at the university cafeteria, and had access to the University's recreation center, health clinic, and library. The curriculum for the training included modules on early childhood education, appropriate classroom practices, child development, and child care issues as well as an assignment to a pre-service, practicum placement at one of four local high quality community child care centers.

The training program resulted in the attainment of four hours of college credit, the North Carolina Early Childhood Credential, and certification in CPR and First Aid. The training was provided by UNCG faculty and staff. In addition, during Year Three training, Corps members were required to participate in three community service activities. The Corps members and the NCCCC staff worked with Habitat for Humanity in Greensboro clearing the grounds for four houses to be built in a "Blitz Build" the following month. Corps members also volunteered at a

Greensboro homeless shelter and extended care facility. The goal for "team" community service in Greensboro was to model a variety of opportunities for volunteering in community programs and to demonstrate the staff's commitment to community volunteer activities. As a result, Year Three Corps members were able to quickly get involved in community volunteer activities and maintain involvement longer than were previous Corps members.

After completion of training, Corps members were placed in community child care centers for a period of nine months to serve in Smart Start counties which had agreed to provide the necessary financial match. Not all counties in North Carolina receive Smart Start funding, nor did the same counties collaborate with NCCCC each year. By the end of the third year of the project, NC Child Care Corps members had served in 17 counties in small to medium-sized cities with the majority of centers serving a high percentage of low income children. Corps members were placed in child care centers sponsored by a variety of community agencies (e.g., churches, hospitals, a community college, and Head Start).

Each Corps member served as an additional teacher, above and beyond the program's current staff-child ratio, to provide supplementary assistance in order to improve the quality of education and care for the children enrolled in the child care centers. Corps members were assigned to a supervising teacher at their child care center who mentored the Corps members. To aid in the supervision of Corps members, each supervising teacher and site director attended an informational meeting designed to orient them to AmeriCorps, NCCCC, and the mentoring process. Corps member not only worked forty hours a week in a child care classroom, but also worked as community volunteers in such activities as tutoring, Hospice support, or community environmental clean up.

PROGRAM EVALUATION

An evaluation of the Corps members' participation in the four-and-a-half weeks of training in child development and appropriate practices with children was assessed in several ways. Corps members were given several written tests of child development and appropriate practices knowledge prior to training, after completion of training, and after completion of their service. In addition, they were videotaped in their classrooms during training, one month after they started their nine-month placement, and shortly before their placement ended, in order to assess the quality of their interactions with children. In all three years, Corps members demonstrated a significant increase in their knowledge of child development as well as their knowledge of appropriate practices with young children from pre-training to post-training. In all three years these gains in knowledge of child development and appropriate practice were maintained from post-training to post-experience. Furthermore, Corps member/child interactions showed an increase in appropriateness (based on a measure of caregiver sensitivity) from pre-training to post-training. Therefore, the four-and-a-half week Corps member training on campus, by UNCG faculty, not only resulted in four hours of college credit and a North Carolina Early Childhood Credential, but also increased knowledge about children and early childhood education as well as improved interaction skills with young children.

Individual personal growth and professional development were also well documented by Corps members in their bi-weekly journal entries. The breadth and intensity of this personal and professional growth was astounding especially in light of the fact that most Corps members served for only one year in the NCCCC. Excerpts from Corps member journals illustrate the impact of the NCCCC volunteer experience on Corps members. A Year One Corps member wrote "I used to consider myself to have a strong work ethic... after doing this program it is even stronger because when you are working with children, you know that everything you do has to be done a certain way. You are not just working around machines that can easily be fixed—children are emotionally and physically fragile." Another wrote "Even though I care about my job very much, and love the children very much, I never thought this service program would become so important to me. I always viewed AmeriCorps as a benefit for me first and others second. I primarily joined to earn money for college and save a little in the bank for the future. I realized how special these kids are to me this week when Jacob moved away."

The North Carolina Child Care Corps also improved child care in the state of North Carolina by providing extra pairs of hands to improve the staff/child ratio. The Corps members' impact on the children and classroom was assessed through questionnaires completed by supervising teachers, center directors, and parents of children enrolled in the child care centers where Corps members were placed. Responses to questionnaires consistently indicated that Corps members had the greatest impact in three specific areas: Children's development, quality of guidance in classrooms, and health and safety procedures used in classrooms.

Comments from supervising teachers illustrate concretely the impact Corps members had in the early childhood classrooms. One supervising teacher wrote, "without her I would not have been able to arrange my room in a way that was developmentally appropriate. She did most of the work, while I interacted with the children." Another supervising teacher noted that "the Corps member has made a large improvement in the amount of activities, one-on-one, art projects, and science experiments that the children have had." Yet another supervising teacher indicated, "One child in our class had a speech problem. Having a Corps member in our room allowed me to work with this child for 10-15 minutes a day. Having a Corps member in our room has been a big plus... The Corps member was there to help calm the kids with separation anxiety while I carried on the lesson, and she freed me up to take a break (use the bathroom) when I needed to." One center director said, "Our Corps member has provided more one-on-one attention with the children, which is very much needed. Also, an extra worker means that there are less chances of injuries and/or conflicts." A Smart Start Executive Director noted, "One Corps member developed a parent involvement project which has benefited many children through greater involvement of their parents in their center's life."

CORPS MEMBER BENEFITS

Not only did Corps members receive the North Carolina Early Childhood Credential, First Aid and CPR certification, and on the job training but they also received a small monthly living allowance, health insurance, and a child care allowance if they were parents. In some cases Smart Start Partnerships supplemented the Corps members living expenses with a housing allowance. At the conclusion of their nine-month experience, the Corps members received an educational voucher to finance college, graduate school, or vocational training or to pay back student loans. AmeriCorps awards all volunteers a $4,725 educational voucher when they successfully complete 1700 hours of community service.

PROSPECTS FOR LONG-TERM SUSTAINABILITY

The National Service Corporation attempted to ensure sustainability of the project by requiring an increasing match over the three years of the project. During the first year, a 20% match was required with a 25% and 33% required match during the successive years. For the North Carolina Child Care Corps, the match was provided by the North Carolina Partnership for Children (Smart Start) and UNCG. Although the match was difficult to achieve, particularly during Year Three, the match requirement did assist in sustaining some of the specific initiatives in the targeted counties beyond the three years of the project. In one county Corps members were used to begin a teacher substitute pool. The substitute pool was continued at the end of the NCCCC project by the local Partnership for Children due to its success while utilizing AmeriCorps participants as teacher substitutes. Furthermore, due to the collaborative arrangement with the NC Smart Start initiative, and the continuation of Smart Start, many of the goals of the NCCCC project remain a focus in the participating counties. Since the collaboration was established during the first year of Smart Start funding it provided an opportunity for child care programs in those communities to experience the benefits of improved staff/child ratios and trained staff during the early stages of program implementation. Fortunately many of the counties continue to focus on improving child care quality, through improving staff/child ratios and educational opportunities for teachers. For example, several of the counties are assisting child care centers in achieving National Association for the Education of Young Children (NAEYC) accreditation, which would require a permanent improvement in staff/child ratios.

A SUCCESSFUL PARTNERSHIP

The North Carolina Child Care Corps was a successful community university collaboration for three reasons: 1) The shared commitment of the community and the university to improving the quality of child care in the state of North Carolina; 2) the willingness of the university to be responsiveness to each community's ideas regarding effective strategies for implementation of the project in that community; and 3) the university's sincere attempt to dissipate the "ivory tower" image often ascribed to it by communities.

The commitment to quality of early childhood educational services has long been a focus of the Department of Human Development and Family Studies at UNCG. With the recent implementation of Smart Start, which allows decisions regarding financial allocations to the discretion of each community, commitment to quality early childhood services has become a strong priority for participating counties. This shared commitment to quality was frequently helpful for university and community project leadership when differences of opinion occurred. With the shared goal of quality education and care as the bottom line, compromise positions were more easily reached.

University personnel did more than pay lip service to soliciting community input. Communities were strongly encouraged to assist project personnel in selecting the participating child care centers, and in all cases the decisions of the counties were respected. When concerns about Corps members were voiced by community supervisors, NCCCC staff never dismissed the issue but initiated a procedure of individual telephone conversations with the supervisor and the Corps member, followed by a conference call, and often a site visit to address the concerns. Every effort was made to honor the input of all community participants as long as their ideas were consistent with the general goals of the project. For example, one community requested that Corps members provide child care for parents while they were enrolled in GED classes. Although this was not the primary intent of the project and did not meet the strict guidelines for community service, it provided an important service to parents of children enrolled in community child care centers and established positive community relations and was readily approved by project staff.

University project staff attacked the "ivory tower" image by *not* requesting community leaders to travel to campus for meetings except for in-service training. Because of the central location of UNCG, campus was the most convenient central location for all counties during training days. In all other cases the Project Director and Project Coordinator traveled to the communities (in some cases several hundred miles from campus) for meetings with child care center staff and supervisors as well as Smart Start administrators. In addition, the Project Coordinator regularly traveled to the communities to meet with Smart Start officials and child care center administrators and teachers to discuss each corps member's performance. Furthermore, during all in-service training sessions supervising teachers and directors were regarded as experts assisting with the training sessions. They were often asked for their input when questions were raised by corps members during the training sessions.

WHY WAS THIS A SUCCESSFUL LEARNING EXPERIENCE?

Although the North Carolina Child Care Corps holds immense promise as an intervention strategy to improve the quality of child care, there are many concerns that must be addressed by university and community collaborators related to the use of AmeriCorps volunteers in child care classrooms. First, the attrition rate must be decreased. Although the rate of attrition did not exceed the national turnover-rate in child care and is comparable to the documented attrition rate in other national service programs, losing one-third of the Corps members originally accepted into the program must be regarded as a significant concern for the program.

The university and community collaborators can perhaps jointly address this concern by better preparing Corps members for their relocation into communities that are often quite different from a Corps member's home community. Although Corps members were placed in communities with a cohort of NCCCC members, there was nonetheless a sense of isolation that resulted for Corps members who were young and inexperienced in coping with moving to a new location and beginning a challenging new job. This process could have been improved by better utilization of community members to assist the project personnel in the adjustment of Corps members to the communities, perhaps by matching Corps members with a family in the community.

For many of the Corps members, the AmeriCorps service project was their first experience away from home and resulted in serious bouts of home-sickness. A family connection in the community could have done much to alleviate the problem. In addition, community child care programs could have benefited from assistance by university personnel in mentoring strategies so that Corps members would not have been expected to do too much too soon.

Often Corps members were more educated than other teachers in the program and, therefore, they were asked to assume responsibility for activities that were beyond their capabilities as novice teachers. Unfortunately, this seemed to result in premature burnout for Corps members. If child care center staff were more formally trained as mentors they could have better understood the importance of bringing the Corps members along slowly and assigning responsibility gradually to the AmeriCorps volunteers.

CONCLUSION

The most important lesson to be learned from the North Carolina Child Care Corps is that National Service is not, and should not attempt to be, a panacea for improving the quality of child care in our country. Although the project administrators believe the project had a significant impact on local communities, created meaningful improvement in the quality of child care services for hundreds of children in NC, and changed the lives of many youth, it is *not* the answer to improving the quality of child care in our country. The Child Care Corps is perhaps an answer and perhaps a piece of a complex puzzle. Without question, AmeriCorps National Service is an important opportunity for American youth and the NCCCC demonstrated that it can be one mechanism to assist in addressing the child care crisis facing young children and their families in the United States.

REFERENCES

Danzig, R., & Szanton, P. (1986). *National service: What would it mean?* Lexington, MA: Lexington Books.

Feeney, S., & Chun, R. (1985). Effective teachers of young children. *Young Children, 41*, 47-52.

Helburn, S. W. (Ed.). (1995). *Cost, quality and child outcomes in child care centers, technical report.* Denver, CO: University of Colorado.

Phillips, D. A., & Howes, C. (1987). Indicators of quality in child care: Review of research. In D. A. Phillips (Ed.), *Quality in child care: What does research tell us?* (pp. 1-19). Washington, DC: NAEYC.

40 SUPPORT OUR STUDENTS: SATURDAY ACADEMY AT EAST CAROLINA UNIVERSITY

Cynthia E. Johnson
Elizabeth A. Carroll
East Carolina University

Jay Faron
Boys and Girls Clubs of Pitt County, Inc.

Support Our Students (SOS) Saturday Academy is an outreach partnership program with the Department of Child Development and Family Relations, School of Human Environmental Sciences at East Carolina University (ECU), the Boys and Girls Clubs of Pitt County, Inc., and the North Carolina Department of Health and Human Services, Youth Services Division. Saturday Academy is an expansion of the SOS concept of improving academic performance among at-risk middle-school students. The SOS Initiative is a public-private partnership that links parents, schools, churches, agencies, and corporations in a collaborative effort to provide mentoring, resources, support and guidance, and safe places for young people.

In its 1994 Special Legislative Session on Crime, the North Carolina General Assembly endorsed the Governor's recommendation to establish the North Carolina Support Our Students (SOS) Initiative to insure success for adolescents (Article 3, Chapter 143B). SOS began as an after-school program for children in grades 4-9. It was designed to help prevent juvenile crime by rallying communities around their young people, thereby helping steer them into positive, constructive activities. During 1994-95, approximately 120 different sites were offering SOS programs to over 6,000 students in 52 of the state's 100 counties. In 1995, the SOS concept was extended to a new concept, Saturday Academies.

The Saturday Academy Program is designed to provide the opportunity for students who are involved in a local SOS program to participate in academic enrichment, social opportunities, and mentoring at one of the three university sites. *ECU Saturday Academy* serves students in the eastern region of 10 rural counties. During the 1996-97 school year, groups of 60 students, at a maximum rate of 20 students per county or 180 students totally, three counties per Saturday, had the opportunity of attending *ECU Saturday Academy*. The volunteer component of the program dealt with issues of culture and diversity, networking, and co-learning. About 90% of the school-agers were black and about 90% of the ECU students were white. All AmeriCorps volunteers were white. All parent volunteers were black and SOS local administrators were about evenly mixed racially.

NATURE OF THE PARTNERSHIPS

Our basic funding partnership was with the Department of Health and Human Services. However, since this was an outreach initiative involving local SOS programs, partnerships expanded to include several university units, volunteers from AmeriCorps and Learn and Serve, and local SOS administrators and volunteers. The two primary partnerships were with two non-profit institutions—the university and the Boys and Girls Clubs of Pitt County, Inc., a local youth organization. Both have successful histories of working together (e.g.,. ECU students volunteer and complete internships at the Boys and Girls Clubs); however, this was the first time both had collaborated on a funded project.

ECU provided administrative support, facilities, and instructional support while the Boys and Girls Clubs provided volunteers, transportation, and supervisory and technical support. University faculty, staff, and graduate students served as instructors, group facilitators, chaperons, and mentors on a pro bono basis. ECU student volunteers represented various backgrounds from athlete to medical student. Undergraduate students enrolled in the department's Middle Childhood and Family and Cultural Diversity courses must have an opportunity to integrate theory and research with experiential learning. Saturday Academy was one vehicle to provide experience working and interacting with middle grade children. Corporations and businesses provided resource speakers and donations to the Saturday Academy. Local SOS volunteers, including parents, provided transportation, logistic support, supervision, and academic assistance. Volunteers from Learn and Serve and AmeriCorps served as group facilitators, supervisors, mentors, and chaperons.

PURPOSE AND GOALS

The purpose of the partnership was to provide academic enrichment, social opportunities, and mentoring to middle-school students. More specifically, students were: 1) provided experiential learning experiences in team building and trust, computer technology, science and medicine, literature and creative writing, culture and art, and development of academic skills; 2) exposed to a university environment and campus life including dining services, athletic activities, classroom instruction, theater productions and visits to the medical center, dormitories, and art center; and 3) afforded opportunities to be mentored by university students and other volunteers.

ANALYSIS OF PROCESS

Saturday Academies contract periods are for three years, subject to renewal and availability of funds each year. Since funds come from federal, state, and local sources, and since each has its own funding cycle, notification of awards varies. However, our funding base has been stable over the past three years.

Universities were notified about funds to start Saturday Academies during late spring of 1996. Invitations were sent to professors, who were known for their work with or interest in young people, to attend an information session. One department (Child Development and Family Relations) from ECU answered the invitation. Before the proposal was written and during the initial stage of the program, numerous hours were spent with state officials and evaluators (Support Our Students Program Director, Youth Voices, Governor's Office of Citizen's Affairs, AmeriCorps representative, corporate leaders, and SOS Technical Assistance and Training Unit).

After a concept paper was approved, the institutional proposal was developed. This step was perhaps the most complicated part of the process since it involved risk management issues—bringing children to campus on weekends (insurance coverage, arranging for lunch, campus security, chaperons, securing tickets to football games, clearance for visits at the medical school, parental approval forms, collaborative arrangements with partners, etc.). The Executive Director of the Boys and Girls Clubs, the Director (and program Manager) of Sponsored Programs at ECU, the ECU Saturday Academy Program Coordinator and Project Director, the Risk Management Officer, and the Dean of the School of Human Environmental Sciences met several times to finalize an activity schedule. We met twice with the staff of the Boys and Girls Clubs for program and facility planning.

ACHIEVEMENT RELATED TO GOALS

During the first year of the project, 90 volunteers (including 64 students) and 11 instructors (including a medical professor, an attorney, an artist, university academic counselors, English and Middle Grade professors, a computer technician, and electrical engineers) were recruited to assist with delivering the program content. We finally limited participation to 150 middle-grade children.

Evaluations from the students and volunteers were positive, mostly 5 on a scale from 1 to 5. Students age 10-12 years comprised the bulk of attendance. The preliminary state evaluations indicated that students who participated in our program improved their academic performance and that their interest in science and writing increased. Students ranked ordered their interests as computer science, arts and creative performance, and science and technology.

ECU students were most satisfied with the experience and were positive about the mentoring and assistance they gave to the children. On a few occasions, ECU students outnumbered the school-agers. ECU students wrote papers about their volunteer experiences. Many were surprised at the maturity level of this age group of children.

The first year concluded with a graduation ceremony where students were given certificates and tee-shirts. Three of our participants received the Governor's Awards for Outstanding School Achievement and one received a college scholarship.

PROSPECTS FOR LONG-TERM SUSTAINABILITY

The prospects for long term sustainability will depend upon financial support and collaborating with regional organizations and youth groups. Corporations and businesses have been most supportive of our program. However, the two major partnerships are both non-profit, the university and the Boys and Girls Clubs. We represent an agricultural/agribusiness, tourism region. The area we serve is rural with a high level of poverty. We will need to seek external support for a long-term project. As this chapter is being completed, the third consecutive year of funding has been obtained.

LEARNINGS FROM THIS PARTNERSHIP

Neither partner to this project was new to collaboration. What surprised us were the steps involved in bringing children to campus on weekends and the logistics of getting anywhere from 60 to 150 children around campus and town each week. Obtaining security coverage, dining cards, insurance, porta toilets for outdoor activities, and tickets to university functions brought out the creativity spirit in us. Keeping pace with children who ran, not walked, sent some of us to bed early each Saturday. Coordinating our schedule with the university and school calendars also challenged us. No two counties had the same school calendar, particularly for spring break!

We provided an opportunity for at-risk students to have experiences unbeknown to them. Some were riding on the vans as early as 7:00 a.m. in order to take advantage of this opportunity. Their days were long but they were eager learners. The middle-school students thought that coming "to college was cool." In the program's beginning, many had no aspirations beyond high school. At the end of the first year, conversations were heard about studying hard to get into college, being a physician or cartoon artist, and living in a dormitory. Their local SOS leaders were committed to the Saturday Academy concept and gave relentlessly to the program, Saturday after Saturday. They were pleased with the change and growth they saw in the children.

ECU students documented their personal growth as they worked with school-agers. A few ECU students were recruited to work with local SOS program during the summer of 1997. One of our recent undergraduates is now a graduate assistant and project co-coordinator for *ECU Saturday Academy.* Professors also indicated how they re-connected to "real students" in middle school and junior high.

Finally, we learned that a "detail person" who is trained in time and resource management and has experience working with children in group situations is needed to run a project of this nature. We were fortunate to have such a person who worked part-time in our department—and who was also a graduate of our Marriage and Family Therapy Program and an attorney.

ADDENDUM

Since we submitted this chapter, *ECU Saturday Academy* was refunded for the 1998 calendar year. Several changes have been made in the program. First, we reduced the age of the children to 10 years, admitting some children who are age 11. These children can stay with the program for three years or longer. We found that this age group best serves the goals of the project. Children of this age are also very receptive to learning and experiential challenges. Second, we limited the number of participants from each county to 5 children and increased the service area from 10 to 13 counties. Sixty-five children are currently enrolled in the program and they will attend for an entire calendar year. Third, we revised our mentoring component by recruiting more African-American male students and resource role models since about 50% of the children are males. The ECU mentor may be a student enrolled in one of our classes, a member of a fraternity, an athlete, or an ECU volunteer. The mentor provides one-on-one academic assistance to a child, assists with supervision, and is basically a "pal" to the child. Mentors provide additional support by writing to the children and sending cards and e-mail messages. Currently, we have more mentors than children. Fourth, we added a parent involvement component. Parents were invited to two information sessions. We shared information about the university, discussed growth and development of elementary-age children, facilitated a tour of the campus, and arranged for recreational activities. Parents can accompany their children to any of the programs. This has been the most rewarding part of the program for parents. Having lunch in a university dining hall with their child is a first for all of our parents. Our department's emphasis on "family" is exemplified in this program. Finally, we increased the emphasis on writing and reading. Each child has been given a journal to write his or her thoughts, stories, and poems for an entire year. A reading program will be implemented during the summer where the children will have a chance to listen to a famous storyteller, purchase a book of their own, and write a book review or report of their book. It is our plan that this will be followed by oral histories and participation in a drama or theater production in the fall.

Since Saturday Academies have received favorable responses, it is expected that state and private funds will be available for 1999. A verbal call for proposals has gone out. Right now, funding prospects for long-term sustainability look bright.

REFERENCES

Jones, B. W. (1996). *Support our students evaluation project: Final Report.* Durham, NC: North Carolina Central University Institute for the Study of Minority Issues.

North Carolina General Statues. (1994). Article 3, Chapter 143B.

Support our students (SOS): Year in review. (1995). Raleigh: N. C. Department of Human Resources.

41 THE DAP*TECH PARTNERSHIP: HELPING CHILDREN WITH DISABILITIES THROUGH TECHNOLOGY

Carol A. Cartwright
Kent State University

NATURE OF PARTNERSHIP

Collaborations between universities and the communities they serve are not new. But, often, they have been consultancies more than true collaborations. Sparked by the broadened definition of scholarship articulated by Ernest Boyer (1990) and by public calls for scholarship that addresses the needs of families and communities, outreach is moving from the service entrance to the front door of the academy, and many campus-community collaborations are marked by a new level of reciprocity.

A promising project to help teachers and parents effectively integrate technology into the lives of young children with disabilities exemplifies a new generation of partnerships based on open communication and shared decision making. The key project goal is to create user-friendly, child-friendly, strategies for using computers and software in home and school environments, and to do so in a manner consistent with the Developmentally Appropriate Practice (DAP) guidelines for working with young children endorsed by the National Association for the Education of Young Children (Bredekamp, 1987).

Funded by a grant from the U.S. Department of Education, the five-year project is a collaboration of Kent State University's School of Speech Pathology and Audiology; the Family-Child Learning Center (FCLC), a nonprofit, training and research facility jointly supported by Children's Hospital Medical Center of Akron and Kent State University; and teachers and parents of children with disabilities in 13 preschool classrooms in which DAP guidelines are followed.

PURPOSES AND GOALS

The project originated in the observation of a faculty researcher in the School of Speech Pathology and Audiology that assistive technologies—particularly computer technologies—are not being used in schools or homes to the maximum benefit of young children with disabilities. She attributed this in part to her observation that when technology is introduced in school or home settings, service providers and caregivers can become uncharacteristically didactic, focusing on device mastery rather than integrating device use into a child's developmental plan.

Research evidence that children with disabilities can increase their independence, communication, and learning through appropriate integration of technology (NAEYC, 1996) reinforced the faculty member's conclusion that a critical, national need exists for guidelines for the use of assistive technologies. She hypothesized that incorporating assistive devices across the everyday routines of children with disabilities in a playful way would yield significant improvement in communication and learning.

ANALYSIS OF THE PROCESS

It was natural for the Kent faculty member and the FCLC to develop a joint grant proposal to develop this "DAP*TECH" (Developmentally Appropriate Practice with Technology) model. The FCLC has collaborated with Kent in numerous training, research, and outreach projects in speech pathology and early-childhood special education. The Kent faculty member's expertise in assistive technology and the FCLC director's expertise in DAP was another logical partnership for the project. By mutual agreement, the FCLC director manages budget and staff matters, while the Kent faculty member oversees daily project operations and the development of print, video, and computer-based training products.

An FCLC speech pathologist with assistive-technology expertise serves as project coordinator. She and a project associate coordinate field-based training, provide technical assistance, conduct workshops, collect and summarize evaluation data, and assist with the refinement of training products. In addition, Kent graduate students in speech pathology participate in data collection and analysis.

Preschools involved in the FCLC's prior technology projects provided a pool of prospective training sites. By choosing schools that already used assistive technologies and had shown interest in technology innovation, project staff avoided the resistance that often accompanies the introduction of technology, as well as the cost of providing computers and other assistive devices. After holding focus groups and soliciting teachers directly via phone and mail, 13 preschool, special education classrooms were chosen as DAP*TECH training sites. Teachers were asked to select target children on whom to test user-friendly, technology-use strategies. The children have a broad range of physical, mental, and developmental disabilities and related communication disorders.

The project was designed to build a sense of ownership in teachers and parents, who were full-fledged members of the project team and essential for developing the DAP*TECH model. Project benefits and expectations were provided verbally and in print prior to training sites' agreement to participate. Teachers were given strong assurances that school administrators could not mandate their participation. This helped convey that the intent of the project was not intrusive or judgmental. To encourage participation, grant funds are appropriated for substitutes, allowing teachers to leave their classrooms to attend workshops. In addition, parents who attend training sessions receive a stipend for mileage and baby-sitters. This action has been very well received, and viewed as further evidence that parent and teacher feedback is valued.

Project staff report that it has been particularly helpful to invite school administrators to attend training sessions. Their participation helps ensure continuing conceptual support for the project, and, in turn, helps build a case for upgrading and expanding technology tools. In another effort to generate support for DAP*TECH, and technology use in general, videotapes of interactions between children and teachers around assistive technology are provided at no cost to schools for use in internal and external training and publicity.

During the first year, project staff visited every classroom weekly for half a day. Subsequently, visits have been held every other week. A drawback emerged quickly: Teachers became over-reliant on project staff, calling them for problems as simple as a computer not working because it was unplugged. Project staff sought a way to decrease dependency on them while remaining supportive. This balance was achieved by identifying, training, and assigning local resource specialists who are assigned to specific schools. These troubleshooters, whose mileage is covered by grant funds, are employees of Ohio's Special Education Regional Resource Centers. Parents and teachers also were invited to contact project staff via e-mail, a communication vehicle that has proven to be efficient and effective.

ACHIEVEMENTS RELATED TO GOALS

In addition to demonstrating and validating the effectiveness of the DAP*TECH model, a primary project goal has been to address the dearth of printed material about the use of assistive technology with young children with disabilities. Field guides, focused on computing and software and on augmentative and alternative communication, were developed and tested during the first four years of the project. The guides contain information, handouts, and extensive resource sections, all emphasizing changes in adult interaction and environmental arrangements that enhance child engagement, enjoyment, and communication. The term "field guide" and a colorful, modern design were chosen to resemble popular, "how-to" books. The guides also will be offered in interactive, CD-ROM format, and in abridged form on the School of Speech Pathology and Audiology's World Wide Web site. Project staff believe that the accessibility of DAP*TECH materials—in terms of cost and format—increases the likelihood that they will be purchased and applied by service providers and caregivers.

PROSPECTS FOR LONG-TERM SUSTAINABILITY

Of course, nothing is a better predictor of sustainability than success. All project activities are subject to evaluation and continuous improvement based on formal and informal data. Results to date show significant improvement in communication behaviors such as rate and initiation of communication using the DAP*TECH model (Mitchell, Mahoney, Porto, & Goldberg, 1997). In addition, pre- and post-participation profiles of 12 children support reported teacher perceptions of improvements such as increased amount of communication, engagement with computer software, and participation in play with adults (Mitchell, Mahoney, Porto, & Goldberg, 1997). Further, 100 percent of teachers contacted in an impact survey said they would recommend the DAP*TECH method to colleagues and parents (Mitchell, Mahoney, Porto, & Goldberg, 1997).

WHY WAS THIS A SUCCESSFUL PARTNERSHIP?

In summary, the DAP*TECH project illustrates the importance of ensuring voluntary participation in community-university collaborations; articulating and reinforcing that all participants' views are valued; enacting practical strategies to allow full participation; and providing opportunities for open and ongoing communication. It is the kind of success that is helping to build a foundation of inclusion, empowerment and mutual respect for community-university collaborations.

REFERENCES

Boyer, E. L. (1990). *Scholarship reconsidered: Priorities of the professoriate.* Princeton, NJ: The Carnegie Foundation for the Advancement of Teaching.

Bredekamp, S. (1987). *Developmentally appropriate practices in early childhood programs serving children from birth through age eight* (expanded edition). Washington, DC: National Association for the Education of Young Children.

Mitchell, P., Mahoney, G., Porto, P., & Goldberg, E. (1997). *DAP*TECH: Using innovative technologies with children with disabilities in developmentally appropriate practice preschool programs* (Year Three Performance Report, Grant Number H024B40054). Washington, DC: Office of Special Education, U.S. Department of Education.

National Association for the Education of Young Children. (1996, September). NAEYC position statement: Technology and young children ages three through eight. *Young Children*, 11-16.

42 CHILD CARE AND HEAD START: COMMUNITY ACTION COMMISSION-UNIVERSITY PARTNERSHIP

Thomas R. Chibucos
Bowling Green State University

Karen Freeman
Jordan Family Development Center

Sally Kilmer
Bowling Green State University

A. Fredericka Larsen
WSOS Child Development and Head Start Programs

Barbara O'Donnel
Bowling Green State University

Don Stricker
WSOS Community Action Commission

INTRODUCTION

The collaboration described in this chapter involves two organizations, the Bowling Green State University (BGSU) School of Family and Consumer Sciences (SFCS) and the Wood, Seneca, Ottawa, and Sandusky Counties Community Action Commission (WSOS). This partnership between a public university and a non-profit community action commission has matured over the past four and one-half years. The SFCS mission emphasizes a multi- and interdisciplinary perspective as essential to understanding the development of individuals, families, and communities in complex human ecological systems. The development of on- and off-campus collaborations and partnerships to address issues of importance to children, youth, and families is a major feature of the SFCS mission. Similarly, WSOS actively develops and engages in partnerships with other non-profit and private sector entities. WSOS serves over 1250 children and operates 21 centers in four counties, and has a 33-year history of providing comprehensive services to low income families and individuals. Since its inception WSOS has been a grantee for the Head Start Program.

NATURE OF THE PARTNERSHIP

Initially, the collaboration received impetus primarily from several related factors. First, there was the desire to provide campus child care (where none had existed) for children of university students, faculty, and staff, as well as the desire of WSOS to locate a Head Start Center in the city of Bowling Green, OH. Each organization was looking for feasible and cost effective ways to achieve these goals. Second, prior positive working relationships had been established between faculty at the university and personnel at WSOS. The interaction had previously centered on grant-writing and other types of (typical) faculty consulting.

It is clear that the partnership described in this chapter had strong roots in familiarity and in the need to maximize potential resources. That is, due to resource constraints, it is highly unlikely that either the university or WSOS would have been able to achieve their individual program and organizational objectives without the development of this (or some) collaborative partnership. Similarly, the previously established (although limited) connection between the SFCS and WSOS provided a starting point on which to build. Because of these factors, the shared commitments to building partnerships (generally) and to carrying out service, education, training, and research to enhance the development of children, youth, and families have been reinforced and facilitated.

PURPOSE AND GOALS

The collaboration had and has a variety of purposes and goals. These include:

1) locating a Head Start program (facility) on the Bowling Green State University campus;
2) offering Campus Child Care to university students, faculty, and staff;
3) building a stronger connection between WSOS and the university;
4) providing enhanced learning, research, and service opportunities to university students and faculty;
5) providing opportunities for continuing learning for personnel in Head Start and child care programs;
6) improving the quality of Head Start and child care programs for children and families, and increasing the quality and availability of infant/toddler care;
7) integrating various Head Start and child care activities to the extent permissible in relation to federal mandates concerning Head Start; and
8) developing an example of the kind of community-university partnership that serves the public interest.

ANALYSIS OF THE PROCESS

History

As noted, members of the faculty in the School of Family and Consumer Sciences (SFCS) and members of WSOS (most notably authors Kilmer and Larsen, respectively) had worked together over a number of years on a range of Head Start and Child Development projects. It was through this network that the SFCS became aware in late 1993 of the fact that WSOS was seeking to build a Head Start facility in the city of Bowling Green, OH. Thus, the more extensive collaboration that emerged indicates continued development of a relationship that already existed because of mutual substantive interests and pragmatic concerns.

The university had been "studying" the need for campus child care for two decades, carrying out at least three surveys of campus constituents to determine need and discussing the matter extensively in the Faculty Senate. For a myriad of reasons the issue of campus child care on the BGSU campus remained in a very static place for a prolonged period of time. Two reasons seem particularly noteworthy: (1) a difficult financial period for higher education institutions in the state of Ohio throughout most of the 1980s and early 1990s had wide-ranging negative effects on potential new initiatives; and (2) child care did not receive high institutional priority or attention from administrative leadership within the university.

Groundwork for the Partnership

With the arrival of a new SFCS (then, the Department of Human Ecology, previously Home Economics) chair, a major SFCS strategic planning process began in the 1993-94 academic year. In late 1993 and early 1994, the department refined and updated its mission statement, key elements of which included an emphasis on multidisciplinarity and the development of partnerships and collaborations to address child, family and community issues. This served both to reinforce the earlier interactions of university faculty with WSOS and to provide a foundation for increased and more formal collaboration. Meetings were held between the partners in early 1994 (some of these meetings included facilities and development personnel from both BGSU and WSOS), a time period during which issues of trust-building, identification of turf issues, and learning each other's cultures were of paramount importance. Three themes about child care, consistent with nationally representative discussions, recurred repeatedly: The cost, quality, and availability of care (e.g., Bridgman & Phillips, 1996; Galinsky, Howes, Kontos, & Shinn, 1994). Although we tried to have all "stakeholders at the table" (Weiss & Greene, 1992) on a regular basis to discuss these and other matters, there were times when this did not occur. Predictably, communication problems tended to surface following those instances. Interestingly, and we think this is probably typical, these instances of less than complete involvement were due to within-institution issues at least as often as they were due to between-partner issues.

After a number of meetings on the BGSU campus it was decided that a rationale for the collaboration had to be clearly articulated in order to justify the collaboration to the university community, and administration. Therefore, Chibucos and Kilmer (1994) wrote a "white paper" that detailed the potential academic relationship between the university and WSOS as well as the kinds of teaching, service, and scholarship activities that might result from the collaboration. The paper also presented a theoretical and empirical rationale for the collaboration. This rationale focused primarily on Head Start but also discussed some essential principles of intervention with families and children. For example, the importance of linking programs and services across developmental periods, the need for multidimensional intervention as well as the need for family capacity-building, and destigmatization of family support efforts were presented. The white paper was discussed with the WSOS community partners and received their imprimatur.

Between early April 1994 and the beginning of the 1994-95 academic year (August 1994) the white paper was shared widely within the university community. During this same time period the facilities people from WSOS and from the university were meeting regularly and began to develop plans for a new facility on the BGSU campus. WSOS had learned in late 1993 that the opportunity existed to apply to the Ohio Department of Education's Early Childhood Division for construction funds. To enhance competitiveness for this funding WSOS required a Bowling Green, Ohio area (though not necessarily BGSU) location and needed land for a new building. The facilities persons at the university and at WSOS discussed land options, the possibility of constructing two connected buildings, and a variety of other matters.

By the beginning of the 1994-95 academic year, then, there was strong momentum to pursue the collaboration. However, major gaps in communication had developed since the facilities people and program people had been operating more or less on parallel tracks. There were two major reasons for this lack of integrated discussion. One concerned the time pressures WSOS was feeling to get a building on track in order to take advantage of a funding opportunity. The other concerned the fact that major administrative changes were occurring throughout the university. Essentially, there was no one at the university in a senior administrative position who was actively involved in or committed to the partnership. This meant that the SFCS was the primary campus unit involved in the process of developing the partnership with WSOS. Substantively this made sense, given the SFCS mission and faculty expertise. However, in terms of ultimate institutional approval, commitment, and support, a vacuum existed. Essentially, therefore, the WSOS acceptance of a university institutional commitment to collaborate and to potential future support was made somewhat on faith. The partnership did receive tacit approval from the vice president for academic affairs in early fall 1994 but, as indicated previously, there was little coordination within the university itself. Nonetheless, strong commitment from the director of the university's office of capital planning (both in working for the new facility and in support of campus child care) gave WSOS and the SFCS hope that funding for a facility to support the programmatic collaboration might be achieved.

Gaining Stability in BGSU Administration

In the fall of 1994 a new dean was hired to head the college (now the College of Education and Human Development) in which the SFCS is located. This appointment began to provide some stability for the context in which the collaboration was taking place. The new dean supported the collaboration and began to voice support for it in meetings and discussions at different administrative levels, including in the university capital planning process. Over the course of the 1994-95 academic year there was on-again, off-again contact and meetings involving the co-authors, essentially due to the fact that the funding mechanism and building plans were somewhat in a state of flux. Through the work of the BGSU and WSOS planning offices a funding plan was finally developed and approved. In the summer of 1995, BGSU was granted a $300,000 capital improvement allocation from the Ohio Board of Regents (half of its $600,000 request). WSOS was awarded the $600,000 it had applied for from the Ohio Department of Education. The agreement was that WSOS would own the building—subject to WSOS providing child care services for children of university faculty, staff, and students for 25 years. In addition, the university would lease the land to WSOS for a nominal yearly fee, and WSOS would move a Head Start program to the BGSU campus.

However, due to the previously noted parallel rather than interactive functioning of facilities and program people (both within the bureaucracies of each partner as well as between partners), a significant number of problems in the building plan were identified when the plan was received by the SFCS in July 1995. The time to review the building plan was very short—a permit to begin the work was to be obtained in several days. WSOS facilities personnel, consulting somewhat with BGSU facilities people, but with little consultation either with their own program persons or with SFCS, had developed a building plan.

The new president of BGSU (who joined the institution in June 1995) and the president and CEO of WSOS responded to the concerns expressed by SFCS faculty about the appropriateness of the planned facility to support a high quality collaboration with commitments to delay proceeding on the building. Formalizing the institutional agreements was delayed until all relevant parties could meet to address the issues of concern. However, the BGSU president made a commitment to support resolution of the problems so that the collaboration could proceed. Such central administration support is critical if community-university partnerships are to be sustained (Lerner & Simon, 1998).

On a practical level, the upshot was that it was not until ground was ready to be broken that serious discussion took place involving program and facilities personnel! The discussions that took place can best be described as a crash course in "learning and accepting the culture of others." It was because of the prior build up of trust, because of shared values about the importance of quality programming for children and families, and because of strong shared commitments at the operational program level that the collaboration survived this occurrence.

Ultimately, with substantial negotiation and modification in the planned facility, reinforced by having worked together to overcome another difficulty, the agreement between WSOS and BGSU was signed in the fall of 1995, ground was broken for the building in December 1995, and the building was licensed in March 1996. Immediately thereafter Head Start services began.

Growing the Partnership

In late 1995 (November), university administrative responsibility was assigned by the BGSU president to the (Interim) Vice President for Human Resources who convened the first formal Campus Child Care Advisory Board (CCAB) meeting. The CCAB included several of the authors of this chapter and other university representatives, notably those for students and staff. The main initial function of the CCAB was to begin to work on the process of application for available Campus Child Care slots as well as on publicizing the pending opening. The CCAB[1] developed a procedure for allotting available child care slots to infants/toddlers and preschoolers, as well as among campus constituents (children of faculty, staff and students), and community members. WSOS began accepting enrollments for child care in April 1996, and child care began in May 1996 (but far below capacity).

The 1996-97 academic year was the first full-year of operation, a year in which a new Provost/Vice President for Academic Affairs joined the university. A major celebration of the opening took place in September 1996, with Dr. James Garbarino delivering a public address and providing perspective about the importance of this kind of collaboration. This activity served to reinforce and uplift everyone involved with bringing the collaboration to the point of development it had attained, and helped to focus university and community attention on it. The center was named the Jordan Family Development Center (JFDC) in recognition of a family that had had children in another WSOS Head Start program over two decades ago. The mother in this family had become President of the National Head Start Association!

Activities and issues during the first year included regular CCAB meetings, the development of plans, policies and procedures for campus constituent research, education, and observational use of the facility, and a wide-range of "growing pains." An example of the latter was the significant misunderstanding within the university by potential users of child care regarding why a full fee was charged. We believe that this was the result of many years of discussion on campus, with many mixed messages sent to the campus community. Similarly, community people assumed that all slots were earmarked only for university people, and thus did not show initial interest.

A major issue during the first year of operation was relatively low enrollment and the associated budget deficit for year one. Given the timing of building completion, the relative scarcity of on-campus people in the summer, and the campus community's perspective on campus child care (i.e., that there was not any!), full enrollment was not expected (by SFCS faculty) at the time of opening. However, expectations about enrollment levels were different for WSOS since this was WSOS' first time providing full day care for fee-paying clients.

Partnership Activities

As the collaboration entered its second year (1997-98), university use of the JFDC (class participation, observation, internship placements, and research) became more frequent. This use reflected the SFCS commitment to allow ample time for program activities to develop before university education, training, observation, and research in the JFDC would proceed. This also allowed time for WSOS to work with its own board and the CCAB to increase enrollments. A critical component was WSOS' work with a consultant to develop management, marketing, and business plans for the campus child care component of the partnership. In addition, a collaborative $60,000 grant (to authors O'Donnel and Freeman) for improving the observation space, equipment, and facilities in the JFDC was received from the

Ohio Board of Regents, with matching monies from the university. Thus, by the end of the year the increase in university activities was more feasible.

Observation equipment was added in the summer and fall of 1998. However, the first-year deficit remained a financial problem producing occasional tension and frustration—not so much between the program level partners as between WSOS and "the university." The provost was invited by the CCAB to a presentation about budget issues, the development of the collaboration to date, the value-added activities brought to the university by the collaboration, and the desirability that the university evidence real resource support for the collaboration. The provost selected a small university committee to make recommendations on the matter of support, but after 8-9 months that committee has not been active. Various tangible types of in-kind support have begun to accrue, however (e.g., snow removal from the JFDC parking lot by BGSU employees; and student participation at the JFDC as support for Head Start funding).

The collaboration (i.e., that part of it since the building of the facility) is now in year three (1998-99 academic year). There has been collaboration to find grant funding and development dollars to support equipment for infants/toddlers as well as to fund the building of a new outdoor playground (the latter being finished as we write). And, 18 months after opening, the Campus Child Care enrollments achieved the financial break-even point of 62 FTE children in preschool or infant/toddler care. At present, campus child care is still underutilized by staff and students due to cost. The CCAB is attempting to work with the university administration to develop some form of subsidy or sliding fee arrangement.

ACHIEVEMENTS RELATED TO GOALS

The Head Start/Campus Child Care aspect of the collaboration is now into year three and the specific collaboration which led to the new building and a campus location is now in year five. Space does not allow further detailed presentation of the growing number of collaborative achievements, but they are plentiful and truly the result of a working and developing partnership. In addition to those examples mentioned in the last section other achievements include ongoing observation activities, internship placements, research, joint grant-writing and fund-raising, and opportunities for professional development, as well as JFDC staff-faculty joint presentations at state and national conferences. Recently, the JFDC Director (author, Freeman) has begun to use the SFCS's Child Development Center[2] (CDC) as a resource for JFDC staff, and as a resource for seeking accreditation for the JFDC from the National Association for the Education of Young Children (NAEYC).

PROSPECTS FOR LONG-TERM STABILITY

The prospects for longer-term stability seem quite good. In general, at the program level, the partners believe that the collaboration is strong and that it continues to develop in very positive directions. Organizationally, WSOS has confidence in the partnership. A key next step is to institutionalize the partnership within the university, a step supported by the exemplary openness of WSOS personnel in the

JFDC to university faculty and student involvement. After the initial semester or two of focusing on the service aspects of the programs (i.e., getting those up and going), the mutual benefits of the collaboration have snowballed in extremely positive directions. Thus, real partnership-building activities, characterized by mutual learning, provide a strong base on which to build.

An ongoing issue exemplifying the need for institutionalizing the partnership concerns the goal of providing quality child care for the children of university faculty, students, and staff. There remains a disjunction between the university's expressed commitment to student service and the reality that students are the least likely to be able to afford to use the facility. For example, after preliminary discussions of resource options, to date there has been no visible institutional movement toward supporting a sliding fee scale or scholarships that cover (at least some portion of) child care costs. WSOS, however, does attempt to access Ohio Department of Human Services funds when possible to support these families. Although the university is not in the direct service business, some level of meaningful resource commitment seems justified on the basis of the value-added nature of the teaching, scholarship, and training that the partnership brings to the university. It is also needed to support the reasonable expectation of university staff and students that Campus Child Care will be affordable.

LEARNINGS FROM THIS PARTNERSHIP

We have again learned that there is no substitute for honest and direct communication, which includes willingness to respect differing perspectives and viewpoints. It is also clear to us that each set of stakeholders operates under the institutional imperatives of its organization. Awareness of this fact facilitates the development of a "comrade in arms" attitude that sustains mutual commitments during times of duress. In addition, full involvement (both within and between organizations) of all major stakeholders from the beginning of the potential collaboration would have facilitated matters substantially.

Although we have demonstrated that a community-university partnership can be accomplished with minimal institutionalized university administrative support, we are quite certain that this approach is not optimal. Indeed, the entire project depended to a large extent on having people in key positions proceed even though there was much future uncertainty. Of course, when a vacuum exists some things can be accomplished that otherwise might not be. Nonetheless, this collaboration demonstrates many of the systemic issues that universities (and other societal institutions for that matter) must address if they are to be believable and useful partners with community members in serving the developmental needs of children and families. It is clear that universities have an extremely important leadership role to play in developing, testing and implementing sustainable partnerships in support of individual, family, and community development.

Although there may be ample evidence to support the view that "universities" can be out of touch with community needs, WSOS learned that this is not always true. WSOS also learned (is learning) about managing and providing full day care in an environment with a different set of expectations and a different rhythm. University faculty and administration have learned (again!) that the oil tanker-like pace of change in universities is neither easy to defend, nor conducive to community-university partnerships, and have been reminded of the special demands on individuals who provide direct services for children and families. Both parties learned that the problem of attracting and retaining high quality professional staff is a problem that demands coordinated and long-term attention.

WHY IS THIS A SUCCESSFUL PARTNERSHIP?

The collaboration described in this chapter has been quite successful for a number of reasons. First, there was fundamental compatibility between the two partners in regard to their individual values about the needs of children, families, and communities, as well as in their missions regarding collaboration. Clearly, the partners did come to the table with somewhat different orientations on a number of matters such as providing a service that is self-supporting versus increasing research and training opportunities. However, essential agreement that families all need support at one time or another, and that the quality of support is of fundamental importance, provided a common basis that has kept this partnership on a successful path over time.

Second, people committed to partnership development, willing to take risks to instigate institutional change, were in key positions within each organization. As a result, cross-organization communication between individuals at corresponding levels of responsibility occurs directly and quickly. Indeed, often the within-institution communication and organizational issues were more difficult than the between-institution issues! For example, making the point in the university setting that outreach service and scholarship are supported by the collaboration, and that, therefore, faculty time put into this effort must be recognized and rewarded is a difficult issue at best.

Third, over an extended period of more than four years there has been mutual respect for the ideas, organizational demands, and the positions and responsibilities of all members involved in the collaboration. For example, as noted, there was a significant first year deficit in operating funds for the Campus Child Care. Despite this, WSOS personnel and the WSOS Board have exhibited remarkable patience (especially since WSOS is an organization, which cannot operate in the red and survive) as the university has moved to develop options for providing resource support for the Center and its programs.

Probably the essential reason that the collaboration is working is that individuals with a common vision simply refused to allow obstacles to prohibit the development of the partnership. As we have said, it is sobering to see the amount of systemic change still required in universities generally if they are to maintain and enhance their connection with and usefulness to society—particularly in collaborations with the aim of serving children, youth, and families. Yet, consistent with the theme of this book, individual institutions are responding positively. As in the present instance, as true institutional and systemic changes to enhance community-university collaboration to support children, youth, and families become more prominent and pervasive, the outcomes will be even more compelling. And, ultimately, a more useful mechanism for addressing the developmental needs of children, families, and communities in our diverse and global society will exist. The task is large, but we are optimistic about its prospects!

ENDNOTES

1. The CCAB continues to meet bi-monthly to discuss: enrollment, planning, fund-raising; WSOS board and university administration support for the collaboration; developing the link between this collaboration and university-wide priorities; development of cash and in-kind support; and other matters. There is a separate Head Start Advisory Board as required by federal law.
2. The CDC, in the SFCS, is the university "model preschool program," used as a training facility for undergraduate majors who engage in observation, practica in child development, program planning, and other learning activities there.

REFERENCES

Bridgman, A. & Phillips, D. (Eds.). (1996). *Child care for low-income families: Directions for research.* Washington, DC: National Academy Press.

Chibucos, T. R. & Kilmer, S. J. (1994). *Integrating Head Start and Campus Child Care with the Missions of the Department of Applied Human Ecology and Bowling Green State University.* Unpublished manuscript, Bowling Green State University: BG, OH.

Galinsky, E., Howes, C., Kontos, S., & Shinn, M. (1994). *The study of children in family child care and relative care: Highlights of findings.* New York: Families and Work Institute.

Lerner, R. M., & Simon, L. A. K. (1998). Directions for the American outreach university in the twenty-first century. In R. M. Lerner & L. A. K. Simon (Eds.), *University-community collaborations for the twenty-first century: Outreach scholarship for youth and families* (pp. 463-481). New York: Garland.

Weiss, H. B., & Greene, J. C. (1992). An empowerment partnership for family support and education programs and evaluations. *Family Science Review, 5*, 131-148.

43 THE GOOD NEIGHBORS PROJECT: A COLLABORATION BETWEEN A NEIGHBORHOOD SOCIAL SERVICE AGENCY, NEIGHBORHOOD RESIDENTS, AND UNIVERSITY FACULTY AND STUDENTS

Golden Jackson
Susan R. Jones
The Ohio State University

NATURE OF THE PARTNERSHIP

The Good Neighbors Project (GNP) represents an innovative and collaborative partnership between a neighborhood social service agency and faculty from the Colleges of Education, and Human Ecology at The Ohio State University. The site of the project is a neighborhood adjacent to the university and within the area targeted for investment by the University. During the early 1990s, the University initiated a planning process and pledged $28 million for neighborhood improvement. A part of the investment is commitment by OSU faculty to a holistic approach to development, engaging neighborhoods, social service agencies, faculty, staff, and students in a teaching/learning community. For faculty, the effort is coordinated by the Campus Collaborative, an interprofessional group of 42 University units providing a structure for faculty and staff to focus on human service aspects of the revitalization of University neighborhoods through community-based teaching, learning, and inquiry. The Good Neighbors Project was funded by the Campus Collaborative Seed Grant program to encourage and support the integration of teaching and learning in University neighborhoods.

PURPOSES AND GOALS

The goal of the Good Neighbors Project is to strengthen the "collective efficacy" of the neighborhood served by the social service agency. Collective efficacy, a term used by Sampson, Raudenbush, and Earls (1997), is a measure of neighborhood responsibility and ability to control certain group level processes. Sampson, et al.

(1997) asked residents of 343 Chicago neighborhoods to rank the likelihood that neighbors would intervene in situations of truancy, vandalism, or violence, their opinion of the level of common help and trust that existed in their neighborhoods, and the frequency of violence in their neighborhoods. Neighborhoods with high levels of intervention and trust were associated with collective efficacy, a condition positively correlated with residential stability and negatively associated with violence. Thus, activities that develop collective efficacy may yield results supportive of neighborhood development (increasing economic opportunity, more investment, increased home ownership).

The purpose of the Good Neighbors Project is to provide building blocks that neighbors can use to develop their own collective efficacy. Through this project, neighbors can know about the number and range of assets present in their neighborhood, the willingness and experience of neighbors to address common problems, and the common goals of residents. A "slogan" coined for the project ("Have you contributed to the GNP?") hints at the link between the social connections in a neighborhood and its economic well-being.

The primary activity of the Good Neighbors Project is the creation of a skills or capacity inventory for the neighborhood. To develop the inventory of the skills or personal assets of the neighborhood, residents from a 15 block area surrounding the social service agency were interviewed using an assets-based approach. The capacity inventory will provide information on household composition, knowledge and use of neighborhood resources, particular skills of residents, willingness to intervene or become involved in the solution of neighborhood problems, beliefs about the willingness of neighbors to become involved, beliefs about common goals, and experiences in neighborhood participation. This project draws on the Kretzmann and McKnight (1993) model of community building emphasizing neighborhood assets rather than deficits and the work of Sampson, Raudenbush, and Earls (1997) on collective efficacy. In addition, the project provides opportunity for neighborhood residents and OSU students to develop relationships and to learn from one another in the accomplishment of project goals.

Resources brought to the partnership by University faculty include teaching and supervision of students, data summary and analysis, and facilitating discussions of ways to use the data for community building. University students at the graduate and undergraduate levels as well as neighborhood residents assisted in development of the capacity inventory instrument. Teams of two students and one resident went door-to-door in the streets adjacent to the Family Center to interview residents. The social service agency provided knowledge of and introduction to neighborhood groups as well as meeting space.

The products of the partnership are an inventory of resident skills or assets, a corps of neighborhood leaders who emerge from the data collection process, a set of processes to foster neighborhood connection, increased communication between OSU students and neighborhood residents, and a photographic essay of the neighborhood. The data base information and the photographic essay on treasures, trouble spots, and potential assets of the neighborhood will be presented at an early summer celebration of neighborhood assets.

ANALYSIS OF THE PROCESS

Sampson, et al. (1997) cited trust as basic to neighborhood viability. Likewise, trust is critical to necessary community partnerships. Establishing trust was especially important in this case because neighborhoods near the University have been the sites of many studies that were perhaps not desired or seen as useful by residents. One of the unique aspects of the Good Neighbors Project—and a key to its success—is that it was initiated by the community through a social service agency rather than by the University. Thus, the project was perceived as a community project, not another study by the University.

A significant lesson from the process is the importance of establishing relationships. The time and trust required to build a relationship necessary for an effective partnership cannot be underestimated. Although we invested time for careful and consistent planning with staff from the social service agency and neighborhood residents, we realized that more one-on-one contact is required to generate and maintain the interest and support of neighborhood residents. A recommendation for others seeking to establish partnerships is to meet individually with each neighborhood organization to discuss the goals of the project and the benefits to the neighborhood and the organization.

Because neighborhood support was less than anticipated, fewer resident-student teams were available for interviewing. We decided to maintain the "partnered" groups rather than assign all-student teams because we wanted to maintain the integrity of our stated commitment to relationship building and understanding of multiple perspectives.

Reflection on the project also focused on the importance of preparation of student participants for the success of the project. We planned and facilitated an orientation and training session for all participants in the Good Neighbors Project which introduced them to the project goals, the neighborhood, the social service agency, and to each other. Topics such as cross-cultural understanding and communication as well as social class need to be included in projects of this nature.

ACHIEVEMENTS RELATED TO GOALS

The Good Neighbors Project has made significant progress toward our goals of facilitating a university/community partnership, developing a capacity and skills inventory for the neighborhood, and planting the seeds for the development of collective efficacy in the neighborhood. Highlights of achievements include:

- Significant time was taken to build relationships with the social service agency. Faculty, students, social service agency staff, and neighborhood residents assisted in development of the instrument for the skills inventory.
- A training session for conducting interviews was held for all participants. Interviews using the inventory instrument were conducted by teams of OSU students and neighborhood residents.
- A photographic essay of the assets, hidden treasures, and areas for improvement in the neighborhood was compiled.

- A celebration of skills and resources in the neighborhood is planned. Part of the celebration includes inviting feedback from neighborhood residents about our findings, the future of the Good Neighbors Project, and future steps.

The Good Neighbors Project has successfully engaged neighborhood residents, staff from the social service agency, OSU faculty, and students (both graduate and undergraduate) in the planning and implementation of the project in a way which models the development of authentic university-community partnerships.

PROSPECTS FOR LONG-TERM SUSTAINABILITY

The Good Neighbors Project has the potential for long term sustainability and capacity building within the neighborhood. The possibility of continued participation in neighborhood projects is enhanced due to the inclusion of service-learning as a central element in three courses associated with the project. One of the present authors (Golden Jackson) teaches a housing course that is part of a specialty area for undergraduate students interested in careers with non-profit organizations. Students learn about the role of housing in effecting family well-being, the range of housing problems faced by families, the solutions embedded in public policy, and problem solving strategies employed by families. The other author (Susan Jones) teaches an undergraduate course on leadership with a service component and graduate courses on service-learning in higher education. Both courses actively engage students in community settings in which they learn about community issues, interact with individuals different from themselves, and develop skills in leadership and citizenship. Thus, the likelihood of continued student assistance with activities such as maintaining and updating the inventory is strong.

LEARNINGS FROM THIS PARTNERSHIP

Engagement in this project has confirmed our knowledge about community partnerships and provided new lessons:

1) Developing partnerships with community groups and working collaboratively requires heavy investment in time to learn each other's value systems, culture, and language. For example, faculty goals focus on design of a "researchable" problem, but community groups seek practical problem solving strategies. Residents may perceive data gathering as interfering with their focus. Residents may view faculty attempts to thoroughly understand a problem as "all talk and no action." In addition, community members may see the University as resource rich, i.e., not needing the grant money associated with the project.
2) Neighborhoods may appear homogeneous, with shared goals and values, to the outside observer. Experience with the Good Neighbors Project neighborhood revealed a number of individual associations and organizations, each with their own leader and agenda. Successful partnerships must expect and build on heterogeneity.

3) The existence of a single social service agency in a relatively small neighborhood provided an interesting dynamic. Resident organizations were very firm in their desire to maintain control of activities in their neighborhood.
4) A lesson learned in the initial months of this project is the importance of a project advisory committee with broad neighborhood representation. Since we, as faculty, were invited into the neighborhood, we yielded to the suggestion to obtain input informally from one organization and from the agency board (many of whom are not neighborhood residents). We now realize the need for a formal and ongoing committee.
5) Students bring to service-learning opportunities their previous experiences, stereotypes, and biases. It is important to address these in advance of, and throughout, the project as many students will come into contact with people and/or neighborhoods different from their own and may be quick to make premature judgments. Students may also express initial reluctance and fear about projects which take them out of more traditional and familiar educational environments. Similarly, neighborhood residents have their own notions and biases about college students. Acknowledging the existence of these preconceived assumptions and dealing with them directly is an important part of the process.

WHY WAS THIS A SUCCESSFUL PARTNERSHIP?

Basic indicators of success of The Good Neighbors Project include completion of planned activities as well as continued participation and commitment by residents. In addition, the partners of the project remained positive about the process and outcomes. The staff of the social service agency were very pleased with the amount of information generated. The staff also observed growth and change in the attitudes of students. Stereotypes about low-income people changed as students participated in interviews with residents. As students engaged in conversations with neighbors, the tensions about completing assignments lessened and the commitment to the project increased.

The following four points are offered as explanation for the success:

1) The project was a community-driven rather than a university-proposed idea. Residents had expressed the need for information about neighborhood assets to the advisory board of the social service agency. This need was then communicated to the Campus Collaborative. The idea fit well with the interest of the authors (Golden Jackson and Susan Jones) in developing a service-learning component in their courses.
2) Broad-based participation continued throughout the project. Neighborhood residents proposed the idea and contributed to initial development. After hearing the idea, the authors wrote a draft proposal for discussion with the social service agency and residents. All participants contributed to development of the questionnaire, interviewing, planning for the celebration, and making recommendations for next steps.
3) The project included orientation and training for all participants. OSU students, social service agency staff, and neighborhood residents participated in a training session. The training included a get-acquainted exercise, exploration

of the neighborhood, reports of assets observed in the neighborhood, discussion of first impressions held by residents and students, review of the instrument, and practice in interviewing. The session provided a setting for open discussion of biases, expectations, hopes, and fears.

4) The project existed within an academic course so that preparation, monitoring, and evaluation continued throughout all parts of the project. Class time was devoted to interview practice, student reflection, and problem solving. Instructors were able to closely monitor student progress and success during weekly class meetings. Assessment of student learning was provided through written assignments and class discussion.

REFERENCES

Kretzmann, J. P., & McKnight, J. L. (1993). *Building communities from the inside out: A path toward finding and mobilizing a community's assets.* Chicago: ACTA Publications.

Sampson, R. J., Raudenbush, S. W., & Earls, F. (1997). Neighborhoods and violent crime: A multilevel study of collective efficacy. *Science, 277*, 918-924.

44 RURAL STUDENT HEALTH CENTERS: A COMMUNITY-UNIVERSITY PARTNERSHIP

Edward A. Smith
The Pennsylvania State University

Daniel Bibeau
The University of North Carolina at Greensboro

Catherine R. DeMason
Rockingham County Student Health Centers

Sylvia Grogan
Morehead Memorial Hospital

NATURE OF PARTNERSHIP

The lack of adequate health care for adolescents in the United States has been well documented. In rural areas the problem is exacerbated by lack of public transportation and an inadequate supply of physicians (Duncan, 1992). Such was the case in Rockingham County, North Carolina, in the spring of 1993. In order for adolescents to receive confidential health care, adolescents had to travel to the county public health department, a distance of ten to fifteen miles from each of the county's four high schools. This chapter will describe the manner in which Rockingham County addressed this problem and how, with the assistance of university faculty, the County was able to overcome some of the obstacles encountered along the way.

In 1993 five people associated with the local hospital, Morehead Memorial, met to discuss the health needs of adolescents. The original group consisted of two physicians, the director of marketing, the community health educator, and the occupational health director. After exploring a variety of issues, the group came to the conclusion that the best way to meet the health care needs of the county's adolescents was to form student health centers located directly in the schools.

A strategic planning session was held to which key community leaders and county officials were invited. In addition to the individuals noted above, other participants included the county directors of mental health, public health, and social services, a cooperative extension agent, the hospital's attorney, and the superintendent of the newly-formed consolidated school district. There was unanimous support to develop the clinics, with the recommendation that all four high schools in the county be included. Recognizing that many students would be unable to pay for services, it was decided that all services should be free. At this point, funding mechanisms were explored, and the decision was made to apply for a grant, with the hospital in the lead role. One of the physicians and the director of marketing met with an official from the Duke Endowment and were encouraged to submit an application for the development of the centers.

Both to assist in securing funding, and to enable the centers to provide better services to the youth, it was decided to engage a professor (Smith) from a local university to assist in the planning process. Dr. Smith was contacted and asked to join in both the writing of the grant and the development of a strategic evaluation plan, including a needs assessment.

A series of meetings was organized to ensure that invested parties were involved in the design of the needs assessment as well as the evaluation procedures. In addition to the stakeholders mentioned above, school principals, student representatives, and school nurses participated. By purposely seeking input from these various constituencies, the effort was made to ensure that all relevant groups bought into the evaluation. Due to cost constraints and the desire to increase the validity of the students' responses, it was decided that the evaluation would consist of a series of annual anonymous surveys, using machine-readable answer sheets, administered to all students at the end of each academic year. It was planned that the first survey would be administered in the year prior to the start of the health centers.

A number of evaluation strategies were proposed by the university faculty. The most scientifically defensible design proposed was quasi-experimental, with two schools having a delayed start-up of the health centers. This design was comparable to that used to evaluate school-linked clinics in Baltimore (Zabin, Hirsch, Smith, Street & Hardy, 1986). School system personnel, however, were concerned that within the newly consolidated school system, unequal treatment would not be accepted within the county.

Recognizing that the definition of success within the stakeholders' perspectives would not require a randomized trial, the evaluation design which emerged consisted of the annual surveys, with two methods of data comparison. Baseline data, collected prior to the start of the health centers, provided the basis for both a needs assessment and a cross sectional view of the health risk status of students prior to the start of the centers. Subsequent surveys could be used to indicate population changes in these indices. The other comparison data were provided by data collected in the nationwide Youth Risk Behavior Survey (YRBS) which is coordinated by the Centers for Disease Control and Prevention (CDC) (Kolbe, Kahn & Collins, 1993). By choosing health measures included on the YRBS, the annual survey could rely on the CDC data to provide benchmarks for secular trends.

After three meetings and several drafts, agreement was reached on the health indices to be included in the survey. The resulting instrument included standardized measures from the YRBS as well as measures developed specifically about the health centers' operations. School principals, having engaged in the process of developing both the strategy and the instrument, agreed to ensure that time would be allotted for administration of the surveys. Further, the principals assured the committee that the schools' teachers would be encouraged to cooperate in the endeavor and, in turn, would encourage the students' honest participation. The support and power of these high school principals in this process was deemed critical.

ANALYSIS OF THE PROCESS

Based on the experience of other communities, the planning group anticipated that some opposition to the health centers would develop. Opposition did surface when a group headed by family practitioners who were opposed to sex education and the provision of condoms to students were informed of the plan. Opposition was further expressed at a school board meeting in which some board members expressed the concern that the centers might promote sexual activity. The school board, however, approved the planning process on a vote of 7-2. The strategy was to avoid publicity until the health centers' plans were further developed; the opposite occurred when the following day's newspaper carried a story about the centers on the front page.

Undaunted by this unwanted publicity, the three months subsequent to the newspaper article were devoted to continued planning for the health centers and the seeking of funds. During this same period, local election campaigns were being held and the health centers became a major campaign issue. In an attempt to meet the political issue head-on, individuals on the centers' planning committee met separately with each of the school board candidates to explain the centers' proposed functions.

Opposition to the centers developed throughout the community. Some of the family practitioners who were opposed, cited both moral concerns regarding potential reproductive services, and financial concerns regarding a potential reduction in business to their practices. In addition, a local chapter of the Christian Coalition was formed with the purpose of opposing the health centers.

In addition to meeting with school board candidates, other strategies to develop community support were employed. Since the main opposition to the centers focused on contraceptive services, and it was anticipated that such services would comprise only about 10% of total services (Scales, 1991), the decision was made to remove contraceptive services from the array of health services to be offered directly at the school health centers. This compromise, while opposed by many on the planning committee, including the faculty, seemed to be the best way to minimize the opposition, while still being able to provide the other 90% of services. The resultant plan for medical services included the administration of medication, neurological care, respiratory care, treatment of gastrointestinal problems, eye exams, and so forth. In consultation with the county family planning services, it was agreed that students with contraceptive needs would be referred to the county public health department.

To foster further community support, a smaller hospital, located on the opposite side of the county, was invited to join in the planning process. In addition, a letter was mailed to all parents of high school students which explained the services to be offered and to give notice that all students would be required to have parental consent in order to receive any service.

At the November 1993 school board election all candidates who voiced public support for the centers were elected. With this signal, an official Student Health

Centers Advisory Board was formed. Members were strategically invited from county-wide vested groups including: County health agencies, schools, students, parents, medical professions, churches, and ministerial associations. In order to minimize future conflict and broaden participation on the Advisory Board, included among those invited were the physicians who initially opposed the centers, and members of the Christian Coalition.

Funding for the centers was granted by the Duke Endowment in December, 1993 and plans were made to open the centers in the fall of 1994. Morehead Memorial Hospital, located in the county's largest town, housed the director's office and assumed oversight responsibilities. With the baseline administration of the evaluation instrument and the needs assessment planned for April, 1994, the final evaluation instrument and procedures for its administration were refined. To ensure continued cooperation in the administration of the surveys and to confirm the group's support for the evaluation process, a four-hour meeting was held with a subset of the advisory board. The resultant instrument and procedures were presented to the full advisory board and the school superintendent for approval. Approval was granted with no changes, due in part to their involvement and consultation in the entire process.

Self-administered questionnaires, in conjunction with machine-readable answer sheets, were distributed during home room sessions. Over 95% of students present the day of administration participated in the survey. Data from the survey were analyzed at the university with attention to understanding the health needs of diverse groups from throughout the county. School, grade, and sex differences were given special attention, since these categories provided natural groupings around which specialized services could be offered. Direct comparisons to YRBS data also provided the ability to ascertain the relative risk of the county's youth in regard to specific health behaviors.

To complete the planning process, prior to the start of the centers in August 1994, the results of the initial survey were presented separately to the advisory board and interested community leaders, and to the newly hired staff of the centers. At the staff meeting the main focus was to inform the staff about the students they would be serving and their health needs. The advisory board/community leader meeting centered largely on comparing county data to national norms, pointing out areas where improvement was needed.

ACHIEVEMENTS RELATED TO GOALS

The student health centers remain in operation as of the publication date of this book. Opposition to the centers has almost completely disappeared, and students, teachers, and school administrators are satisfied with the services provided. During the initial school year of operation (1994-95), the centers experienced over 10,000 visits, serving an average of 784 students per month, reinforcing the advisory group's original perception of the need for health services. Approximately 55% of the high school students received parental permission to receive services during that year.

As an indicator of the health centers' acceptance within the community, almost 16,000 visits, often involving multiple diagnoses, were made during 1996-97, an increase of 60% from 1994-95. The most frequent use of the centers was for medication (9,000), 3,300 visits involved respiratory services, 2,400 addressed neurological problems (mostly headaches), 2,000 were for genitourinary problems, 2,000 were for musculoskeletal needs, and 1,200 were classified as gastrointestinal visits. Parental consent has also increased, climbing to 88% of the student body in 1996-97. The overwhelming growth in the demand for services resulted in the hiring of clerical assistance at each school to supplement the nurse practitioners and a rotating health educator who alternates between schools.

The university has continued to play an important role in the evaluation and monitoring of the centers' performance. While the initial survey served as a stimulus to the community regarding the students' needs for services, subsequent surveys have been used to pinpoint where additional services were needed (e.g., mental health counseling) or to stimulate new health promotion campaigns (e.g., seat belt use). Prior to the start of each school year, survey results and utilization data are discussed at staff meetings. These discussions provide the opportunity to take stock of changes, positive and negative, and to openly assess the previous year's initiatives.

LEARNINGS FROM THIS PARTNERSHIP

The university's role in the success of the student health centers has been as an important player, but not as the star. This initiative required community leaders and institutions to take lead roles and assume the responsibility for the program's development and endurance. Given the political process that unfolded community ownership and support was critical to the evolution of the centers and to their continued support. Had university faculty attempted to engage in these roles, health center opponents would have been able to apply an "outsider" label to the project and it would have been doomed.

From the beginning community leaders recognized the need to involve stakeholders in both the planning process and as advisors to the centers' operation. These stakeholders were from throughout the county and represented all potential groups to be affected by the health centers' implementation. Involvement of key people from the schools, county health departments, churches, hospitals, and social services department was deliberate and methodical. In addition, the advisory board embraced the political process and met it head on.

WHY WAS THIS A SUCCESSFUL PARTNERSHIP?

The university partnership in this endeavor has been a key part of the project's success. The university is perceived as a neutral party which brings scientific credibility to the evaluation process. Data collection, analysis, and interpretation are perceived by all stakeholders, including grantors, as independent of the system which provides the health services. In addition to the evaluation role, the faculty serve as a direct source of up-to-date knowledge and techniques regarding adolescent health promotion. In this latter role, the university faculty have provided the role of a critical listener to new ideas or strategies, and have suggested appropriate program objectives and mechanisms for achieving change.

REFERENCES

Duncan, E. (Ed.). (1992). *Rural poverty in America.* Glenville, IL; Auburn House, Greenwood Publishers.

Kolbe, L. J., Kahn, L. & Collins, J. L. (1993). Overview of the youth risk behavior surveillance system. *Public Health Reports, 108,* 2-10.

Scales, P. (1991). *A portrait of young adolescents in the 1990s: Implications for promoting healthy growth and development.* Chapel Hill, NC: Center for Early Adolescence.

Zabin, L. S., Hirsch, M., Smith, E., Street, R., & Hardy, J. (1986). Evaluation of a pregnancy prevention program for urban teenagers. *Family Planning Perspectives, 16*, 119-126.

45 MULTIPLE PARTNERS AND MULTIPLE VOICES: THE CREATION OF A STATEWIDE PRENATAL CARE COLLABORATION

Lynne Vernon-Feagans
The Pennsylvania State University

Robert P. Haigh
Department of Public Welfare

Margaret M. Petruska
Howard Heinz Endowment

There has been a growing recognition in this country and others that the major societal problems have complex and multiple causes. In order to better address these problems, large scale multifaceted and long-term prevention efforts that coordinate public and private community intellectual and monetary resources must be mobilized. This realization has led to some recent large scale prevention efforts that have benefited communities in need by the formation of partnerships between the public and private sectors.

The Carnegie Corporation of New York forged partnerships in the middle 1980s with industry, institutions of higher education, and schools to promote better science education for children (Hamburg, 1996). The Heinz Endowments in Pittsburgh, Pennsylvania have encouraged the development of new programs that are grounded in the grassroots efforts of the community and that include "opportunities for leverage" such that the foundation seeks to "amplify resources by forming partnerships with other grant makers, organizations of government and the private sector" (The Heinz Endowments, 1998). They underwrote the design of a child-care effort that would pool the resources of foundations, local and state government, and the United Way (Stehle, 1997). Up to $59 million in private funds will be raised. According to Stehle, "Child care advocates nationwide are watching to see if the collaboration works, in the hope that Pittsburgh will develop a model for the way business, philanthropy, and government can work together to insure that poor children get the education and attention they need in their preschool years" (p. 8).

As the federal government has shifted more of the responsibility of social programs to the states, state governments have been looking for partners in developing innovative programs that can serve as models for future funding priorities. In the late 1980s, the Pennsylvania Department of Public Welfare recognized the need for support for service innovation and enfranchised a senior staff person to seek public/private partnerships. Over the past eight years, these government/foundation partnerships in Pennsylvania have resulted in over $60 million in grants and a strong relationship with foundation leaders at many levels.

Institutions of higher education have not been on the forefront in these collaborations because of slowly changing priorities for rewards of faculty members who engage in outreach efforts. Recently, William Richardson as the new President of the Kellogg Foundation, issued a challenge to major research universities "to redirect our knowledge and our resources in the service of rural communities and urban neighborhoods." This challenge to universities has been taken up by the new President at Penn State University, Graham Spanier (1997), who has set a tone for outreach scholarship to be valued and rewarded. His vision stresses the importance of long-term partnerships with communities within the state of Pennsylvania that would blend the expertise of the university with the complex and changing needs of communities.

These shifts over the last 10 to 20 years and the recent interest by universities in these partnerships have not been without their growing pains. At the beginning, there were not many guidelines on how best to develop trust among partners that had not worked together. Recently, studies have analyzed the key elements of such partnerships to help others in the future by positing keys for successful collaboration. One such work (Riggan, Cavicchio, & Cook, 1992), prepared for a national conference on partnerships, listed five important aspects of collaborations between states and private foundations. They included (1) shared vision, (2) skilled leadership, (3) equality among partners, (4) diversity among collaborators, and (5) accountability. These aspects of successful collaboration are presented later in this chapter in order to analyze the present collaboration; a collaboration that involved foundations, state government, three major research universities, and eight healthcare institutions.

A PENNSYLVANIA EXAMPLE: PURPOSES AND GOALS

A Better Start is the story of a complex partnership among two state government agencies, three foundations, three universities, and eight healthcare communities. The goal of the partnership was to improve the health of pregnant low-income women, and ultimately the health of their babies, through more accessible and sensitive prenatal care programs in diverse communities around the state of Pennsylvania.

Background

In the early 1990s, there was concern about the lack of timely prenatal care among low income and minority women, because of the negative outcomes for the mothers and their babies. For many young and minority pregnant women and their babies the outlook was becoming worse. According to the National Center for Health Statistics, between 1985 and 1986 the U.S. infant mortality rate remained virtually unchanged at 10.4 deaths per 1,000 live births. However, for black infants, the mortality rate continued at a level more than twice that of whites. Among blacks the infant mortality actually increased. In addition, the percentage of babies born to women who received late or no prenatal care rose 5 percent for all races and 6 percent for blacks.

According to the National Governor's report (1990), lack of prenatal care was clearly associated with poor birth outcomes. At the beginning of the 1980's 20% of women who failed to receive prenatal care gave birth to low-birthweight babies, while only 5.9% of women starting prenatal care in the first or second month of their pregnancy gave birth to low-birthweight babies.

Pennsylvania, like many other states, was experiencing severe problems with infant mortality and low-birthweight among low-income families. In Philadelphia, 17 of 1,000 babies did not reach the age of one, and nonwhite babies died at nearly double the rate of white babies. Nationally, the incidence of low birthweight in non-white babies was nearly double the rate of white babies. Between 1984 and 1987, the number of mothers of low-birthweight babies in Philadelphia who had received no prenatal care almost tripled.

To address the problem of better prenatal care for low income women, the state of Pennsylvania established a new innovative Medicaid program called "Healthy Beginnings Plus (HBP)." This program, built on the client centered approach, emphasized: (1) Client empowerment; (2) early detection and treatment of complications; (3) care coordination; and (4) continuity of care. To ensure that the health care system was fully responsive to the client, the care coordinator was designated as having the pivotal role. However, there were problems inherent in converting from a traditional fee-for-service to a more innovative care system and a concern that HBP did not go far enough in enfranchising the women in prenatal care. Thus, a partnership program was aimed at supplementing HBP to make it as effective as possible.

The enhancement to HBP in Pennsylvania that was funded by the three foundations was called "A Better Start (ABS)." Each of the eight sites, competitively selected from among more than 43 HBP programs, was given $150,000 a year for four years to accomplish the goals of the initiative. The specific goals were to: (1) Reach and bring into the healthcare system low-income women in the first trimester of their pregnancy; (2) provide these low-income pregnant women an array of physical, mental health, and daily living services that were easily accessible and sensitive to their needs; (3) aggressively provide linkages for these women to other services such as treatment for alcohol and drug abuse; and (4) ensure that the women continued participation in prenatal care throughout their pregnancies.

ANALYSIS OF THE PROCESS

The initial history of the formation of the partnership for "A Better Start" is chronicled in Improving Public Policy: States and Grantmakers Working Together (Riggan et al., 1992) and we will summarize some of the major points in that document. The initial impetus for this program came from The Pew Charitable

Trusts based on the prior New Jersey state government experience of their then-director of Health and Human services. Pew planned to partner with state government to set up four model programs in eastern Pennsylvania where Pew was located and to use Penn State University to help monitor the implementation of the program at the four sites. At the same time, the Howard Heinz Endowments became interested in this program and agreed to fund the addition of four sites in the western part of Pennsylvania. At one site, a local foundation matched the Heinz grant. The Health Department, through the support of a senior staff administrator, committed considerable monies for the evaluation of ABS which supplemented the monies from the Heinz Endowments. Further, within the Department of Public Welfare there was a senior staff person whose functions included state level fostering of collaborations within and across a number of units. This key person facilitated relationships among the partners and helped to coordinate a multitude of state-wide services for these pregnant women.

Differing expectations, culture, and experience among the partners resulted in a number of initial communication problems about the roles and responsibilities of each partner. The Pew program officer who spawned ABS departed before it became operational. As a result, a senior program officer at the Heinz Endowments took the lead in the partnership. The stable and strong leadership ability at Heinz was critical in the management of the project. The University of Pittsburgh was chosen to manage the daily functioning of all the sites because Heinz had a strong working relationship with the University of Pittsburgh. Penn State's role became one of monitoring the implementation of the programs at each of the eight sites and overseeing the budgeting at the four Pew sites.

The evaluator for ABS was chosen in consultation with the partners who had a clear vision of the goal of such an evaluation, but were unable to pose precise evaluative questions to be answered. Thus, the selection of Johns Hopkins University as evaluator was complicated because the questions and the actual products of the evaluation were not framed well for the evaluators.

ACHIEVEMENTS RELATED TO THE GOALS

The challenge for a project this large ($6.7 million) was to support the different strategies for success at each of the eight sites and also to maintain the enthusiasm and support of the program over the entire course of the project. Some sites served a wide range of inner-city poor women with a variety of ethnic and language barriers to good care. Other sites were more rural and Caucasian, with women living up to 60 miles from the nearest prenatal care site. At some sites outreach workers of the same ethnic and language background were critical to the success of the goals while at others a mobile van with key healthcare personnel on board was critical to success in very rural areas.

The success of ABS was due to the partners allowing sites to vary considerably in their approach and to be able to change strategies as new information emerged from the women themselves. Lerner and Fisher (1994) have stressed "collaboration must be sought in order to gain knowledge needed for adequate application. However, collaboration here involves the true 'experts' of life in a particular community: the people in the community!" (p. 507).

The description of two contrasting sites might be helpful before we discuss the key components of a successful partnership. One site was located in a medium-sized city that had seen a tremendous growth in the Latino population, without concomitant changes taking place in the healthcare system to provide this new population with the best care. This city had a hospital board that was very responsive to the project goals and a local foundation that was willing to add even more resources to help improve the prenatal care for the Latino women. In addition, the original "A Better Start" director at that site was able to recruit indigenous Latino women, who lived in the community, as outreach workers. Until the intervention by the partners, the hospital planned to hire the outreach workers for a number of hours per week below the benefits threshold but the partners made sure this did not happen. These women were very successful in recruiting women into care and providing the support needed at prenatal visits so that quickly they were recruiting almost all Latino women into care in the first trimester and keeping them in care. One woman commented, "I was an older mother and this was my first child. I was so scared because my English wasn't that good and I was also afraid some of my family who did not have papers could be sent back to Puerto Rico if I went to the hospital for care."

The hospital at the site began publishing their information in Spanish and classes were set up for physicians and nurses to learn the basics of Spanish and the Latino culture of childbirth. The combination of the support of the hospital administration, with the support of a local foundation, and a strong director made this site extremely successful.

On the other hand, there was another site with some strengths but the program fell apart over the 4+ years of ABS. In this small city there were few external resources except for the hospital itself and many pregnant women with multiple health problems. ABS initially hired a male van driver who would transport the women to and from their appointments. This man was well respected as a minister and also a former resident of these poor communities. He turned out to be a key player in the initial success of this site but he moved on to become a state legislator for the community. Unfortunately, other staff left ABS as cutbacks at the hospital necessitated the elimination of key personnel.

As the site's success diminished dramatically, Penn State University met with key extension personnel and designed a series of meetings in the community with the former van driver (now a legislator), the regional director of extension, and other key players at ABS and Pew. Although the meetings seemed hopeful, without the clear support of a strong community institution, this site disappeared before the end of ABS, having to give back money in the last year of the project. One of the former directors of this site commented, "There just isn't any infrastructure in our community that can take leadership in all this. All our human services efforts seem to fail here and people are moving out of the city."

PROSPECTS FOR LONG-TERM SUSTAINABILITY

The initial expectation for "A Better Start" was that it would generate a groundswell of state support for women-focused enhancements to prenatal care throughout the state Medicaid program. In the course of the project, the Medicaid emphasis shifted from fee-for-service to managed care. The high visibility of A Better Start and the vigor of many of the eight sites gave the program sustainability across state gubernatorial administrations. Senior and mid-level staff in the Pennsylvania Department of Public Welfare were able to get the involvement of the new Secretary of Public Welfare in 1995 and to assure that the lessons learned permeated policy thinking about maternal and child health programs. A direct result was the involvement of national MCH experts in the development of the Philadelphia area managed care call for proposals. The RFP reflected ABS's commitment to women friendly prenatal care.

SEVEN STEPS TO A SUCCESSFUL PARTNERSHIP

So what have we learned about this complex partnership? We will try to answer this question by using the five aspects of successful collaborations mentioned earlier in this chapter (Riggan et al., 1992) and adding several other aspects that we believe are also important. We will try to combine these into what we can call "seven steps to a successful partnership."

1) Shared Vision

Shared vision was absolutely key to the successful implementation of the project at the eight sites. An initial delay in choosing the sites forced extended talk on priorities. This initial close contact and meetings over the first year were influential in achieving shared purpose. Since the evaluation team was selected late in the initial formative year they were not as involved in the development of the vision over the first year and, with lack of clarity in evaluation outcomes from partners, produced an evaluation document that contained excellent data, but not the tools to clearly change policy at the state level. In retrospect, a shared vision that resulted in a clear "theory" of change in prenatal care might have enhanced the communication between the other partners and the evaluation team.

2) Skilled Leadership

"A Better Start" was fortunate in having strong leadership at the state level and at the Howard Heinz Endowments. The leadership turnover at The Pew Charitable Trusts made for more uneven influence of The Trusts, even though some of the players had major impact at various times during the project. By design, the participation of Penn State University faculty was consultative, although they did participate fully in the monitoring of the implementation of the ABS program at each site.

Leadership was an issue at the sites and this made a difference in the success at the sites. Initially, all the sites had strong leaders, but as some of them left the sites, it was clear that the programs suffered. The overall ABS director at the University of Pittsburgh provided strong support for the sites and made sure they understood her commitment to them. She would make trips for any ABS crisis that arose for staff and/or clients. In addition, she set up regular regional and state meetings for key ABS staff and the partners to discuss critical issues and to help with training.

3) Equality Among Partners

The equality among partners varied over time and was difficult to maintain when key people left. The partners did an excellent job of empowering the sites and making each feel that their input was valuable. The periodic site visits and biennial meetings helped to validate the important programs at each of the sites. This contact also helped the overall project coordinator make changes in training and resources based on site directors' input.

4) Diversity and Power Among Collaborators

Strength can come from diversity but the number of players in this collaboration were many and it took effort to understand each perspective. The key element in success with diversity is the realization that each player contributes in a different way and not all players can play equal roles across elements or across time. With so many players actively involved, there had to be some hierarchy of the importance of the diversity, especially after the initial decisions had been made. It was critically important as the implementation of strategies was taking place at the eight sites that the foundation and state partners played a lesser minor in leadership. The foundations and the major state players allowed the empowerment of the overall ABS director and the individual staff at the sites during the implementation that worked extraordinarily well.

5) Accountability and Impact

Although the major partners agreed somewhat on the kind of data to be collected, this was not clearly articulated in the evaluation. The partners had wanted process data that would document who was receiving services and the kind of services being received. These data were not being systematically collected by the evaluation. In order to supplement the evaluation to gather these data, a computer monitoring program was designed to track the characteristics of the women being served at each site and the services they were receiving. Unfortunately, the firm hired for this was in Philadelphia and the program office was at the University of Pittsburgh. Although extraordinary effort was given to this initiative in the middle of the project, the monitoring piece failed to be completed successfully. Although ABS had a large effect on state practices, the evaluation itself failed to provide the kind of policy implications that had been hoped for.

6) Adaptability and Flexibility

It was difficult to predict system change at the outset of a multi-year project, particularly since other dynamics were evolving. Thus, it was important to make mid-course corrections and changes that were inevitably part of a large collaborative project. For instance, at the outset of this project it was expected that ABS would lead to enhanced Medicaid fees for creative prenatal interventions, not realizing that Medicaid would embrace managed care as the only approach. Thus, this portion of the project became somewhat less important. Still, ABS did create a climate in Pennsylvania State Government that valued woman-focused prenatal care resulting in a significantly stronger component to the managed care state requests for services. Also at the outset, Pew strongly proposed that the 23 separate Medicaid fees for Healthy Beginnings Plus be bundled into a global fee per trimester. The State agreed for the first time to bundle fees and was able to demonstrate the efficiency of this approach.

Over the course of the project, a number of components of the project changed and different strengths and weaknesses became more apparent. The partners allowed evolving programs that were better than the initial ones. This freedom to evolve was reflected in the adaptability of the sites to perceived needs and to crisis management that create strong and sustainable programs.

7) Established Relationships Work

Although many of the partners in "A Better Start" had not worked together before, there had been a long-term relationship among three of the partners. The Heinz Endowments, the key person at the state, and the University of Pittsburgh had forged relationships on other projects. With the many staff changes at Pew and with the changing role and relationships of the other two university partners, it was critical to have a core of three diverse partners that could keep the project going through critical periods. Further, the third foundation which is from one site, continues to have significant partnerships with DPW.

In summary, ABS was a very successful project in spite of the number of problems that arose among partners and at the diverse sites. Our reflection on the five years led us to our Seven Steps to Success. Hopefully, these steps may help other potential community/university partnerships.

REFERENCES

Hamburg, D. A. (1996). *A perspective on Carnegie Corporation's program 1983-1997: President's essay*. New York: Carnegie Corporation.

The Heinz Endowments. (1998). *Goals and strategies: Health and human services*. Pittsburgh: The Heinz Endowments.

Lerner, R. M., & Fisher, C. B. (1994). From applied developmental psychology to applied developmental science: Community coalitions and collaborative careers. In R. M. Lerner & C. B. Fisher (Eds.), *Applied developmental psychology* (pp. 505-522). New York: McGraw-Hill.

Richardson, W. C. (1996). *A new calling for higher education*. University Park, PA: The Pennsylvania State University.

Riggan, J., Cavicchio, C., & Cook, L. (1992). *Improving public policy: States and grantmakers working together*. Washington, DC: Council of Governors' Policy Advisors.

Spanier, G. B. (1997). *Enhancing the quality of life for children, youth and families*. University Park, PA: The Pennsylvania State University.

Stehle, V. (1997, August). For Pittsburgh's children. *The Chronicle of Philanthropy*, pp. 8-11.

46 THE HEALTHY NEIGHBORHOOD PROJECT

Nancy J. Bell
Elizabeth G. Haley
Ginny Felstehausen
Charlie Adams
Texas Tech University

NATURE OF PARTNERSHIP

The Healthy Neighborhood project is a collaborative effort involving community residents and school personnel in the target community, the College of Human Sciences at Texas Tech University, a city-wide Neighborhood Association, St. Mary Hospital, the United Way, the Texas Tech Health Sciences Center, and from time to time, other community organizations. The project was inspired and initiated during 1994 by a steering committee composed of the Dean of the College of Human Sciences, the Vice President and Major Gifts Director of United Way, the Assistant Superintendent of the local school district, two representatives of the city's United Neighborhood Association, and a Vice President of St. Mary Hospital. Later joining this original group were representatives from the Texas Tech Health Sciences Center, School of Nursing, and from the Texas Agricultural Extension Service.

PURPOSES AND GOALS

The project integrates outreach to a local community with graduate and undergraduate instruction and research. Guided by developmental and ecological principles (e.g., Lerner, 1995; Perkins, Ferrari, Covey, & Keith, 1996), its overriding philosophy is one of partnerships and collaboration; its outreach goals are to draw together scholars, practitioners, community agencies, and community residents to derive strategies and engage a broad base of the community in united efforts to assist children and families. Its specific community-level objectives are based upon community action tools for building healthy communities and healthy youth (Search Institute, 1998). Its university-level educational goals are to involve students in community collaborations during their undergraduate and graduate education. It was anticipated that students would both learn from and contribute to the collaboration, gaining an appreciation of the importance of university-community partnerships as they assisted with resource development, research, and specific projects. Finally, the project's research goals are to provide ongoing needs assessment and evaluation data to be used for future planning, modifying existing programs, and securing funding for community initiatives.

THE PROCESS

The steering committee described above first helped to establish a Neighborhood Association in the target neighborhood, a neighborhood characterized by low-income families and a high crime rate. They then served in an advisory capacity to a Human Sciences doctoral level course which enrolls students from all majors within the college—Human Development and Family Studies; Marriage and Family Therapy; Food and Nutrition; Family and Consumer Sciences Education; Consumer Economics and Environmental Design; and Clothing, Textiles, and Merchandising. Students in this course initially discussed social, environmental, and economic issues which impact individuals and families at national, state, and local levels. They then conducted discussion groups at a meeting of the Neighborhood Association in the target community. From this dialogue came the need for a neighborhood assessment and also the specific topics to be covered in a questionnaire designed to document neighborhood strengths and problems.

Representatives of the Agricultural Extension Service prepared students to train neighborhood volunteers to conduct the survey. A random sample of neighborhood households was identified, and volunteers from within the neighborhood conducted the survey with these residents. Additional responses were obtained through the neighborhood elementary school and senior citizens program. Recommendations derived from the survey included a need for increased community awareness and understanding about community problems, partnerships to support the public schools, prevention programs within the public schools and within the community, job training opportunities, better publicity of community center activities, and street and alley clean-up, repair, and lighting.

Each doctoral student also selected a neighborhood issue for in-depth study and prepared a final report and executive summary. Neighborhood issues selected for in-depth study included community leaders' perceptions of the target neighborhood, factors associated with participation in neighborhood associations, strategies for implementing change by neighborhood associations, youth violence and gang activity, teen pregnancy, child care, access to health care, reforming education, high school dropouts, and adult literacy.

ACHIEVEMENTS RELATED TO GOALS

Community Assistance Goals

Growing out of discussions with the neighborhood was the need to develop projects for visible, short-term results in addition to those expected to have a longer-term impact in the neighborhood. Consequently, graduate students from Human Sciences worked with the neighborhood and with local businesses to organize and hold an alley clean-up day followed by a cookout at the community center. They assisted in the development of a neighborhood newsletter and with a garage sale to raise funds for the community organization. In subsequent years, students have worked with community members to conduct a safety fiesta, a health fair, and to plan a community garden plot. They have assisted parents, students, and teachers on a reading night at the elementary school to promote family reading activities. They have taught computer classes for neighborhood families. They have helped in accessing community development funds through the city, in compiling a list of resources for community residents, and in conducting a follow-up needs assessment survey. Undergraduate Human Sciences students also have contributed to this effort, volunteering in a HOSTS (Helping One Student to Succeed) program and other activities within the elementary school. Students and faculty in the Texas Tech Health Sciences School of Nursing have sponsored health fairs and have provided other health-related assistance at the school. Safety and health fairs also have been sponsored by the city, in cooperation with the Texas Agricultural Extension Service.

Community contributions to this joint effort have been substantial. St. Mary Hospital, in collaboration with the elementary school, Boys & Girls Club, and the Community Center, developed an after-school sports program for area youth. The hospital also has employed a Coordinator for Healthy Community Initiatives, purchased playground equipment, funded the establishment of a Family Center and a "Project Fit America" program at the elementary school, and provided to the school consultative services of a health educator and psychologist. Other sources of support include local foundation funding for community and university representatives to attend a national conference on Healthy Communities, and city Community Development Block Grant funds for repairs and improvements.

Student Goals

Since the project's initiation in 1994, doctoral students have been involved in community initiatives. Course work, involving reading, literature reviews, and presentations from community leaders, has given them a conceptual grounding for community partnerships. Through hands-on participation in the community collaboration, they have seen how concepts are translated into action. Based upon their evaluations of the experience, many are enthusiastic about the potential of collaborative community action, e.g., "It's a great initiative because it involves all aspects of the community—the village approach, " and, "...our youth are one of our most important resources and the initiative can help them to actualize their potential." In response to a question about the need for continuing the project, one student wrote, "Our profession is involved in helping to better the lives of families, individuals, and communities. It is impossible to do that well without collaborating. While we are students we need to get involved in people's lives. The university also needs to be involved in outreach. I also think it gives graduate students from the various departments an opportunity to collaborate with each other."

Research Goals

In the fall of 1996, a follow-up to the initial 1994 needs assessment survey was conducted. The College of Human Sciences provided funds for questionnaires to be mailed to every address in the target neighborhood. Between 30% and 52% of respondents reported improvements in some areas targeted by the project: cleaning up of graffiti, home improvements, recreational activities for children and youth, and involvement in the community center. The majority of those reporting changes associated the changes with the activities of the Neighborhood Association.

PROSPECTS FOR LONG-TERM SUSTAINABILITY

Prospects for sustainability of the project are positive due to the commitment and continuing involvement of representatives of the initial core group—the community, St. Mary Hospital, the university, and the United Neighborhood Association. The long-term vision that has come from this partnership is of a community that is stable, safe, aesthetically pleasing, and conducive to healthier lifestyles, with more home ownership, better education, and an effective leadership base.

LEARNINGS FROM THIS PARTNERSHIP

University-community partnerships of this sort inevitably present a number of challenges. In the Healthy Neighborhoods Project, major challenges have been (a) building relationships within the community and insuring that initiatives grew from needs as perceived by neighborhood residents; (b) appropriately utilizing the different skills of all participants in the collaboration; (c) communication and organizational issues; and (d) maintaining continuity over time, since different groups of university students are involved with the project each year.

Meeting these challenges is an ongoing process, but over time participants have developed effective strategies for avoiding or resolving problems in these areas. First, community residents were, from the beginning, a major voice in project planning and implementation. The establishment and maintenance of relationships between community residents and Texas Tech students and faculty have been facilitated by the active support of several leaders of the city-wide United Neighborhood Association which promotes and nurtures neighborhood organizational and self-help activities. Further, several of the doctoral students as well as the course instructor have spent many extra hours in nurturing these relationships.

Appropriate skill utilization has been addressed in several ways. Within the community, a variety of different projects—alley clean up; garden planning; community center activities; fund raising; community surveys; newsletter writing, production, and dissemination—involve a range of people with different skills. Community leaders within the neighborhood association are instrumental in recruiting those with special skills for these projects. Graduate students, because they are enrolled in different programs throughout the college, also represent a range of interests and skills. For example, some can offer expertise in health and nutritional programs, others in the development of parenting programs and prevention, and still others in mapping the neighborhood home owners, renters, and business locations.

Project participants continue to work toward improvement in the areas of communication, organization, and continuity over time. At Texas Tech, the person primarily responsible for maintaining ongoing contact is the instructor of the graduate course in which students enroll for the community experience. As additional faculty and students become involved in program development and research in this neighborhood, a coordinating committee involving others within the College may be needed. Also, the city-wide United Neighborhood Association has been helpful in serving as a liaison to maintain contact between project periods, as has the principal of the neighborhood elementary school, the Outreach Coordinator at St. Mary Hospital, and the Dean of the College of Human Sciences.

WHY WAS THIS A SUCCESSFUL PARTNERSHIP?

The project has been successful because of the commitment and dedication of key individuals within the neighborhood, the community at large, and the university. It has benefited both the neighborhood and graduate education within the College in a number of ways, many of which are listed above. These accomplishments have been recognized by an award from the National Urban Neighborhood Association to the Dean of the College of Human Sciences and a 1998 Lubbock Independent School District "Adopt-A-School" award for four years of collaboration. Perhaps the most important accomplishment, in the long term, is the realization on the part of all participants that these kinds cooperative efforts can make a difference in a community, even with very limited funds.

REFERENCES

Healthy communities healthy youth tool kit. (1998). Minneapolis, MN: Search Institute.

Lerner, R. M. (1995). *America's youth in crisis. Challenges and options for programs and policies.* Thousand Oaks, CA: Sage.

Perkins, D. F., Ferrari, T. M., Covey, M. A., & Keith, J. G. (1996). Getting dinosaurs to dance: Community collaborations as applications of ecological theory. In C. B. Simerly, H. Light, & D. I. Mitstifer (Eds.), *A book of readings: The context for professionals in human, family, and consumer sciences* (pp. 31-39). Alexandria, VA: American Association of Family and Consumer Sciences.

47 SEIZING THE OPPORTUNITY TO FULFILL A MISSION

Gladys J. Hildreth
Joyce Armstrong
Texas Woman's University

"Outreach," "collaboration," and "partnership" are key terms embedded deeply into the mission statement of Texas Woman's University and are in keeping with the renewed emphasis of American higher education to engage in partnerships and collaborations. As universities and colleges aim for excellence across their mission and determine the best way to meet the needs of society in the twenty-first century, university faculty will be expected to articulate and assess their outreach agendas (Outreach Program at Michigan State University, 1996). When a request for assistance came from a local elementary school to the College of Education and Human Ecology, the response was overwhelming and encouraging. The invitation was viewed as an opportunity for administrators, faculty, and staff to engage in outreach activities that would enhance the mission of the university and at the same time assist the elementary school in achieving its goals of educating families and children.

The request was channeled through the office of the dean and disseminated to appropriate faculty in the college. Within weeks, initiatives, faculty resources, and directions had been identified to begin the process of forming a partnership with the local elementary school which has the potential for many positive results. The discussion that follows briefly describes the nature, need, purpose, key players, expected outcomes, and other aspects of the new partnership.

PURPOSES AND GOALS

According to the information received, the local elementary school had experienced various problems in the last few years. Some of the challenges which needed to be addressed included a lack of parental involvement and concern for student academic interest and accomplishments. The school is located in a neighborhood that is known to be one of the poorest in the city, with high unemployment rates. Ninety percent of the students are designated at risk. The school's ethnic population is 96% Hispanic, 1% Black, and 3% Caucasian, with a total population of 840 in the 1991 year. Historically student test scores have been low. The average yearly income per household is below the poverty level. Many parents hold multiple jobs which result in very little extra time to become involved in their children's education. A substantial percentage of parents are illiterate in their native language.

Since 1995, the faculty of the elementary school has engaged in efforts to involve the community in planning and implementing school programs that would meet the educational, physical, and social development needs of the student population. After-school programs and academic enrichment and extracurricular activities are supported through various community groups. However, the school staff recognizes and places much confidence in parents and their roles as partners in their children's education. "Education is too important to leave up to our schools. Ideally, parents, guardians and other family members are children's first and most important teachers-at home, in the community, and as partners with the school" (Louv, 1997a).

The stated need of the elementary school included in the request for assistance from the university was to form a partnership to achieve the following objectives: 1) To provide education and training to parents that would further the goal of making every parent feel welcomed, wanted, and comfortable. In return the parent(s) would be able to assist their children in achieving self-confidence, physical and social maturity, and in becoming academically successful; and 2) to provide, and assist with, academic programs through tutoring and other support services.

Shelby J. Maier (1996), a family life educator with the University of Wisconsin-Extension, believes that traditional planning for a model community program begins with focusing on community needs, deficiencies, and problems. This approach often results in a nearly endless list of problems and needs and leads directly to a fragmentation of efforts to provide solutions. Maier suggests that an alternative pathway is to begin with a commitment to discovering a community's capabilities and assets. Members of this newly formed partnership will focus on helping the school community identify its own local assets to address community needs.

ANALYSIS OF THE PROCESS

This first step in developing a collaborative plan was a discussion among the stakeholders. Such discussion should focus on outreach as scholarship, its relationship to the mission of the university and its benefits for each partner (Outreach Program at Michigan State University, 1996).

To facilitate the beginning of a working relationship between the university and the elementary school, an invitation was issued to interested potential participants. The initial process involved a university professor who had a deep interest in university/community relations, and an elementary school staff member. Through a series of telephone calls, e-mail, and office visits, the two professionals organized the first round table discussion. The group consisted of the dean of the college, five university professors, two graduate students, the elementary school principal, the after-school coordinator, two elementary school teachers, the school technical assistant, a major airline representative, a volunteer, and two parents. The 17-member group was identified as being composed of key people who would have the responsibilities of ensuring the success of the partnership. Involving volunteers and parents creates an organizational structure for parental involvement. The absence of parents at the planning stage may cause parents to feel at a loss about how they can help, and teachers can sometimes feel burdened by parents whose skills may not match the classroom's needs (Louv, 1997b). The round table discussion provided an opportunity for the elementary school administrator and teachers to describe their needs and to listen to the university personnel indicate how their teaching, research, and service programs could assist in meeting the needs of the elementary school. Each participant at the meeting was committed to a particular aspect or task necessary for an effective partnership. These roles and responsibilities are briefly described below.

The University

a. *The Dean of the College* provided the leadership by inviting interested faculty to participate in the partnership. A presentation made by the dean included a discussion of available opportunities and possibilities within the college which would promote scholarship for faculty and students and at the same time meet the needs of the elementary school. The dean created an environment that assured the group that the college was committed and interested in establishing an effective partnership.

b. *Faculty from the Department of Family Sciences* with expertise in family and parent education agreed to develop strategies and implement procedures for addressing parent education and involvement. This process would involve although not be limited to: 1) Conducting parenting workshops; 2) providing resources and a referral network through which the school can seek assistance from other agencies such as cooperative extension, the Parenting Center, the Family Place, and other organizations that offer education on parenting and involvement; and 3) encouraging or requiring students enrolled in undergraduate and graduate parenting classes at the university to develop new strategies and conduct research on parent involvement.

c. *Faculty from the Department of Reading and Bilingual Education.* Eighteen students in the College of Education and Human Ecology have applied to conduct their field experience at the local elementary school. According to the coordinator of field experience, students are required to complete 12 credits of professional education for elementary certification to become teachers. During these 12 credit hours, the students must fulfill 90 hours of field experience within an elementary school setting. Two students are already placed in classrooms helping teachers. At the request of the school, their primary focus will be on reading and language arts. Most of the students will have completed six hours of course work related to teaching reading and involving one-to-one tutoring and in-class small group reading instruction. It is expected that the field experience of the University student will play a fundamental role in assisting elementary school students to raise their test scores in reading.

d. *Librarians from the University Library.* Two librarians in the University library have participated in the Literacy Week program by reading to six Second and Third Grade classes. They will continue to offer story-time opportunities and consultation about library enrichment programs. Six award-winning children's books were presented to the Library during Literacy Week.

e. *Staff from the Elementary School* will be responsible for much of the implementation and day-to-day activities of the partnership. They will collaborate with the university staff in: 1) Arranging seminars; 2) coordinating and supervising the experiences of students who are enrolled in the early field experience classes and have field placements in the school; and 3) consulting with university faculty for assistance in securing resources through writing grants and networking with other family service agencies.

f. *Airline Representative.* A major airline has adopted the elementary school as a partner and expects to continue active involvement with the new partnership. In the past the airline has: 1) Provided transportation to students to visit NASA facilities and to state-level competitions; 2) provided outer wear and school uniforms for students in need; 3) provided school supplies; and 4) assisted with tutors and mentors. The airline will provide additional assistance by providing transportation to university students who assist as tutors and mentors. A major clothing manufacturer is also contributing to the partnership by adopting families for holiday celebration and donating fabric for parental skills workshops.

g. *Volunteers.* The school's volunteer program lags behind those of many schools. Recent efforts have resulted in developing a volunteer program involving teachers, parents, community members, businesses, and church volunteers. Volunteers will enhance the partnership by strengthening the overall educational program at the school by generating additional resources, and by providing educational equipment and supplies. Examples of activities conducted by volunteers include teaching in the after-school program. Some of the courses taught are fine arts, chess, computer with desktop publishing, media presentation, and crocheting.

h. *Parents.* As reported by Louv (1997a) parent-school partnerships must begin developing before the child reaches school age. Parents will play a leading role in the success of the partnership. They will be invited to attend and participate in every activity in which the partnership will be engaged. This will include volunteering in the classroom activities, helping teachers prepare materials for future lessons, going on field trips with students, working in the parenting resource center, and participating in the library programs and other after-school events. Parental participation in professional education of their children will be encouraged at all levels of the partnership.

PROSPECTS FOR LONG-TERM SUSTAINABILITY

Expected Outcomes

Measurable and expected outcomes are already being realized. Members of the newly formed partnership are planning and collaborating in activities that will accomplish the mission of the university and elementary school. Specific activities currently underway include:

- Students who are enrolled in early field experience classes at the university have been assigned to the elementary school. The teacher education program provides an opportunity for students to become mentors and role models to school children, to serve as tutors, and to assist with school work. In addition, the college students develop a new awareness of the issues and situations facing many school educators.

- Two parent workshops are planned and will be held in late afternoon to accommodate working parents. The workshops will focus on recommendations for parent involvement in assisting their children with reading, social skills, study habits, test taking skills, and in learning ways in which they can help out at school. The workshop will be conducted by university faculty with opportunities for parents to participate.
- Expectations for future activities include identifying opportunities that will encourage university faculty to use their teaching, research, and service areas to match the needs of the elementary school. According to the Michigan State University Outreach Program (1997), much can be gained through faculty members acting as broad-service partners. "A faculty member participating in a broad service partnership can expect to be matched with a community initiative in an administratively cohesive way designed to result in scholarly work that will have benefits for all involved. In pursuing outreach scholarship as a part of a broad-service partnership, faculty members realize the value added benefit provided by the partnership team" (p. 9).
- A state agency is seeking small grant applications to fund innovative school programs. University staff and elementary school staff members are in the process of preparing a grant which would provide a learning and resource center for parents which will be located in the elementary school. The center will provide educational resources and support to parents in the form of books, audio tapes, videos, referral information, and leadership.

The parenting resource center will be patterned after the Drake University program. A brief description of Drake University's Outreach activities in the School of Education includes: a) Teachers as partners program; b) adult literacy center; c) career opportunity program; d) students at risk conference; and e) a resource center and other school and community partnership efforts (Drake University, 1997). As pointed out by the Michigan State University Outreach Project (1997), the amount and consistency of available resources can influence the role and importance of outreach in a unit (p. 9). The partnership will be enhanced by collaborative commitments in the form of service and materials from additional community businesses and agencies. Members of the team from the University and the elementary school will meet regularly to assess and evaluate the progress of the partnership. It is expected that these collaborative efforts will address and begin to meet the needs of the elementary school.

WHY THIS WAS A SUCCESSFUL PARTNERSHIP

Although the partnership is in its beginning stage, it can be identified as a success. As a result of the two parent workshops taught by University personnel, parents are already more involved in the school life of their children. This is evidenced by the numbers of parents who attended the workshop and made request for opportunities to volunteer in the classrooms. Parents also requested materials and books on specific topics relating to their children's development. They were interested in information about effective methods for assisting children with homework, developing good study habits, positive discipline, good nutrition, and assisting children with academic skills. The University partners and school administrators are negotiating plans to purchase an existing building which will be moved to the campus of the elementary school. The building will be used to house different aspects of the partnership such as a learning resource center for parents.

REFERENCES

Drake University School of Education, School and community partnership. (1997, September 29). [On-line] Available: http://www.educ.drake.edu/soe/general/outreach.html.

Louv, R. (1997a, September 29). *Families and learning: What we can do at home, at school, in our neighborhoods, and with new technologies* [On-line]. Available: http://www.kidscampaigns.org/hot/reunion-louvl.html. Benton Foundation.

Louv, R. (1997b, September 29). *Parents as teachers,* from "Childhood Future" (Anchor Books) [On-line]. Available: http://www.kidscampaigns.org/hot/louv-parentsteach.html. Benton Foundation.

Maier, S. (1997, September 29). *Family living program* [On-line]. Available: http://www. walworth-county.com/uwex%20Living0/220Programs.html.

Sandmann, L. (1996). *Points of distinction: A guidebook for planning and evaluating quality outreach.* Michigan State University.

48 DEVELOPING EFFECTIVE UNIVERSITY-COMMUNITY COLLABORATION THROUGH GRANTWRITING

Richard Nader
Greg Muller
Charles Johnson
Craig Blakely
Texas A&M University

Communities have problems, universities have departments.
(OECD, 1982)

INTRODUCTION

America's research universities, having become institutions of specialized knowledge creation, are now being called upon to change direction, to pull specialized knowledge out of the labs and lecture halls and translate it into know-how. As pointed out by Daniel Yankelovich, "For years, our institutions of higher education had remained exempt from these [public] criticisms" (Walshok, 1994), and leaders in higher education were unprepared to respond to what the public claimed was wasteful, self-serving and indulgent behavior on the part of research universities.

At the same time, higher education leaders in Texas have witnessed an increasing interest at the state level to identify ways in which university resources can be used to benefit the community. This resurgence is partly driven by the need for accountability to state legislatures who are, in turn, responding to the demographic shifts taking place in Texas and across the nation. But this resurgence also is reflective of a realization on the part of many in higher education that, in an age of rapid social change, the university must develop innovative ways to respond to society's needs.

Despite an appreciation by many in education for an expanded university role in providing more tangible services to the community, formidable barriers remain in place in most four-year institutions. For instance, faculty reward systems continue to focus on scholarship through publications or research grants. In the case of the land grant college, extension systems are often ill equipped to effectively respond to an expanded role in the community due to a traditional focus on agriculture. In fact, few university-community collaboratives have had the staying power to capture, over time, the knowledge and skills of the university's faculty and staff, a human resources reservoir that could potentially contribute more to community development efforts than any other institution in our culture (Boyer, 1994). Finding ways to capitalize on these resources and apply them to the community setting without detracting from traditional functions of the university has been a persistent challenge for many inside and outside higher education.

The problem facing university-community partnerships is a basic one: where does the university draw the line on its responsibility for service? It is inherently difficult for a university to define its role or measure its success in meeting the needs of a diverse statewide community, but it is even more problematic to make partnerships viable and sustainable. Clearly the university should not undertake any activity at the expense of its values, which include preserving academic freedom and maintaining high standards. But when possible, the university should actively promote programming that considers the needs of those who stand to benefit from the intellectual services that a university can perform (Bok, 1986).

In this chapter we review the features and outcomes of the Community Grant Support Initiative (CGSI). We begin by detailing the rationale and structure of the CGSI and review the institutional basis for its emergence and continued development. We then explain the processes that portray CGSI partnership activities. Finally, we review the benefits that accrue both to the university and to the community as a result of the initiative.

NATURE OF THE PARTNERSHIP

Improving quality of life is the driving force behind most community service initiatives. People staffing local community-based non-profits are responding to national and state funding opportunities spanning the spectrum from juvenile delinquency to substance abuse to unemployment. However, many barriers exist for well-intended local efforts. Impediments faced by non-profits include a lack of management skills such as budgeting, accounting, fundraising, and data information systems for improving decisions about efficiently running service programs. But, according to our experience with non-profit leaders, one of the biggest barriers impeding the success of innovative efforts at the local level is inadequate funding. Proposal development knowledge is a specific university skill that can readily be applied in the community setting.

In discussing higher education's role, James C. Votruba, President of Northern Kentucky University, states that "while universities cannot and should not be expected to solve community problems, it is legitimate to expect them to inform the problem-solving process through responsible extension and the application of their expertise" (Votruba, 1994). Building upon Ernest Boyer's idea of the scholarship of application (Boyer, 1990), connecting theory and practice is part of a vision that higher education shall play an increasingly facilitative role in helping local leaders establish programs to serve their local constituencies.

Derek Bok (1992) states in *Beyond the Ivory Tower* that universities have a clear obligation to take into account societal needs. Fulfillment of this obligation provides the underpinnings of the land-grant institution. Justin Morrill spoke of enriching the liberal education model with practical education concepts in presenting The Morrill Act of 1862. This Act institutionalized Thomas Jefferson's concept of the university as a place where every branch of knowledge useful to society is taught. Enarson (1989) described the uniqueness of the land-grant mission as responding to "people's problems." Corrigan (1997) described community building as "acting on scholarship," or "shortening the distance between thought and action."

One of the Community Grant Support Initiative's (CGSI) greatest strengths is that services provided to communities draw from the work of faculty without detracting from, or impinging upon, academic freedom or the quality of scholarship. Further, the CGSI preserves the independent missions of both the community organization and the university, and plays a significant role in bridging institutional communication barriers inherent in different organizational cultures. The Community Grant Support Initiative provides a link between the "academic" and "real" worlds.

THE COMMUNITY GRANT SUPPORT INITIATIVE

The Community Grant Support Initiative (CGSI) is a university-based center that is supported by state appropriation to provide a broad range of grantwriting services for Texas communities at no cost. The initiative is located within the Public Policy Research Institute, a multi-disciplinary academic research center at Texas A&M University. CGSI draws upon policy and evaluative research expertise from the institute and from faculty throughout the university. Proposal development staff at the Initiative provide a community-friendly interface that in turn serves as a conduit through which university resources can be focused to strengthen community applications for funding. Services target programs designed to improve the quality of life and promote safe and healthy lifestyles among children, families, and the community at large. In an effort to expand existing state resources, emphasis is placed on attracting new funds from federal and private sources.

THE COMMUNITY GRANT DEVELOPMENT PROCESS

In this section, we will discuss the three general phases in delivering the services: monitoring grants and high need areas of the state; technical assistance; and grantwriting. While these steps are chronologically representative of activities, it should be noted that each community organization has unique attributes and needs for CGSI services. Services are structured so that each community that contacts CGSI for help can receive proposal development assistance anywhere along the spectrum of need.

Monitoring and referring grant opportunities

A common request by communities involves suggesting funding mobilization strategies. Here one of the primary roles of CGSI is steering communities to potential funding sources. CGSI conducts keyword searches on a variety of funding data bases to locate appropriate sources of funds.

CGSI monitors the availability of federal and state funding opportunities through grant alert subscriptions, by forecasts of upcoming legislation affecting the availability of funds, and by tracking a variety of print and electronic resources. Concurrently, CGSI assesses high need areas of the state to effectively target available and upcoming funding to organizations operating in those areas of the state.

Technical Assistance

A second service dimension involves technical assistance. CGSI identifies and interprets data in support of proposals and provides research-based literature reviews for communities on request. To respond to this demand, CGSI developed the Texas Quality of Life Database, which holds data from disparate state and national agencies that collect variables relevant to assessing need. Responding to the needs of the community, other services include conducting key-leader or client interviews to collect qualitative data and assisting with technical and conceptual program evaluation issues.

Program evaluation is sorely needed, yet all too often remains a neglected method of assisting programs to be competitive for grant funding at the local level. The Community Grant Support Initiative utilizes the Public Policy Research Institute's Survey Research Lab, and the various policy research programs (public health, education, substance abuse, government policy innovation and technology transfer) to assist community organizations in developing client tracking and outcome-based evaluation systems.

The CGSI also assists non-profits gather new data through the development of local surveys based on national standardized instruments in order to generate complementary data specifically geared toward each program's unique attributes.

Grantwriting

By far, the most popular service is proposal writing and proposal review. Early on in the process, CGSI conducts an assessment to determine how best to efficiently and effectively meet the needs of the community organization. Community organizations are selected to receive proposal writing assistance based on the following considerations:

- Is there a high level of documented need?
- Do local needs align with the stated objectives of the funding source?
- Is there strong community commitment to the proposed project?
- Are local resources insufficient to prepare competitive grants independently?
- Is local capability sufficient to manage the grant if awarded?

During the proposal development process, each entity shares responsibility in developing the proposal to ensure that a quality grant application is achieved. Whether or not the proposal is funded, CGSI will provide a post-submission evaluation of the proposal, assessing the strengths and weaknesses of the proposal, as well as assist the non-profit with final budget negotiations or site visit preparation for community organizations that have never had such experience.

Each partner contributes in the following ways:

Role of the university

1. Interpret the funder's priorities
2. Help mobilize community support
3. Gather data and research related to the proposal
4. Write the proposal

Role of the community

1. Fully participate in project planning
2. Help gather information and mobilize support
3. Review and edit-check for accuracy and appropriateness of proposal content
4. Provide on-going feedback

University and community contact is focused and short term. But it is designed to be intensive. Mentoring takes place between the university's proposal developers and the leaders of the community non-profit organization. The partnership is geared toward being non-intrusive and is locally controlled. CGSI strives to build capacity through the development of positive, short-term working relationships between university and community representatives. Neither side is required to sustain the collaboration beyond the proposal submission period.

ANALYSIS OF THE COLLABORATIVE

Experience has shown that a great deal can be accomplished in a short period of time. Deadlines provide the urgency for action, funding priorities produce the common purpose, and the trust is built through complementary, interdependent tasks. The focused nature of the partnership, while not ruling out long-term involvement, reduces risks associated with prolonged university-community associations such as the complications that invariably arise when attempting to establish shared governance procedures and when competing over scare resources.

Could another entity, or the private sector, better perform this function? First, the expertise base of the university is broad, while the expertise of many consultants is narrow. It is thus unlikely that another type of organization could mobilize the broad array of expertise needed to respond to such diverse priorities, especially when services are provided pro bono. The CGSI does not impact on private consultants or other grant writing services for several other important reasons. Social and human services (i.e., people) grants do not present an economically viable private sector opportunity. The university is not crowding out private sector consultants, who often target more lucrative technical proposals specializing in municipal infrastructure, economic development, or engineering services, for example.

Second, the CGSI, through its screening criteria, targets start-up non-profits with innovative ideas looking for seed money. The large majority of these organizations can not afford to purchase the services of a professional writer and are left to struggle with both the programmatic details and the responsibility for finding the funds. Non-profit assistance centers are not in an ideal position to assist with community-based grant development. Both state-supported and private non-profit assistance centers can successfully hold grant-writing seminars and training, but they have no ready access to research literature, academic expertise, data, or skills in manipulating and utilizing data. In addition, they do not have any incentive or mandate to serve the public good.

A third consideration in analyzing the Initiative's viability involves whether or not the community agency would have applied for the grant without the assistance provided by CGSI. Surveys of non-profit directors who have received CGSI assistance indicate that most would never have even applied without CGSI involvement. In fact, 88% said that the fact that CGSI was able to directly assist in writing the proposal was "very critical" in their decision to apply for the grant. Are community-based non-profits satisfied? In surveys of organizations that received assistance, 95% of non-profit directors said they highly valued the hands-on experience they received in developing the actual proposal, whether or not it culminated in a funded grant.

BENEFITS

The program over time represents not only an obvious return on investment for the state ($12:1), but also exemplifies a successful model for university-community partnering for capturing available federal funds essential to the implementation of community-based prevention, intervention, and coalition-building efforts. CGSI has demonstrated that the state can make a focused investment in universities pay big dividends for non-profit organizations within its communities.

Community Benefits

The initiative benefits communities by developing proposal, data, and evaluation skills at the local level. These capacity building activities have a longer-term impact than sporadic and low stakes training. Through the partnerships, CGSI helps Texas communities compete on a national level, successfully securing funding for "innovative" ideas. The process encourages community non-profit leaders to set aside time to strategically plan and evaluate their own, as well as research-based alternatives to current programming. Taking the time to reflect, to share ideas and discuss methodology provides both the university and community with valuable insight. In essence, writing skills don't impede the conveyance of local ideas that work, research and data skills of the university inform the local planning process, and the university enriches the non-profit's array of research-based program intervention options.

The dollar amounts and funded proposal ratio is an easy and expected measure of benefit to the community. To date, over the life of the collaborative, CGSI has had an 85% success rate. Grants that have been awarded have ranged from $7,000 to $1.7 million. CGSI has also served a broad variety of organizations within the non-profit sector including, health (30%), education (30%), social welfare and community service (18%), criminal justice (15%), and others including non-profits that promote personal growth and development, self-help and minority serving groups (7%). It is important to note that although the university officially collaborates with one community organization on a grant (the applicant), many organizations partner with the applicant agency to provide coordinated services. Therefore, the university's involvement often impacts a broader range of organizations within one community than is reflected by working with the actual applicant, especially in rural areas.

University Benefits

Just as there is no quid pro quo for the university to fulfill its teaching and research mission, service by definition, should not be bound by the expectation that students, faculty, or any other sub-community within the university directly benefit from partnership activities. Be that as it may, the university accrues many benefits in addition to the intrinsic benefit of extending the fruits of teaching and research into its service mission.

First, the initiative provides a vehicle for faculty from many departments to become engaged by informing the grant process. The arena of substance abuse prevention provides one example. Competitive programs derive ideas not only from the theories of sociology and psychology, but also engineering technology, advances in telecommunications, and even tourism science, through new developments in parks and recreation. With the community as a focus, faculty members gain interdisciplinary perspectives through dialogue with faculty and researchers in other departments. In addition, faculty and research staff acquire an entrée to community level projects, as well as the opportunity for long-term relationships with communities. The Initiative also provides funding for several graduate assistants who work on proposals and conduct research on broadening the university's ability to extend the university-community partnership experience.

Second, personal contact or first-hand experience with an institution was identified by the National Center for Postsecondary Governance and Finance as the single most influential factor in an individual's perception of a university. The CGSI allows the university almost limitless geographic penetration across all 254 counties in the state. Through the grant development model, the university can directly expand its contribution to the non-profit sector and do so in a way that extends the ability of the university to disseminate knowledge to professionals in both small towns and large urban settings.

But perhaps the greatest single benefit to the status of the institution is the university's increased stock of goodwill. The university is able to touch people who otherwise would not have any contact with the university. CGSI is a vehicle by which the university can make a direct impact on communities by helping them do what works according to local priorities. In return the university's service reputation is enhanced and media coverage of successful local programs, in turn, increases another influential factor affecting institutional reputation: Positive press.

CONCLUSION

The efforts of the Community Grant Support Initiative are unique for several reasons. Typically, the technical assistance of most publicly sponsored grants-assistance programs stops at a very crucial point—actually writing the proposal. Where their assistance stops, Community Grant Support Initiative assistance continues, helping community-based organizations write and submit competitive applications. Another reason the Initiative is valuable to local communities is its commitment to serve organizations that otherwise would not have the resources with which to construct a competitive grant application.

Through the Community Grant Support Initiative, Texas A&M University is responsive to the needs of both community and national priorities. The CGSI partnership is a vehicle for reformulating the needs of communities into clear and programmatic solutions suitable for federal funding. Program designs are data driven and projects are innovative for the community and coordinated with best-practices research from many disciplines. Community-based leaders receive hands-on experience with proposal development that is more effective than grant writing training in opening up new vistas for sustaining or implementing projects. The ultimate benefit of CGSI efforts is realized as community leaders who may not have believed they could compete for federal grants find themselves the developers of nationally acclaimed programs serving children and families, which has occurred in several communities that received CGSI assistance.

REFERENCES

Bok, D. (1982). *Beyond the ivory tower: Social responsibilities of the modern university.* London: Harvard University Press.

Bok, D. (1986). *Higher learning.* London: Harvard University Press.

Boyer, E. L. (1990). *Scholarship reconsidered: Priorities of the professoriate*. Princeton: The Carnegie Foundation for the Advancement of Teaching.

Boyer, E. L. (1994, March). Creating a new American college. *The Chronicle of Higher Education*, p. A48.

Center for Educational Research and Innovation. (1982). *The university and the community: The problems of changing relationships*. Paris: OECD.

Corrigan, D. (1997). The role of the university in community building, *The Educational Forum*, *62*, 14-24.

Enarson, H. (1989). *Revitalizing the land-grant mission.* Blacksburg: Virginia Polytech Institute and State University.

Theus, K. (1990). Academic reputations: Hard to come by, easy to loose. *Centerpiece*, *5*, 2. National Center for Postsecondary Governance and Finance.

Votruba, J. (1994). *Role of outreach in higher education.* Paper presented internally for strategic planning, Michigan State University.

Walshok, M. (1995). Knowledge without boundaries: *What America's research universities can do for the economy, the workplace and the community.* San Francisco: Jossey-Bass.

49 PARTNERS IN SUCCESSFUL PARENTING

Cathy Nathan
Texas Tech University

Quincy White
Housing Authority of Lubbock

La Nelle Ethridge
Parents as Teachers

NATURE OF THE PARTNERSHIP

The Lubbock Housing Authority and Texas Tech University College of Human Sciences have undertaken a collaborative effort to utilize the expertise and resources of both entities to help families in subsidized housing move toward self-sufficiency. One way to do this is to provide parent education and support to parents of children from birth to three years of age so that these children enter school with optimal growth in cognitive, language, social, emotional, and physical development which are critical to their success. Recent research has indicated that the first three years are crucial in the development of the brain, and that experiences during this period are quite influential in determining the future success of children in school and in life (Shore, 1997).

PURPOSES AND GOALS

The Housing Authority has as its goal not only to provide public assistance to those who need housing, but also to help families in public housing to move toward self-sufficiency. Approximately 60% of the parents who are in subsidized housing have not completed school and do not have the job skills necessary to support themselves without assistance. A major long-term goal of the project is to provide early intervention with the very youngest children to help them develop a sense of competency which will eventually help to prevent the perpetuation of the cycle of poverty. A short-term goal is to give parents the information and support to help them feel competent and capable as parents, helping to reduce the risks of child abuse and neglect and facilitating the development of their children. Goals for the university include providing opportunities for faculty and undergraduate and graduate students to apply their knowledge base to help solve existing problems in the community and to evaluate programs to determine their efficacy in solving these problems.

THE PROCESS

The targeted population for this program is residents in a subsidized housing project in Lubbock, Texas. The parenting model which has been selected is the Parents as Teachers program. This parenting program, which was developed in Missouri in 1981, is based upon the work of Burton White as a result of his 13 year study of early development in the Harvard University Preschool Project. The Parents as Teachers program has been adopted statewide in the state of Missouri and has over 100 sites in Texas. In independent research studies, Parents as Teachers has proven to be an effective early intervention model for working with families across the socioeconomic spectrum, but especially for low income, at-risk families (Miller, 1995). It is a model which recognizes that outcomes for children cannot be improved without involving parents in the process. Positive outcomes for children include significant increases in:

- language development;
- problem solving skills and cognitive functioning; and
- coping skills and emotional development in children.

Outcomes for parents include improvements in:

- knowledge of child development;
- self esteem and competency as parents;
- relationships between parents and the school system when the children enter school; and
- the number and quality of relationships among parents of children in the same age group.

Parents as Teachers is particularly well-suited for young children because it involves the home and the family, the places and people with whom young children develop their primary attachments. Parent educators with a background in child development make periodic (beginning weekly and moving to monthly) home visits to talk to parents about the development of their child, to introduce developmentally appropriate toys and books, and to model developmentally appropriate interactions. Monthly group parent meetings and child play groups provide opportunities for parent educators and families to discuss developmental issues and for parents of young children to meet and to provide support for each other.

The partnership between the College of Human Sciences and the Lubbock Housing Authority provides the opportunity to expand the scope of the traditional Parents as Teachers program. Faculty and doctoral students in Marriage and Family Therapy, and faculty as well as graduate and undergraduate practicum students in Nutrition, Child Development, and Family Financial Planning provide resources and services beyond the parenting and child development information in the Parents as Teachers curriculum. Graduate teaching assistants and undergraduate practicum students in Human Development and Family Studies are directly involved with parent educators in program planning and direct service delivery. Graduate interns in Marriage and Family Therapy assist in facilitating parenting groups, and families are referred to the Marriage and Family Therapy Clinic for mental health services as needed. Community nutrition classes conduct needs assessments and design nutrition programs for families. Graduate research assistants in Human Development will conduct both short-term and long-term program evaluations to establish the efficacy of the program for children, for parents, and for the university students involved in the program.

Other community agencies also are involved in the project. Developmental Education Birth Through Two (DEBT), an early intervention program for children with developmental delays and disorders in the local school district, will screen children in the Parents as Teachers program and will refer children who need special services to the appropriate programs. DEBT and Parents as Teachers will also provide cross training between early intervention teachers and parent educators. A local health clinic will provide check-ups and immunizations to prevent health problems. Proposed but not yet in place are adult literacy and GED programs to be provided to families at the parenting center. An advisory committee consisting of Housing Authority personnel, university faculty, and community leaders will oversee the project.

Through a five year federal grant, the Lubbock Housing Authority has contracted with the College of Human Sciences to provide a full-time Parents as Teachers Coordinator, two half-time parent educators, and a half-time secretary. The administrative offices, parent group meetings, and the children's play group are housed in a community facility owned by the Housing Authority. The Housing Authority has also provided office machines, furnishings, and utilities. Provided by the university are the graduate teaching assistants, the practicum students, and faculty expertise as well as supervision of students. External funding from foundations provides additional funds for toys and books for children and parent education materials. Our goal is to establish a lending library of developmentally appropriate toys and books and to provide gift books for children on each home visit. Parents will be encouraged to read to their children regularly and to increase their own reading time, since reading research indicates that reading to children within the first five years and parental modeling of reading are important for children's later acquisition of reading skills (Kraschen, 1993).

ACHIEVEMENTS RELATED TO GOALS

Because this program is in the start-up phase, we do not yet have outcomes related to our goals. However, we do have a faculty member and a graduate student who are designing a comprehensive evaluation component which will measure outcomes for children, for parents, for students, and for the agencies involved. This evaluation will include measures of growth in the cognitive, language, physical, and social/emotional development of children as compared with a control group, for self-esteem and competency of parents as compared with a control group, for parent satisfaction with the program, and for growth in the abilities of college students to work with families. Logs are being kept to record degree of participation in the various components of the program. Since a focus in this program is to help parents to learn to read to their children and to interact with the children in book-reading experiences, instruments will be included to measure growth in both parents' abilities and attitudes toward reading to children and children's growth in responsiveness to book-reading experiences. An open-ended questionnaire will be used to determine if the Housing Authority's goals for the program have been met as well.

PROSPECTS FOR LONG-TERM SUSTAINABILITY

The prospects for long-term sustainability for the project are good for several reasons. One is the commitment of the Housing Authority of Lubbock and the College of Human Sciences to the project. Both entities are committed to the premise that early childhood intervention and support to parents of young children have long-term outcomes for both children and parents. In addition, the Parents as Teachers project and the partnership with the Housing Authority have formed the basis for a grant proposal for an Early Head Start program which was submitted by faculty in the Department of Human Development and Family Studies in the summer of 1998. If this proposal is funded, the Housing Authority will provide the facility for a full-time child care center, and the existing Parents as Teachers program, as well as the mental health services provided by the Marriage and Family Therapy Clinic, the nutrition component provided by the Nutrition Department, and the Family Financial Planning program, all housed in the College of Human Sciences, will be expanded to serve low income families who qualify for Head Start but who do not necessarily live in public housing. A second site in a predominately Hispanic neighborhood as well as additional health services provided by the Texas Tech University Health Sciences Center and St. Mary of the Plains Hospital will also be added. Adult education, economic self-sufficiency, and English as a Second Language will also be emphasized.

LEARNINGS FROM THIS PARTNERSHIP

A vital lesson we have learned about building community partnerships from this project is the importance of persistence and patience. Discussions about a Parents as Teachers Program for teen parents, initiated by a faculty member within the College of Human Sciences, began approximately ten years ago, initially with the board of the public schools. During the discussion stage which lasted about a year, the composition of the school board changed and the school superintendent retired. Unfortunately, the new board and new superintendent were not interested in pursuing collaborative work on the project. In the early 1990's, the city mayor became interested in early intervention and brought together a committee of university and community leaders including the Dean and faculty members in the College of Human Sciences. After several years of meetings and discussion of various proposals, all participants agreed to move forward on a Parents as Teachers program to be conducted collaboratively by the city, the local school district, and the university. However, when the mayor resigned to pursue another public office in the fall of 1996, the proposal again died.

In the spring of 1997, at a public forum for the "I Am Your Child" public awareness campaign, the idea was resurrected during an informal conversation between the executive director of the Housing Authority and two faculty members from the College of Human Sciences. A partnership was born based upon the mutual conviction that early intervention for children and support for parents utilizing the combined resources of a variety of entities is the most effective way to make long-term differences in the lives of at risk families. Thus, in this instance, refusal to give up on an idea paid off. The current partnership is attributable primarily to the persistence of a faculty member and the dean who remained committed to the importance of establishing an early intervention program in the community.

Not only were persistence and patience necessary to bring the parties together in this collaboration effort, but they were also necessary in the project planning stages. The original concept called for the program to be conducted by university students on a voluntary basis. Faculty, however, argued that an effective program required: (1) Personnel with a strong background in child development; (2) continuity of relationships between staff and families; and (3) effective leadership. While college students can and do provide excellent assistance, they need supervision by trained professionals. Therefore, persistence in pursuing a commitment to quality resulted in the hiring of a director with a master's degree in child development and experience in working with children, families, and college students to oversee the operation of the program.

Merging the talents and resources of two public institutions, the Housing Authority and the university, each with its own bureaucratic rules and regulations as well as its expertise and experience, also presented a challenge. In order to ensure that the procedures and policies of each were protected and that the responsibilities and contributions of each of the parties were clearly stipulated, a written contract was negotiated by the legal counsels of the two entities. Many collaborations fail because the roles and responsibilities of the parties are assumed rather than defined or because one of the parties drops out of the project because a formal commitment has not been made. While this process was time-consuming and somewhat tedious, it eventually resulted in a contract which formalized the relationship and the joint commitment to the project, thereby providing protection against future misunderstandings.

Mutual respect and trust are basic to effective partnerships. These develop over time in negotiations in which all parties are heard, all issues are discussed, and agreements are reached based on consensus. Sometimes in our haste to get a project underway, we rush through these critical steps and compromise basic ideals which are crucial to the success of the project. Patience and persistence are needed to maintain a focus which will lead to a successful partnership.

WHY IS THIS A SUCCESSFUL PARTNERSHIP?

In his book, *The Vulnerable Child: What Really Hurts America's Children and What We Can Do About It*, Richard Weissbourd (1996) states that programs which are the most successful in producing positive outcomes for children who are at risk are those that combine resources to provide comprehensive services to families in their own communities and have consistent staff who develop relationships with the families. Services which are fragmented and address only one area of need are much less successful than programs which consider the family and its needs as a whole and try to coordinate services to meet those needs. The Housing Authority of Lubbock and the College of Human Sciences have combined their resources to provide services to families in public housing. The parent educators in the Parents as Teachers program develop personal relationships with families within their own homes and act as case managers to refer and to facilitate access of families to health, mental health, and social services. According to Weissbourd, programs also need to focus on the strengths of parents and to empower them to help their children rather than focusing on their deficits. The main goal of the Parents as Teachers program is to support parents in their roles as the first and primary teachers of their children. By providing child development, health and safety, and nutrition information, and by helping parents to access health, mental health, and social services, parent educators facilitate feelings of competency in parents.

This partnership not only benefits the families involved, but it benefits the university and the Housing Authority as well. The knowledge and expertise of university faculty is taken out of the ivory tower and into the community to help solve real problems. Not only do faculty benefit by testing their knowledge in a real world setting, but undergraduate and graduate students also benefit by applying what they have learned in the classroom while also providing a service. A primary goal of the Housing Authority is to help its residents move toward self-sufficiency and away from dependency on public assistance. As the Executive Director of the Housing Authority has stated, his goal is to put his agency out of business. While the Parents as Teachers program alone will not end the need for public assistance, it is part of an overall strategy on the part of the Housing Authority to develop competency and self-sufficiency in both the current generation of public housing residents and in their children as well. While it is our hope that the parents and children in the Parents and Teachers program are the primary beneficiaries, all participants in this partnership have gained from this collaborative effort.

REFERENCES

Kraschen, S. D. (1993). *The power of reading: Insights from the research.* Englewood, CO: Libraries, Unlimited, Inc.

Miller, S. H. (1995). *A select review of past and current evaluations of the Parents as Teachers program.* St. Louis, MO: Parents as Teachers National Center.

Shore, R. (1997). *Rethinking the brain: New insights into early development.* New York: Families and Work Institute.

Weissbourd, R. (1996). *The vulnerable child: What really hurts America's children and what we can do about it.* Reading, MA: Addison-Wesley Publishing Co., Inc.

50 THE TEEN ASSESSMENT PROJECT COMMUNITY-BASED COLLABORATIVE RESEARCH

Kathleen Boyce Rodgers
Washington State University

Stephen A. Small
University of Wisconsin, Madison

At public universities across the nation, scholars are increasingly being called upon to address community needs while also meeting the expectation for rigorous and sound research. For the scholar unfamiliar with action-research, accomplishing these tasks may seem difficult if not impossible. The Teen Assessment Project (TAP) demonstrates how collaborative research can be a rewarding process for both researchers and community partners, while also advancing scholarship in the area of adolescent development. Meeting these dual goals requires building trust and cooperation at the community level, sensitivity to the idiosyncracies and politics of a particular community, and employing a research design that is perceived as valid and relevant to the community while also being consistent with sound scientific methods.

Since its inception in 1989, TAP has been conducted in over 225 communities and 13 states throughout the U.S., and has been a catalyst for community action on behalf of youth. The project differs from most traditional research in that it utilizes a collaborative research model to both empower local citizens and advance scholarly knowledge about adolescent development (Small, 1996). Youth are anonymously surveyed during a standard classroom period to assess their behaviors and perceptions regarding personal concerns, drugs, alcohol and sexuality, indicators of positive youth development and mental and physical health, and attitudes toward home, school and community. The researcher works with a local steering committee to develop the survey instrument and determine survey questions that are most relevant and that will best inform local policy and practice. The researcher also provides guidance on data collection procedures, strategies for gaining community based support, and dissemination of findings. Descriptive data and simple relational analyses are reported to the community through a variety of means such as parent-focused newsletters, community forums, press releases, fact-sheets, presentations to local organizations and governing bodies, and a comprehensive written report targeted to professionals and policy makers.

ESSENTIAL COMPONENTS OF TAP

The Stakeholders

Communities that conduct TAP have a local coordinator who serves as the liaison between the university-based researcher and the local steering committee. In Wisconsin, county Extension 4-H and Family Living faculty typically serve this function. In other instances, the liaison may be a representative of a sponsoring agency such as the county health department or a prevention coalition. A steering committee is formed through a process of identifying and soliciting the involvement of key community leaders and individuals concerned about youth. Steering committees typically comprise local policy makers, parents, social service personnel, law enforcement representatives, educators, and members of the clergy. Sometimes youth are also included. The diversity of the steering committee membership is critical to the success of the program. The steering committee is instrumental in gaining entrance into the schools, gaining community support, and ensuring that the research findings are used and acted upon.

Because TAP assesses risk behaviors and attitudes of adolescents toward their family, it has the potential for controversy. Some community factions may perceive the survey to be intrusive in the lives of the teens and their families, may fear that survey questions will cause harm to teens who participate, or are afraid the survey may lead to a change of the status quo. A representative steering committee can gain community support because it knows the political climate, values, and tolerances of their community. For example, some communities include questions on sexual abstinence as well as sexual intercourse to provide a balance among political factions.

Trust

Trust between the researcher and the community, and among involved community members is paramount to community-based action research. Building a relationship of trust takes time and skill on the part of the researcher and the local coordinator to effectively facilitate communication and maintain balance between the needs of the researcher and each partner in the project (McHale et al., 1996; Wandersman, Chavis & Stucky, 1983). For the TAP project, trust is built primarily through the process of developing the survey instrument. Stakeholders in the project often feel very strongly about issues and will debate at length the inclusion or omission of questions in the survey. Through debate and discussion they learn from each other, develop a collective ownership of the project, and begin the process of changing political agendas into community action. Among the many surveys that have been developed, we find about 70-80% consistency in the questions and issues addressed by communities across the U.S. Each survey, however, reflects particular interests or concerns that are unique to the social, economic, ethnic, and historical context of the community. For example, communities with a high rate of gang involvement might address issues concerning violence, criminal behavior, or community monitoring; whereas, communities experiencing racial tensions might wish to assess students' perceptions of racial discrimination, tension, or attitudes toward other cultures.

Balancing Research and Action Agendas

The process of survey development is one in which there exists some degree of tension between the breadth and depth of measures used. Steering committees frequently want to address a wide variety of issues. In contrast, social science researchers are typically interested in a more focused investigation of behaviors or phenomena to explain human behavior and development (Small, 1995; 1996). Balancing the need for breadth and depth requires that the researcher let go of some control, and that the community members trust the integrity and expertise of the researcher to advise them on use of reliable and valid measures.

Having a conceptual framework around which survey questions can be developed is particularly useful because it provides community partners a rationale for certain measures in the survey. TAP is based on an ecological framework that assumes factors related to adolescent development are multidimensional and interrelated (Bronfenbrenner, 1979). Sensitive questions, such as those concerning sexuality or mental health, are less likely to be perceived as intrusive by the community when they are understood as important in the context of adolescents' lives. In addition, with a sound conceptual framework, measures that have practical use to the community can also answer empirical research questions. For example, Small and his associates have reported on multiple risk factors associated with sexual initiation and risk-taking behavior among adolescents (Luster & Small, 1994; Small & Luster, 1994), on sexual abuse and related adolescent problem behaviors (Luster & Small, 1997), and on determinants of parental competence (Bogenschneider, Small, & Tsay, 1997).

FUNDING

The TAP project requires minimal funding because of the involvement of the community. Steering committee members and other volunteers donate their time and often provide in-kind donations for services such as the printing of survey booklets, parent newsletters, and reports. The fixed costs of the project involve costs for development of the survey instrument, the computer scan sheets used for data collection, and data processing. Additional expenditures may include funds to support a graduate student and/or travel for the researcher. In almost every case, small local grants are used to cover project costs which typically run between $2,000-$5,000. Because the research addresses questions that are important to the community, community organizations are usually generous about providing financial support for the project.

EVALUATION AND IMPACTS OF TAP

To date, over 125,000 Wisconsin adolescents have been surveyed in more than 225 communities. In 1993, an evaluation was conducted by an independent researcher to assess the impact of TAP in Wisconsin communities (Lande, 1994). In-depth interviews with over 40 county extension faculty, community leaders, and others who had utilized TAP data revealed that the TAP process was a stimulus for a wide variety of community action. At least 45 new school or community policies have been enacted in response to TAP data. For example, law enforcement agencies have responded by creating uniform policies for youth regarding curfew violations, underage alcohol consumption, and tobacco use. TAP data have been used by schools in health education and family life classes and to develop student counseling programs to address depression and low self-esteem. School boards have been more responsive to requests for prevention programming as a result of local TAP data.

At least 43 community programs have been credited as resulting from TAP data. Parent groups have responded to local data by developing parent networks and support groups to promote parent-adolescent communication, to organize awareness campaigns about youth needs and risk behaviors, and to establish curfew norms. Adolescents themselves have also responded to TAP data. In one community, for example, junior high students formed the MOO (Make Other Options) Club. They developed a super-hero cow character, logo, and cartoons depicting the cow rescuing students from alcohol and other drug abuse (Lande, 1994).

The data have been particularly useful for documenting need in rural areas, thus making grant funds more attainable. TAP data have been cited in at least 112 funded grant proposals, totaling more than $1,000,000. Funds have been used for activities such as mental health screening, the development of a family resource center, to assist schools in helping high-risk families, and to develop a parent network to reduce underage drinking. In addition, the TAP process has led to the formation of over 24 community coalitions or task forces concerned with addressing some of the issues identified in the data (Lande, 1994; Small, 1996).

The Teen Assessment Project empowers citizens to effect change by actively involving them in the research process. Citizens who are involved in TAP gain a better understanding of and appreciation for utilizing social science research as a tool for community action. This appreciation is evident in Wisconsin where TAP continues to be self-funded and driven by community interest in collaborating with the university. In addition, the TAP process rewards academicians professionally by providing them opportunities to gather quality data that can contribute to the scientific knowledge base, and personally by knowing that their research makes a difference in the lives of adolescents and their families. Successful implementation of TAP requires active community involvement and a researcher who values community partnership. When these elements are present, TAP has the capacity to inform local policy and practice, affect social change on behalf of youth, and contribute to our understanding of adolescent development.

REFERENCES

Bogenschneider, K. Small, S. A, & Tsay, J. C. (1997). Child, parent, and contextual influences on perceived parental competence. *Journal of Marriage and the Family, 59*(2), 345-362.

Bronfrenbrenner, U. (1979). *The ecology of human development.* Cambridge, MA: Harvard University Press.

Lande, J. (1994). *Teen Assessment Project Five Year Impact Study, 1989-1994.* Madison: Department of Sociology, University of Wisconsin-Madison.

Luster, T., & Small, S. A. (1997). Sexual abuse history and problems in adolescence: Exploring the effects of moderating variables. *Journal of Marriage and the Family, 59*(1), 131-142.

Luster, T., & Small, S. A. (1994). Factors associated with sexual risk-taking behaviors. *Journal of Marriage and the Family, 56*(3), 622-632.

McHale, S. M., Crouter, A. C., Fennelly, K., Tomascik, C. A., Updegraff, K. A., Graham, J. E., Baker, A. E., Dreisbach, L., Ferry, N., Manlove, E. E., McGroder, S. M., Mulkeen, P., & Obeidallah, D. A. (1996). Community-based interventions for young adolescents: The Penn State PRIDE project. *Journal of Research on Adolescence, 6*(1), 23-26.

Small, S. A. (1996). Collaborative, community-based research on adolescents: Using research for community change. *Journal of Research on Adolescence, 6*(1), 9-22.

Small, S. A. (1995). Action oriented research: Models and methods. *Journal of Marriage and the Family, 57*(4), 941-955.

Small, S. A., & Luster, T. (1994). Adolescent sexual activity: An ecological approach. *Journal of Marriage and the Family, 56*(1), 181-192.

Wandersman, A., Chavis, D., & Stucky, P. (1983). Involving citizens in research. In R. F. Kidd & M. J. Saks (Eds.), *Advances in applied social psychology, Vol. 2* (pp. 189-212). Hillsdale, NJ: Lawrence Erlbaum Associates, Inc.

AFTERWORD

Sidney A. Ribeau
Bowling Green State University

THE IMPACT OF VOLUNTEER SERVICE

Today in America, one hundred million citizens participate in service to others. Roughly speaking, that is one out of every two people over the age of thirteen (O'Connell, 1998). It has become a hallmark within our country that "we the people" care about collaborating and making a difference in the lives of others. Building individual and group partnerships has become one of the most distinguishing features of American society. It is these partnerships that have shaped the lives of many and bettered the world in which we live.

Perhaps one of the strongest partnerships in our society today is that between the university and the community. Through this collaboration, universities and communities are positioned to capitalize on the national momentum of volunteer service by forging productive partnerships resulting in meaningful service to others. This collaboration has resulted in the voices of our involved citizens resonating a chorus of "we are not afraid," even when they were. And when the strength of these partnerships was realized, the chorus echoed, "we shall overcome." And they did.

Finally, when almost one out of two Americans regularly works to improve our communities (O'Connell, 1998), the entire country benefits. When you add up all the outcomes of meaningful service through partnerships, the results are potentially astounding. The modern university must be a leader in this movement.

THE APPLICATION OF RESEARCH, TEACHING, AND SERVICE FOR HUMAN BETTERMENT

As a result of successful community-university partnerships (which can and should be applied to a variety of disciplines in numerous contexts) we see tremendous citizen participation focused on societal problems that could not be solved by individuals alone. This volume of best practices in university-community partnering illustrates the significant impact applying institutional research, teaching, and service has on addressing many of the issues facing children and their families within our local communities and throughout the nation at large.

Graham Spanier, President of Penn State, spoke of the importance of these partnerships when he stated that:

> The new model for land grant universities must center on the idea of fuller integration and engagement with the larger society—in short, a renewal and revitalization of our commitment to service... That model must integrate the larger society, addressing societal issues and integrating the University's three missions: research, teaching and service. And in so doing, reaching out and partnering with communities to improve the quality of life for all Americans...from birth to old age (Spanier, 1997, pp. 1-2).

Young (1997) further emphasized the importance of applying the three institutional missions to addressing community and societal problems when he asserted that:

> The functions of teaching, research and service serve a larger purpose than the perpetuation of the academy and academicians... the goal of academic service is an applied ideal of human betterment... all academic values, rights and responsibilities are based on the value of service to humankind (pp. 11-12).

The old adage "it is better to give than to receive" rings true here as clearly the giver gets back as much as he or she gives. This includes a sense of satisfaction in feeling needed and the heightened awareness that service to others, indeed, makes a difference. Boyer (1990), as cited in Young (1997), suggested that: "The functions of scholarship need to be applied for human betterment, otherwise the altruistic value of the academy is unfulfilled" (p.21).

BEST PRACTICES AT A GLANCE

We see the fruits of community-university partnerships through the many best practices illuminated throughout this publication.

At Texas Woman's University, the university has partnered with a local elementary school to increase adult involvement and increase student academic interest and accomplishment. We also see that outreach activities have benefited the Lubbock, Texas Housing Authority and Texas Tech University. In collaboration, these partners have aided subsidized-housing families move toward self-sufficiency by providing parent education in all areas of child development. The Teen Assessment Project, represented in over thirteen states throughout the U.S., is innovative in that it draws on a collaborative research model empowering local citizens and advancing scholarly knowledge about adolescent development. In Alabama, some visionaries dreamed of a world-class child care facility, and in 1994, they made their dream a reality.

In Phoenix, Arizona scholarly outreach has involved a group of university child development researchers and community physicians who have worked to bring together services and interventions for autistic children and their families. Kent State University (Ohio) and teachers and parents of children with disabilities have joined forces in thirteen preschool classrooms in their efforts to help children with disabilities learn by using technology. Connecticut's general assembly has teamed up with the University of Connecticut to present a Family Impact Seminar focusing on youth violence. Florida State University is committed, along with their community school system, to enhancing the literacy of elementary school children.

Recognizing that not all college students fit the profile of the eighteen to twenty-two year old, unmarried, unemployed, full-time residential college student, Eastern Illinois University has developed a program designed to create a different and responsive Child and Family Studies degree program. This program is designed to enhance opportunities for persons for whom it might be difficult to complete degree requirements. Working in collaboration with social services agencies, Western Michigan University has created a partnership designed to provide support to custodial grandparents. And the University of Missouri and a number of regional Human Development Extension specialists, along with a judicial circuit court in central Missouri, have joined together to provide research-based education for divorced parents.

Few would argue with the statement that these programs are making a difference in the lives of those affected by them. It is also important to note that one of the most fundamental elements of any successful university-community partnership is the reciprocity that exists between the involved organizations.

RECIPROCITY

Research indicates that when people work for the betterment of humanity, not only are others helped, but those engaged in serving others gain a sense of personal satisfaction and contentment. And when many are involved in building partnerships by serving others, there is an increased respect for community, a high awareness of shared hopes, and an increased degree of civility. For obvious reasons, it is of paramount importance that these relationships be reciprocal.

The idea of reciprocity asserts that the University does not only serve as "missionary," an institution that will seek to "save" the community, but rather, the university has something to gain. As Professors Chibucos and Lerner state directly in Chapter 1 of this volume (p. 4), and as the rest of their book reinforces and makes clear time and time again, the community can teach the university about real life experiences and the impact those experiences have on the lives of people. Once universities recognize and value the legitimacy of the experiences of our external communities, we can better understand the world in which we live. Without question, the university must work closely with the community to identify local issues of concern, and develop intervention strategies centered on prevention through education. The reciprocal nature of this relationship is evident as the academy's primary goal must be not to do things "for" the community, but to do things "with" the community.

At Bowling Green State University (BGSU) in Ohio, such reciprocity is illuminated in the mission statement for the Partnerships for Community Action (PCA) program:

> BGSU Partnerships for Community Action (PCA) is dedicated to redefining the relationship between the University and the broader community through building and supporting campus/community projects based on reciprocity, co-equal participation, and mutual benefit. PCA is responsible for mobilizing ideas and resources from the University and the

community that enhance equal educational opportunity, economic development, health and wellness, and cultural awareness for areas including, but not limited to northwest Ohio.

Many major social breakthroughs in America have originated in the volunteer sector. If volunteers and the causes they represent were to vanish from the national spotlight, we would, without question, be less distinctly American. Service to others enhances our creativity, enlivens our communities, nurtures individual responsibility and growth, and reminds us of the reciprocity involved in giving.

THE INCREASING COMPLEXITY OF OUR WORLD

As institutions of higher education and their local communities reach out to one another, there must be an understanding that the context of our environments is constantly changing. With the blitz of technological advancements as well as the growing diversity of our nation, the university in the twenty-first century will exist in a far more complex world than the university of the past. Our partnerships with others must be formed with this in mind. Consider these facts regarding the world in which we work:

- Already an estimated two-thirds of U.S. employees work in the services sector, and "knowledge" is becoming our most important "product." This calls for different organizations, as well as different kinds of workers.
- In 1991, for the first time ever, companies spent more money on computing and communication gear than the combined moneys spent on industrial mining, farm, and construction equipment. This spending pattern offers hard proof that we have entered a new era. The Industrial Age has given way to the Information Age.
- Since 1983, the U.S. work world has added 25,000,000 computers. The number of cellular telephone subscribers has jumped from zero in 1983 to 16,000,000 by the end of 1993. Close to 19,000,000 people now carry pagers, and almost 12,000,000,000 messages were left in voice mailboxes in 1993 alone.
- Since 1987, homes and offices have added 10,000,000 fax machines, while E-mail addresses have increased by over 26,000,000. Communication technology is radically changing the speed, direction, and amount of information flow, even as it alters work roles all across organizations. As a case in point, the number of secretaries is down 521,000 just since 1987 (Pritchett, 1998).

Like our work world, the society in which we live is also radically changing. Consider these demographic trends:

- The U.S. Census projects that the current population of the United States is approximately 269 million. It will rise to 286 million in 2005, 298 million in 2010, and 323 million in 2020. Of the more than 50 million who will be added to our national population in the next few decades, about 60% will result from more births than deaths and about 40% from immigration. Immigrants and their children will account for more than one-half of our population growth.

- The U.S. population will show significant increases in racial and ethnic diversity in the coming years. The Latino population nationally will more than double between now and 2025 and will be the largest minority group by 2005. European-Americans will be a minority in the under-eighteen population by 2030 and in the entire U.S. population by 2050.

The economic stratification and social problems facing our nation will require the university to adapt research, teaching, and service to meet the emergent needs of our technologically sophisticated, demographically changing communities and society.

Universities are stewards of information, charged with collecting, maintaining and protecting the information-base that grounds the academic community. However, in addition to maintaining our existing knowledge base, institutions of higher education are also responsible for discovering new artistic and intellectual vistas, within the context of an ever changing world. These new discoveries can be made through collaborative efforts with our community partners. In extending the resources unique to universities and communities, we must advance our collaborative strategies, with the ultimate goal of helping individuals, families, and communities develop or strengthen their own ability to make sound decisions based on greater knowledge.

A CLOSING THOUGHT

This book illustrates a variety of best practices in community-university partnerships focused on bettering the lives of children, families, and the communities in which they live. It is these partnerships that are transforming higher education through outreach scholarship which, in effect, is contributing to and advancing the lifeblood of our communities.

It is of paramount importance that administrators and community officials engage in significant collaborative initiatives. These leaders must be invested in paving the way to promote the positive development of children, families, and communities as it is their collective "word, deed and action" that will ensure successful partnerships between institutions of higher education and the communities that host them.

Volunteers come together to impact positive change. There are more than a million volunteer organizations in America today, ranging from small community groups to massive national initiatives (O'Connell, 1998). They organize to serve every imaginable human condition and ambition and to affect almost every public issue.

No matter how one describes how or why Americans are involved, the central message is that millions of people serve in thousands of ways. Within all of their causes, they perform an inordinate amounts of service. They assist, heal, teach, inform, protest, comfort, build, advocate, testify, demonstrate, support, guide, solicit, feed, organize, criticize, contribute, appeal, and, in hundreds of others ways, serve people, their communities, and their causes. The nearly fifty community-university partnerships illustrated in this book chronicle the adage that "anything is possible" when universities, by applying their three institutional missions of research, teaching, and service, work together with their communities to address issues impacting children and their families. Within the context of these partnerships forged in an ever changing world, universities both impact and are impacted by their communities. With the continuation of community-campus partnerships, universities and the cities and towns that host them will be able to effect positive change for future generations.

REFERENCES

Chibucos, T. R., & Lerner, R. M. (1999) Serving children and families through community-university partnerships: A view of the issues. In T. R. Chibucos & R. M. Lerner (Eds.), *Serving children and families through community-university partnerships: Success stories* (pp. 1-12). Norwood, MA: Kluwer Academic Publishers.

O'Connell, B. (1998). *Voices from the heart: In celebration of America's volunteers.* San Francisco, CA: Jossey-Bass Publishers.

Pritchett, P. (1998). *New work habits for a radically changing world* Dallas, TX: Pritchett & Associates, Inc.

Spanier, G. B. (1997). *Enhancing the quality of life for children, youth and families.* Unpublished manuscript. University Park, PA: The Pennsylvania State University.

Young, R. B. (1997). *No neutral ground: Standing by the values we prize in higher education.* San Francisco, CA: Jossey Bass Publishers.

Author/Subject Index

—A—

—Q—

—R—

—T—

—U—

—V—

Printed in the United States
99695LV00001B/202/A

9 780792 385400